A synopsis of
Haematology

A synopsis of
Haematology

John D M Richards MA MD FRCP(Edin) FRCPath
David C Linch BA MB BChir MRCP
Anthony H Goldstone MA FRCP(Edin) MRCPath

Department of Haematology, University College Hospital London

WRIGHT·PSG

1983 Bristol . London . Boston

Published by:
John Wright & Sons Ltd, 823–825 Bath Road, Bristol BS4 5NU, England.
John Wright PSG Inc, 545 Great Road, Littleton, Massachusetts 01460, U.S.A.

British Library Cataloguing in Publication Data

Richards, John D. M.
  A synopsis of haematology.—(Synopsis series)
  1. Haematology
  I. Title II. Linch, David C.
  III. Goldstone, Anthony H.
  616.1′5 R145

ISBN 0 7236 0650 1

Library of Congress Catalog Card Number:

Typeset and printed in Great Britain by
John Wright & Sons (Printing) Ltd, at The Stonebridge Press, Bristol BS4 5NU.

Preface

Haematology has expanded rapidly in the past decade; perhaps more so than any other specialty within internal medicine. Major advances in molecular genetics, cell cloning, immunology, transplantation, prostaglandin metabolism and other areas of biochemistry have all been applicable to the study and management of haematological disease. This book is intended to cover all the main subjects in outline and include accounts of these recent developments. We believe that haematology should be essentially a clinical discipline, practised by physicians with a sound knowledge and understanding of the laboratory aspects of the subject and a clinical emphasis has been given throughout this 'Synopsis'.

This book largely follows the traditional style of the Synopsis Series, though the writing is a little less telegraphic. As with all brief texts some dogmatism has been unavoidable in the interests of clarity. The text has not been referenced but a brief selected bibliography is given where appropriate at the end of individual chapters. A list of some of the major textbooks of haematology which contain extensive bibliographies follows this preface.

We hope this small text will fulfil the requirements of senior undergraduates and postgraduates involved in the clinical management of haematological disease or studying for higher qualifications.

J D M R   D C L   A H G

General reference texts

Clinical Haematology in Medical Practice	De Gruchy G. C. et al. 4th ed. (1978) Oxford, Blackwell Scientific Publications.
Blood and its Disorders	Hardisty R. M. and Weatherall D. J. 2nd ed. (1982) Oxford, Blackwell Scientific Publications.
Haematology of Infancy and Childhood	Nathan D. G. and Oski F. A. 2nd ed. (1981) Philadelphia, Saunders.
Haematology	Williams W. J. et al. 2nd ed. (1977) New York, McGraw-Hill.
Clinical Haematology	Wintrobe M. M. 8th ed. (1981) Philadelphia, Lea & Febiger.

Contents

Chapter 1   Classification and diagnosis of anaemia   1
2   Examination of the peripheral film   6
3   Examination of the bone marrow   16
4   Iron metabolism and associated disorders   27
5   Megaloblastic anaemia   40
6   Aplastic anaemia and bone marrow failure   51
7   General features of haemolytic anaemia   61
8   Hereditary haemolytic anaemias   66
9   Haemoglobin and the thalassaemia syndromes   75
10   Haemoglobinopathies   84
11   Acquired haemolytic anaemias   92
12   The anaemia of chronic disorders   102
13   Disorders of granulocytes and monocytes   109
14   Myeloproliferative and allied disorders   116
15   Acute leukaemia   126
16   The lymphoreticular system   139
17   Malignant lymphoreticular disorders   150
18   Immunoproliferative disorders   169
19   Normal haemostasis and its laboratory evaluation   179
20   Platelet disorders   191
21   Hereditary coagulation disorders   202
22   Acquired coagulation disorders   208
23   Hypercoagulability   213
24   Anticoagulants and antithrombotic drugs   220
25   Blood groups, antibodies and compatibility testing   230
26   Use of blood products   238
27   Hazards and complications of blood transfusion   245
28   Useful investigations   255
29   Cytotoxic drugs in haematology   278
   Appendix   291
   Index   293

Every attempt has been made by the authors to verify details in the text regarding the use and dosage of drugs. However, no responsibility can be accepted by the authors or publishers for any errors which may be present in the text.

Chapter I
The Classification and Diagnosis of Anaemia

Definition. Anaemia is a haemoglobin (Hb) level falling below the 'normal' value for that individual—less than 13 g/dl for men and 12·0 g/dl for women. Children and infants have lower levels, except at birth when the haemoglobin level may be 21 g/dl (*Table* 1.1).

Table 1.1. Variation of Hb and red cell indices with age

	Hb	MCV	MCH
Birth (cord blood)	14–18 g/dl	98–118 fl	31–37 pg
First 3 days of life	13–21 g/dl	96–120 fl	31–37 pg
Neonatal period	10–18 g/dl	85–110 fl	28–40 pg
1–12 months	10–13·5 g/dl	70–105 fl	23–35 pg
1–12 years	11·5–15·5 g/dl	75–95 fl	24–33 pg
Post-puberty males	13·0–18·0 g/dl	80–98 fl	28–34 pg
Post-puberty females	12·0–16·0 g/dl	80–98 fl	28–34 pg

Knowledge of a previous haemoglobin level is helpful as the level is normally very constant. Living at a high altitude raises the 'normal' haemoglobin level. True anaemia results from an imbalance between red cell production and loss: a relative anaemia is due to an increase in plasma volume (associated with pregnancy, hypoproteinaemia, macroglobulinaemia or splenomegaly) and there is no reduction in the total red cell mass.

CLASSIFICATION OF ANAEMIA

Impaired Red Cell Formation

1. Impaired haemoglobin synthesis occurs:

    1.1 With iron deficiency (*see* Chapter 4).

    1.2 With impaired iron utilization as occurs in chronic disease (*see* Chapter 12).

    1.3 With impaired haemoglobin synthesis as occurs in sideroblastic anaemia, lead poisoning, pyridoxine deficiency and porphyria erythropoietica.

    1.4 With impaired globin synthesis which occurs in thalassaemia and severe protein malnutrition.

2. Impaired deoxyribose nucleic acid (DNA) synthesis occurs:

    2.1 With vitamin B_{12} deficiency.

    2.2 In folate deficiency.

    2.3 With megaloblastic anaemia refractory to vitamin B_{12} and folate therapy (*see* Chapter 5).

3. Pure red cell aplasia (*see* Chapter 6).
4. Aplastic anaemia (*see* Chapter 6).
5. Marrow infiltration in which the marrow is replaced by bone, fibrous tissue, malignant cells or abnormal cells in storage disorders. The anaemia is often associated with nucleated red cells and granulocyte precursors in the peripheral blood (leuco-erythroblastic anaemia).
6. Toxic dyshaemopoiesis as occurs in infections, collagenoses and malignant disorders. The mechanism is complex and often involves poor iron utilization, erythroid hypoplasia and ineffective erythropoiesis.
7. Metabolic disorders such as:

> 7.1 Hypothyroidism.
> 7.2 Hypopituitarism.
> 7.3 Hypoadrenalism (anaemia may be marked by a low plasma volume).
> 7.4 Liver disease.
> 7.5 Renal failure (*see* Chapter 12).

Blood Loss

1. Acute blood loss does not cause a fall in haemoglobin for several hours. The anaemia of haemorrhage is initially normocytic and normochromic (or macrocytic and normochromic if there is a marked reticulocytosis); if chronic, iron deficiency frequently coexists and the anaemia then is microcytic and hypochromic in type.
2. Idiopathic pulmonary haemosiderosis is associated with a refractory iron deficient type of anaemia caused by pulmonary capillary rupture and haemorrhage into the pulmonary alveoli.
3. Goodpasture's syndrome is associated with a refractory iron deficiency type of anaemia caused by expectoration of iron-laden macrophages in the sputum and the renal failure complicating the acute glomerulonephritis.

Haemolysis

1. Congenital red cell disorders may be classified thus:

> 1.1 Affecting the red cell membrane are hereditary spherocytosis, elliptocytosis, stomatocytosis and acanthocytosis.
> 1.2 Enzyme defects, such as glucose-6-phosphate dehydrogenase deficiency, pyruvate-kinase deficiency and methaemoglobin reductase deficiency.
> 1.3 Abnormal or defective haemoglobin synthesis, such as occur in the haemoglobinopathies and thalassaemia syndromes.
> 1.4 Erythropoietic porphyria which is associated with circulating normoblasts as well as a reticulocytosis with considerable abnormalities of red cell morphology. The haemolytic effects tend to be clinically minor compared to the consequences of the skin sensitivity to ultraviolet light.

2. Immune red cell destruction may be (*see* Chapter 11):

> 2.1 Associated with idiopathic antibody production.
> 2.2 Secondary to lymphoproliferative and other neoplasms, autoimmune disorders and infections.

2.3 Associated with drug therapy.

2.4 A complication of blood transfusion.

2.5 Associated with haemolytic disease of the newborn.

3. Acquired non-immune red cell disorders may be classified thus:

3.1 An acquired abnormality of the red cell membrane (e.g. paroxysmal nocturnal haemoglobinuria).

3.2 The dyserythropoiesis of megaloblastic anaemias may be associated with a haemolytic element.

3.3 Mechanical trauma occurs with some diseased heart valves, cardiac valve prosthesis and in march haemoglobinuria; fragmentation of red cells also occurs in disseminated intravascular coagulation.

3.4 Severe burns may be associated with haemolysis due to thermal injury to red cells.

3.5 Chemical red cell injury occurs in lead poisoning, which interferes with normal red cell maturation and defective stippled cells have a shortened life span; arsine, naphthalene, nitrobenzene and trinitrotoluene may cause haemolysis.

3.6 Metabolic disorders may be associated with haemolysis, e.g. uraemia.

3.6 Infections, such as malaria and bartonellosis (Oroya fever), are associated with marked haemolysis; clostridial infections and occasionally streptococcal septicaemia may also be associated with haemolysis.

4. Hypersplenism which may be associated with:

4.1 Red cell sequestration in the spleen.

4.2 Premature red cell destruction.

4.3 An increase in plasma volume producing a relative anaemia.

Multiple Mechanisms

This is very common; for example the anaemia of acute leukaemia may be due to marrow replacement, ineffective erythropoiesis due to the leukaemic process, toxic dyserythropoiesis secondary to infection, folate deficiency, blood loss secondary to thrombocytopenia, and hypersplenism.

DIAGNOSIS OF ANAEMIA

The diagnosis of anaemia begins with clinical suspicion followed by analysis of an automated counter printout. The possibility of an increase or decrease in the plasma volume must be considered when evaluating the absolute haemoglobin level.

The type and cause of the anaemia may be apparent from the history and examination.

In other cases, the red cell indices may indicate the cause or point to further appropriate investigations.

As well as the haemoglobin level, the automated counters measure directly the red cell count and the mean cell volume. The other indices are then calculated as shown:

$$\text{Haematocrit or packed cell volume} = \frac{\text{MCV (fl)} \times \text{rbc count} \times 10^{12}/\text{l}}{1000}$$

$$\text{Mean cell haemoglobin (MCH)} = \frac{\text{Hb (g/dl)} \times 10}{\text{rbc count} \times 10^{12}/\text{l}} = \text{(pg)}$$

$$\text{Mean cell haemoglobin concentration (MCHC)} = \frac{\text{Hb (g/dl)}}{\text{Packed cell volume (per dl)}} = \text{(g/dl)}$$

The mean cell volume (MCV) is the most useful index in classifying the anaemias.

Microcytic Anaemia

Microcytic anaemia is usually associated with hypochromia and is found in:
1. Iron deficiency.
2. Thalassaemia.
3. Sideroblastic anaemia.
4. Chronic disease.
A microcytic anaemia which is hyperchromic may be found in spherocytosis.

Normocytic Anaemia

This type of anaemia is usually normochromic and is seen:
1. Following haemorrhage.
2. Haemolytic conditions.
3. In chronic disease in which there is impaired red cell production, such as pure red cell aplasia, aplastic anaemia, marrow infiltration, toxic and metabolic dyserythropoiesis.
4. Combined deficiencies, e.g. iron and folate deficiency in coeliac disease.
Following haemorrhage and haemolysis the anaemia may be macrocytic if there is a marked reticulocytosis; the MCV of a reticulocyte is approximately 110 fl.

Macrocytic Anaemias

1. Megaloblastic erythropoiesis (the red cells will show considerable abnormalities of morphology and the white cells and platelets will also show quantitative and morphological changes), due to vitamin B_{12}, folic acid deficiency or refractory megaloblastic anaemia.
2. Normoblastic erythropoiesis
    2.1 With increased erythroid marrow activity; post-haemorrhagic and haemolytic due to the raised reticulocyte count.
    2.2 With impaired erythroid marrow activity (i) leukaemia (especially acute), (ii) marrow infiltration with metastatic carcinoma, lymphoma, myelomas, myelofibrosis and osteopetrosis, (iii) aplastic anaemia, (iv) endocrine disorders,

myxoedema and hypopituitarism, (v) liver disease, (vi) scurvy, (vii) alcohol, (viii) protein malnutrition.

The next stage is the careful examination of the peripheral blood film. The cause of the anaemia may be apparent or highly suspected in which case appropriate further investigations can be requested.

Selected Further Reading

Izak G. and Lewis S. M. (ed.) (1972) Haemocytometry. In: *Modern Concepts in Haematology.* New York, Academic Press.
Williams W. J. et al. (ed.) (1977) Examination of the peripheral blood. In: *Haematology,* 2nd ed. New York, McGraw-Hill.

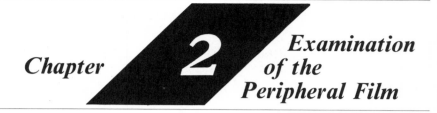

Chapter 2 — Examination of the Peripheral Film

PREPARATION AND STAINING OF BLOOD FILMS

It is essential that satisfactory films be made with a smooth-edged spreader that does not cause distortion of cells or irregular distribution. The blood samples must be fresh otherwise morphological changes will occur.

A small drop of blood placed 0·5 cm from the end of a clean slide is spread; the film being made trailing behind the spreader which is held at an angle of 45°. The dried smear should be 'fixed' as soon as possible in absolute alcohol if the film smear is not 'fixed and stained' immediately. Romanowsky stains using combinations of eosin and methylene blue are routinely employed, e.g. Leishman's, Wright's, May–Grünwald–Giemsa (*see* Chapter 28).

GENERAL EXAMINATION

With a low power objective the number and distribution of the white cells can be assessed and an area selected where the red cells are evenly distributed, not touching each other and not distorted. In every film the red cells, white cells and platelets must be examined systematically.

RED CELL MORPHOLOGY

The following appearances should be noted—size, shape, staining intensity, distribution of staining and the possible presence of inclusions.

Normal Appearance. Reference can be made to the white cells to help in assessing red cell size, but nothing can replace the observer using the same microscope all the time so that comparison of one film with the next becomes reliable. In health there is some variation in size of the red cells (6–8·5 μm) which mostly have a round contour, though up to 10 per cent may appear slightly oval in outline. Normal cells stain deeply at the periphery with a pale zone in the centre (*Fig. 2.1*).

Variation in Size (Anisocytosis). Anisocytosis is an increase in the variation of the size of the red cell population, and reflects dyserythropoiesis or fragmentation. The commonest cause is iron deficiency and it is particularly apparent after blood transfusion.

Some modern electronic cell counters (e.g. Coulter-S plus) calculate the individual red cell volume directly and, as well as determining the mean cell volume

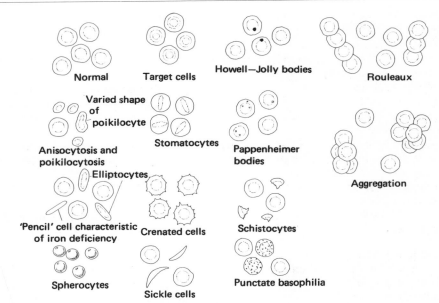

Fig. 2.1. Red cell abnormalities.

(MCV), estimate the red cell distribution width (RDW) which is a measure of anisocytosis.

Abnormalities of Shape (*Fig. 2.1*)

Poikilocytes. Variation in shape occurs due to similar causes which produce anisocytosis, hence these variations occur together though in differing degrees.

Elliptocytes. Oval cells occur in hereditary elliptocytosis, when over 90 per cent of cells may be affected or acquired in megaloblastic anaemia and also in iron deficiency when very narrow cells may be present—'pencil cells'.

Spherocytes. These cells are of smaller diameter, but of greater thickness than normal. Their presence may be due to:

1. A congenital abnormality as in hereditary spherocytosis.
2. An acquired abnormality associated with a positive direct antiglobulin test (DAT) test.
3. In association with hypertriglyceridaemia in acute alcoholic hepatitis (Zieve's syndrome).
4. Due to the action of bacterial lecithinases in clostridial infections.

Leptocytes. Abnormally thin cells occur in:

1. Iron deficiency.
2. Thalassaemia.
3. Some haemoglobinopathies, e.g. HbC.
4. Liver disease.
5. Sideroblastic anaemias.

Target Cells. These are a variety of leptocytes which, in addition to the thin rim of haemoglobin around the circumference of the cell, have also a small disc area of haemoglobin in the cell centre. These cells are found after splenectomy, in liver disease, thalassaemia, HbC disease, HbE disease, combinations of these haemoglobinopathies, and in some cases of severe iron deficiency.

Stomatocytes. As the name suggests these have the appearance of a stoma or mouth. Stomatocytosis may be hereditary, or associated with alcoholism and liver disease.

Crenated Cells. The surface is irregular and projections occur. These cells are found in uraemia, but may be artefactual.

Acanthocytes. These are a variety of crenated cells with marked irregularity of the surface, occurring in abetalipoproteinaemia, liver disease associated with haemolysis, pyruvate–kinase deficiency, malabsorption, kwashiorkor and sometimes following splenectomy.

Burr Cells. These are small cells or cell fragments with only a few spines. They are also to be found in uraemia, with bleeding peptic ulcer, carcinoma of the stomach, pyruvate–kinase deficiency and following transfusion with aged blood.

Schistocytes or fragmented cells occur in microangiopathic haemolytic anaemias (*see* Chapter 10).

Drepanocytes or sickle cells may be found in freshly-made films from patients with sickle disease.

Variation and Abnormalities of Staining and Inclusions

Polychromasia is due to ribonucleic acid (RNA) in the red cells being stained by the blue component as well as the red component of the Romanowsky stain and appear a purplish-grey colour on the film indicating the presence of a reticulocytosis. A deep intensity, referred to as 'blue polychromasia', occurs sometimes in the presence of extramedullary erythropoiesis.

Punctate basophilia causes the appearance of stippled red cells (probably due to degenerate mitochondria and siderosomes) and is associated with lead poisoning, thalassaemia and toxic conditions, including infections and intoxications.

Siderocytes are reticulocytes containing iron granules which are confirmed by the Prussian blue reaction and are seen especially after splenectomy and in hereditary spherocytosis, thalassaemia, lead poisoning, pernicious anaemia, haemochromatosis and also in infections and burns.

Howell–Jolly bodies are nuclear remnants and occur following splenectomy, in hyposplenic states such as coeliac disease and in folate-deficient megaloblastic anaemia.

Normoblasts may be found in many severe anaemias and sometimes in cyanotic heart disease. Very high normoblast counts usually reflect extramedullary erythropoiesis such as occurs in haemolytic disease of the newborn, thalassaemia major and myeloid metaplasia. In myeloid metaplasia and in bone marrow replacement syndromes (e.g. carcinomatosis, myelofibrosis, osteopetrosis) a leuco-erythroblastic condition occurs (immature white cells, in addition to nucleated red cell precursors).

Variation in Cell Distribution

Rouleaux formation is due to the red cell forming together 'like a stack of coins' and is associated with a high sedimentation rate.

Aggregation of red cells or 'clumping' is due to the presence of warm and cold agglutinins.

Malarial Parasites. These may be more readily apparent on a thick film. Romanowsky stains should be performed with a buffer at pH 7·2 (usually pH 6·8) as Shüffner dots are more readily demonstrated at a higher pH.

WHITE CELLS

Neutrophils

Structure. Size slightly smaller than the metamyelocyte, about 10–14 µm in diameter. The nucleus has coarse chromatin with 2–4 lobes. Sex chromatin, Barr bodies, appear as 'drumsticks' projecting from one of the lobes in about 3 per cent of female neutrophils; there is a single fine strand with a densely stained round knob at the end (*Fig. 2.2*). Sessile nodules, attached to the nucleus, are also a female sex characteristic. Drumsticks and sessile nodules are found in males with Klinefelter's syndrome and absent in females with Turner's syndrome. The cytoplasm is pale pink containing fine violet granules. There are three types of granules: azurophil granules which contain myeloperoxidase, cationic proteins and some lysozyme, specific granules containing some lysozyme, lactoferrin and vitamin B_{12}-binding protein, and lysosomes containing the digestive acid hydrolases.

Fig. 2.2.
Granulocytes.

Neutrophil with female 'drumstick'

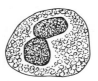

Eosinophil

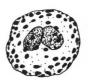

Basophil

Normal Levels and Physiological Variation. At birth the neutrophil count ranges from 5·0 to 13·0 × 10^9/l but by 1 week the level falls to about 2·0 to 7·0 × 10^9/l and remains constant throughout infancy, childhood and adult life. There is a slight diurnal variation, with a slight rise in the afternoon. A rise in the neutrophil count occurs physiologically during exercise, following a heavy meal, with anxiety or fear (sympathetic activity), in late pregnancy and during labour, returning to normal within 1 week of the puerperium.

Neutrophilia. This occurs in a number of pathological states:

1. Infections, especially with pyogenic organisms, but also in spirochaetal, rickettsial and viral infections, e.g. poliomyelitis, herpes zoster.

2. Tissue injury as with fractures, crush injury, burns, myocardial infarction and pulmonary embolism.

3. Connective-tissue diseases and other inflammatory disorders.

4. Metabolic disorders, such as diabetic ketosis, starvation, eclampsia, acute gout, uraemia, Cushing's disease and acute poisoning.

5. Myeloproliferative disorders—chronic myeloid leukaemia, polycythaemia rubra vera, myeloid metaplasia and myelofibrosis.

6. Rapidly growing malignant tumours.

Neutropenia. This occurs in:

1. Certain bacterial infections, typhoid, paratyphoid and brucella and sometimes in miliary TB.

2. Many protozoal, fungal, viral or rickettsial infections.

3. Bone marrow infiltration due to myelofibrosis, leukaemia, lymphoma, myeloma and carcinoma.

4. Total marrow depression in aplastic anaemia.

5. Hypersensitivity of drugs with immune destruction of myeloid cells.

6. Collagen disorders as with systemic lupus erythematosus, and rheumatoid arthritis with splenomegaly (Still's disease and Felty's syndrome).

7. Splenomegaly of other causes.

8. Association with megaloblastic anaemia.

9. Endocrine disorders of hypopituitarism and hypoadrenalism.

10. Cyclical neutropenia (*see* Chapter 13).

11. Kostmann's syndrome (severity of neutropenia usually declines with age).

Fig. 2.3. Neutrophil abnormalities.

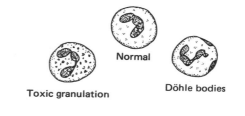

Normal

Toxic granulation

Döhle bodies

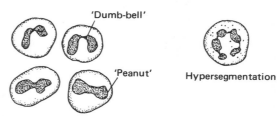

'Dumb-bell'

'Peanut'

Hypersegmentation

Pegler—Huët anomaly
with associated lack of granulation

Morphological Changes (*Fig. 2.3*). An increase in cells with few lobes is referred to as a 'shift to the left' and occurs in acute infections. The autosomal dominant condition of the Pelger–Huët anomaly is associated with the presence of neutrophils with not more than two lobes, about 30 per cent of the cells appearing as band forms. Appearances similar to Pelger–Huët anomaly may be found in acquired conditions such as leukaemia, severe infections and metastases affecting the bones. Also the anomaly may be induced by drugs, especially sulphonamides. A 'shift to the right' occurs in vitamin B_{12} and also folic acid deficiency. A hereditary disorder of hypersegmentation occurs as a Mendelian dominant; it is unassociated with any other anomaly.

Heavy granulation occurs in toxic conditions associated with bacterial infections. Large reddish granules may be found in aplastic anaemia and sometimes in myeloproliferative diseases. Decreased granulation frequently occurs in acute leukaemia and may occur in severe infections.

Döhle bodies are deeply staining and are 2–3 μ in diameter, being oval or round and are found in severe infections, burns, leukaemia, other malignancies and occasionally are seen during pregnancy.

The May–Hegglin anomaly is an inherited disorder associated with 'Döhle-like bodies', leucopenia and giant platelets. The anomaly is seldom associated with clinical symptoms although occasionally there is a bleeding tendency.

The Alder–Reilly anomaly is the presence of large granules in neutrophils (and sometimes in the other types of cells in the peripheral blood) due to a metabolic defect of polysaccharides and may be associated with gargoylism; it is an autosomal recessive condition.

In the Chédiak–Higashi syndrome there are giant lysosomes which appear as eosinophilic inclusions in neutrophils and other cells (*see* Chapter 13).

Eosinophils

Structure. Size 10–15 μm in diameter; usually two lobes to the nucleus. Granules are intensely eosinophilic and have a high content of peroxidase and numerous other enzymes, including a PAS-reactive mucopolysaccharide (*see Fig. 2.2*).

Normal Levels and Physiological Variation. The absolute eosinophil count varies from 0.04 to $0.4 \times 10^9/l$. The maximum count occurs between midnight and 3 a.m. and the minimum count at about noon. The rhythm is reversed in night workers.

Eosinophilia. This occurs in:

1. Allergic conditions such as asthma, urticaria, hay fever, serum sickness, angioneurotic oedema, food and drug allergies.

2. Drug ingestion without overt evidence of allergy, e.g. penicillin, sulphonamides and streptomycin.

3. Parasitic infections; ankylostoma duodenale, ascaris lumbricoides, bilharzia, filaria, hydatid, toxicara and trichuris—the eosinophilia is more marked when parasites invade tissues than with intestinal infestation.

4. Occasional bacterial infections, e.g. scarlet fever and tuberculosis.

5. Many skin diseases including eczema, exfoliative dermatitis, dermatitis herpetiformis, scabies and sometimes psoriasis.

6. Pulmonary eosinophilia (Loeffler's syndrome) which may or may not be associated with parasitic infections or allergy.

7. Loeffler's endocarditis.

8. Gastrointestinal disorders including eosinophilic gastroenteritis, protein-losing enteropathy and inflammatory bowel disease.

9. Idiopathic histiocytosis including eosinophilic granuloma of bone, Letterer–Siwe disease and Hand–Schüller–Christian disease.

10. Malignant haematological disorders; eosinophilic leukaemia (eosinophils may be deficient in granules), chronic myeloid leukaemia when eosinophilic myelocytes may be present, polycythaemia rubra vera, Hodgkin's disease and non-Hodgkin's lymphomas (especially of T cell origin).

11. Non-haematological malignancies including metastatic carcinoma, melanoma and other epithelial tumours.

12. Miscellaneous disorders including polyarteritis nodosa, sarcoidosis, Goodpasture's syndrome, hypoadrenalism and familial eosinophilia.

Eosinopenia. This may occur:
1. In the intermenstrual period.
2. Associated with stress.
3. Following the administration of adrenocorticosteroids and sympathomimetic amines (adrenaline, noradrenaline and ephedrine) and also insulin.
4. Endocrine disorders such as Cushing's disease and acromegaly.
5. Systemic lupus erythematosus.

Basophils

Structure. Size 10–15 μm in diameter. Coarse, large purplish-black granules in the cytoplasm overlie the nucleus which contains 2–3 lobes (*Fig. 2.2*). The granules contain heparin and histamine. Similar cells found in the tissues are called mast cells.

Normal Levels. The absolute basophil count varies from $0 \cdot 01$ to $0 \cdot 1 \times 10^9/l$.

Basophilia. This occurs in:
1. Chronic myeloid leukaemia. A rise in the basophil count is a serious prognostic sign and may herald the transition to a 'blastic' phase of the disease.
2. Myelofibrosis, myeloid metaplasia and also in polycythaemia rubra vera if there is a leucocytosis.
3. Myxoedema. The basophil absolute count varies inversely with thyroid function.
4. Chronic infections occasionally and rarely in some viral infections.

Basopenia. This can only be detected with difficulty.
1. Commonly occurs in association with a neutrophil leucocytosis associated with infection, neoplasia and tissue necrosis.
2. Follows the administration of steroids.
3. Occurs in thyrotoxicosis.
4. May occur in urticaria.

Lymphocytes

Normal Levels and Physiological Variation. The normal lymphocyte count varies with age. At birth, the count is $3 \cdot 5 – 8 \cdot 5 \times 10^9/l$ and although the upper limit remains constant during the early years, at 6 years the upper limit is taken at $5 \cdot 5 \times 10^9/l$, then the absolute count gradually falls until at the age of 12 years the adult range of $1 \cdot 5 – 3 \cdot 5 \times 10^9/l$ is attained.

Many subpopulations of lymphocytes are recognized by phenotypic and functional analysis (*Table 2.1*).

T cells are comprised of at least two subgroups: a 'helper' subset and a 'suppressor' subset. These subgroups can be identified with specific monoclonal antisera and the ratio of helper : suppressor cells is approximately 2 : 1.

Table 2.1. Phenotype of peripheral blood lymphocytes

	Sheep red blood cell rosette receptor	Surface immunoglobulin	Percentage
T cells	+	—	60–80
B cells	—	+	10–30
Non T non B cells	—	—	2–10

B cells carry surface immunoglobulin. The approximate incidence of the specific surface immunoglobulin is as follows: IgG 33 per cent, IgA 10 per cent, IgM 40 per cent and IgD 30 per cent. Many cells have both IgM and IgD. Any one cell is restricted to expression of only one light chain type. The ratio of $\kappa : \lambda$ light chain bearing B cells is approximately $2 : 1$.

Lymphocytosis. This occurs in:

1. Infections.

    1.1 Viral infections.

    1.2 Young children often respond with a lymphocytosis to an infection which would produce a neutrophilia in adults.

    1.3 Certain acute bacterial infections such as pertussis and acute infectious lymphocytosis.

    1.4 Chronic bacterial infections, brucellosis, tuberculosis and secondary syphilis.

    1.5 Parasitic infections, such as toxoplasmosis.

2. Malignant haematological disorders, chronic lymphatic leukaemia, lymphocytic lymphoma (if haematological spread), multiple myeloma.

3. Auto-immune conditions, rheumatoid arthritis, thyrotoxicosis, Hashimoto's disease.

4. Endocrine disorders, myxoedema and hypopituitarism.

5. Carcinoma.

Lymphocytopenia. This occurs in:

1. Decreased production.

    1.1 Congenital: thymic aplasia, Wiskott–Aldrich syndrome, Di George's syndrome and the agammaglobulinaemia syndromes (associated with thymoma, Swiss-type, sex-linked and dwarfism ectodermal dysplastic type).

    1.2 Acquired, in severe pancytopenia, lymphocyte-depleted Hodgkin's disease and also in some cases of non-Hodgkin's lymphoma, sarcoidosis, renal failure.

2. Increased lymphocyte destruction.

    2.1 X-rays.

    2.2 Cytotoxic drugs.

    2.3 Steroid administration and ACTH administration, also Cushing's disease and syndrome.

    2.4 Following administration of antilymphocyte globulin.

3. Intestinal lymphocyte loss in intestinal lymphangiectasis, mesenteric lymphatic obstruction, Whipple's disease.

The lymphopenia associated with some infections is partly due to decreased production and partly due to increased destruction.

Morphological Changes. Atypical lymphocytes are moderately enlarged with an eccentric nucleus, oval or kidney-shaped, with coarsely stranded nuclear chromatin occasionally showing nucleoli and a deep blue staining cytoplasm which may contain vacuoles and azurophil granules. These cells are most commonly found in glandular fever, infective hepatitis, cytomegalovirus infection, toxoplasmosis and in drug hypersensitivity reactions. In glandular fever and some other disorders these cells are of the suppressor T cell type. Alder–Reilly bodies or granules occur in the metabolic disorder of polysaccharides associated with azurophilic inclusions. Binucleate lymphocytes are found in the peripheral blood following irradiation.

Plasma Cells

These cells are found only rarely in the peripheral blood in health. May be present in small numbers in:
1. Serum sickness.
2. Sarcoidosis.
3. Viral infections such as measles, rubella, chicken pox, mumps and infectious mononucleosis.
4. Bacterial infections such as typhoid, streptococcal cellulitis and subacute bacterial endocarditis.
5. Gaucher's disease.
6. Heavy chain disease.
7. In myeloma occasional atypical plasma cells may be found in the peripheral blood; rarely large numbers may be present—plasma-cell leukaemia.

Atypical Plasma Cells. These may be found:
1. In myeloma and plasma-cell leukaemia; the cells may be immature with vacuolation of cytoplasm and the presence of Russell bodies (granular and hyaline bodies staining red with Romanowsky stains).
2. During treatment with stilbamidine and with pentamidine, 'Snapper–Schneid' basophilic inclusions may be present.

Monocytes

Normal Range and Physiological Variation. In the first week of life, the count may be as high as $4 \times 10^9/l$, but rapidly falls during the first week so that the maximum count is about $1·2 \times 10^9/l$ between 1 week and 6 months. At 4 years the monocyte count assumes the normal adult range of $0·2–0·8 \times 10^9/l$.

Monocytosis. This occurs in:
1. Convalescence from many acute infections.
2. Some chronic bacterial infections such as tuberculosis, brucellosis, subacute bacterial endocarditis.
3. Viral infections, especially in young children (also in older children and adults).
4. Protozoal infections, malaria, kala-azar and trypanosomiasis.
5. Ulcerative colitis and Crohn's disease.
6. Sarcoidosis.
7. Collagen vascular diseases.
8. Hodgkin's disease.
9. Monocytic leukaemia.
10. Some preleukaemic states.

PLATELETS

Normal Appearance and Quantitative Variations. Platelets appears as round or oval bodies, 2–4 μm in diameter with a light blue background, but packed with azurophilic granules. The ratio of the number of platelets to red cells is about 1 : 20, but there is great normal variation in the peripheral film due to clumping and margination. However, in thrombocytopenia, the platelets are scanty and in thrombocythaemia they may appear very numerous.

Morphological Variation. It is often difficult to make a satisfactory assessment of variations in morphology because of changes which occur as a result of storage in anticoagulant before the smear is made and because of variations in technique of the specimen collection and smear preparation. If films are made directly from the peripheral blood without the addition of an anticoagulant some small clumps will be seen. Neonates have greater morphological variation of platelets than older infants, children and adults.

Abnormal Platelet Appearances

Immune Thrombocytopenia. Reduced numbers associated with giant platelets and marked anisocytosis.

Myeloproliferative Disorders. Increased numbers associated with giant and bizarre forms.

Post-splenectomy. Similar appearances to those found in the myeloproliferative disorders may occur following splenectomy, although the count usually returns to normal within a few months.

Bernard–Soulier Syndrome. A familial bleeding disorder associated with dense granules present in large platelets.

May–Hegglin Anomaly. A familial condition with the presence of giant platelets and Döhle bodies in the granulocytes; occasionally there may be thrombocytopenia. Clinical symptoms are rare.

Glanzmann's Diseases. A thrombasthenic disorder in which absence of platelet clumping may be noted in the peripheral blood.

'Storage Pool' Disease. This is associated with a deficit of adenosine diphosphate (ADP) release; small platelets are found in the peripheral films of some patients.

Wiskott–Aldrich Syndrome. This is a sex-linked recessive disorder characterized by abnormally small platelets, thrombocytopenia, bleeding tendency, recurrent pyogenic infections (due to an immunological deficiency) and eczema.

Selected Further Reading

Begemann H. and Rastetter J. (1979) *Atlas of Clinical Haematology*, 3rd ed. Berlin, Springer-Verlag.
Dacie J. V. and Lewis S. M. (1975) *Practical Haematology*, 5th ed. Edinburgh, Churchill Livingstone.

3

DESCRIPTION OF THE MARROW

At birth the volume of the bone marrow is some 80 ml and it is all 'red'. It is composed of a supporting structure of reticulin cells whose fibres form a network, vascular ramifications, and haemopoietic cells clustered around venous sinuses. From the age of 6 years the 'red' marrow is slowly replaced by 'yellow' marrow composed of fat cells occupying the interstices of the reticulum network, in the shafts of the long bones. In adults 'red' marrow occurs only in small zones at the upper ends of the femora and humeri and the flat bones, notably vertebrae, ribs, sternum, clavicles, scapulae, pelvis and skull, occupying some $1\frac{1}{2}$–2 litres of the total marrow volume of 3–4 litres.

The development of haemopoietic cells is summarized in *Fig. 3.1.*

TECHNIQUES OF OBTAINING BONE MARROW

Bone marrow may be obtained either by aspiration or by biopsy. The only absolute contraindication to the procedure is a severe uncontrolled bleeding tendency.

Aspirates are obtained, usually using a Klima (guard adjustable by threaded shaft) or Salah (guard fixed by side screw) from the sternum, anterior or posterior iliac crests or, rarely, from a lumbar vertebral spine. Sternal aspirates are the most cellular and are taken just to the side of the midline, as the median raphe is hypocellular, below the level of the second costal cartilage. In infants under the age of 12 months, samples may be obtained from the medial aspect of the tibia, distal to the level of the tubercle. After that age, the posterior iliac crest is used. The sternum is very thin in a child and this site should not be used until after puberty. Biopsies are usually performed with a Jamshidi needle from the posterior iliac crest. A cone of marrow is obtained which is examined after fixation, decalcification, wax embedding and section. Where there has been a dry aspirate, dab preparations of the biopsy onto a slide can be made before the biopsy core is placed into fixative.

STAINING OF MARROW SPECIMENS

Smears are routinely stained by the May–Grünwald–Giemsa technique and Perl's Prussian blue stain for iron. Additional stains which are sometimes performed

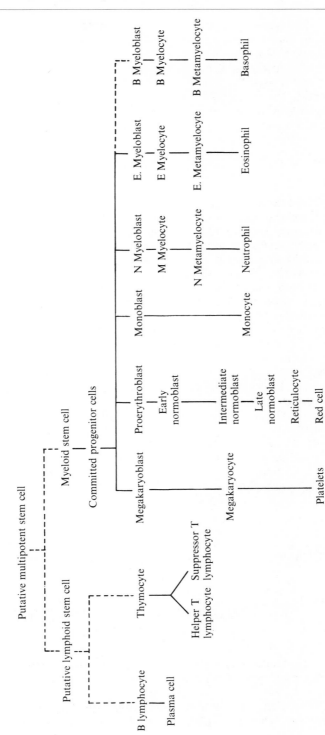

Fig. 3.1. Differentiation of blood cells.

include:

1. Sudan black or peroxidase stains to facilitate the identification of myeloid cells in acute leukaemia.
2. Periodic acid–Schiff reaction which stains granules containing glycogen magenta and is used to identify lymphoblasts and abnormal normoblasts.
3. Esterase stains are used to differentiate monocytes from granulocytic cells.
4. Haematoxylin stain of biopsy specimens to detect the architectural pattern.
5. Reticulin stain of biopsy specimens to detect myelofibrosis.

TECHNIQUE OF EXAMINATION

Smears are examined under the low power objective to determine that a satisfactory smear has been made. Almost all the cells should be touching one another except in the fragments of unspread marrow to be found in the trails of the smear. The fragments of normal marrow from the sternum and posterior iliac crest contain fat cells comprising between 40 and 70 per cent; if haematological cells comprise less than 25 per cent of the volume of fragment, the marrow is 'hypo-cellular', if more than 70 per cent, it is 'hypercellular'. The number of fragments also help in assessing cellularity; in a 'hypoplastic' marrow, the fragments may be absent. Under low power the number of megakaryocytes which tend to be carried into the trails can be assessed as can the presence of abnormal clumps of cells which may be found in myeloma and secondary carcinoma.

Under an oil-immersion lens the ratio of myeloid to erythroid precursor cells is determined—normally between 2·5 : 1 and 10 : 1 in adults. At birth the ratio is about 2 : 1 but by 2 weeks of age the ratio increases to about 10 : 1. Lymphocytes are more numerous in infants than adults and may account for up to 50 per cent of the nucleated cells. An aspirate from the vicinity of a lymphoid aggregate present in the marrow cavity may be responsible for great variation in the lymphocyte count. After the age of 5 years, the lymphocyte count comprises less than 20 per cent of the nucleated cells. Pregnancy is associated with increased marrow activity; the number of immature cells is also increased, the myeloid series being more affected than the lymphoid. The hypercellularity of pregnancy does not return to normal until about the sixth week of the puerperium.

Marrow Differential Count

At least 500 cells should be counted. Dilution with peripheral blood may distort the count.

MORPHOLOGY AND PHENOTYPE OF NORMAL CELLS

The following descriptions relate to May–Grünwald–Giemsa-stained preparations unless otherwise stated. The percentages relate to normal marrows (*Figs. 3.2, 3.3, 3.4*).

Putative Stem Cell. The putative multipotent stem cell has not been identified microscopically. These cells probably do not carry the Ia antigen (Ia − ve).

Fig. 3.2. Development of a neutrophil.

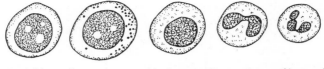

Myeloblast   Promyelocyte   Myelocyte   Metamyelocyte   Neutrophil

Fig. 3.3. Lymphoid cells.

Lymphoblast   Small lymphocyte

Fig. 3.4. Development of a red cell.

Proerythroblast   Early   Middle   Late   Mature
                                                        red cell

                            normoblasts

Committed Myeloid Progenitor Cells. These can be enumerated by in vitro colony-forming assays. The cells vary in size between 10 and 25 µm, have a high nuclear to cytoplasmic ratio, with little nuclear condensation and several ill-defined nucleoli. The cytoplasm is basophilic and contains no granules. Electron microscopy reveals large numbers of mitochondria and ribosomes in the cytoplasm. These cells carry the Ia antigen but not the marker seen in most cases of acute lymphoblastic leukaemia (cALL negative).

Myeloblast (0·1–3 per cent). Vary in size from 10 to 25 µm. They contain a large nucleus and have relatively little cytoplasm. The nucleus is round or slightly oval with a fine chromatin pattern with little condensation around nucleoli or nuclear membrane. Nucleoli are 2–5 in number and pale blue. The cytoplasm is blue, usually uniform in colour, though sometimes foamy. A perinuclear clear zone is rarely present.

Auer rods result from abnormal alignment of azurophil granules in cytoplasm of leukaemia cells and occur in acute myeloblastic leukaemia. Reider cells occur in acute leukaemia—the nuclei of myeloblasts or lymphoblasts show deep indentations or cleavages.

Promyelocyte (0·5–5 per cent). Slightly larger, on average, than a myeloblast, with more abundant cytoplasm containing primary granules; the nucleus still contains nucleoli.

Myelocyte (5–20 per cent). Similar in size to the promyelocyte. The nucleus is eccentric, the chromatin pattern is more coarse than its precursor cells, and no nucleoli are present. Identifiable as neutrophilic, eosinophilic or basophilic from the colour of the granules. Eosinophil myelocytes have blue cytoplasm present between eosinophilic granules. Eosinophil granules are large, coarse and orange-red in colour. Basophil granules are large, intensely blue-black; some of the granules overlie the nucleus. The neutrophil granules are fine pink-mauve and, like eosinophilic granules, do not overlie the nucleus.

Metamyelocyte (1–30 per cent). Characterized by a horseshoe-shaped nucleus but otherwise similar in nuclear features and cell size to a myelocyte. There are more granules present in the cytoplasm. The metamyelocyte develops into a band form with a nucleus of uniform thickness.

Mature Granulocytes. Described in Chapter 2.

Lymphoblasts. Normally absent but sometimes seen in infants, children and in regenerating marrows. They are 10–15 μm in diameter. The nuclear chromatin is more coarse than myeloblasts and shows condensation around the nuclear membrane and nucleoli of which there are usually one or two. The cytoplasm is more scanty than that of myeloblasts and there is often a perinuclear clear zone.

Lymphocytes (5–20 per cent in adults). Small lymphocytes are approximately 8–10 μm in diameter, large lymphocytes up to 20 μm in diameter. The round nucleus has a heavily clumped coarse chromatin pattern. The cytoplasm is pale blue, sometimes containing a few magenta granules. Most T lymphocytes have a single cytoplasmic dot staining with non-specific esterase and acid phosphatase.

Plasma Cells (0·1–3·5 per cent). Size approximately 12–20 μm in diameter. Nucleus is round and eccentrically placed, chromatin is coarse and clumped. Binucleated forms sometimes occur. Cytoplasm is deep blue, often with a perinuclear clear zone; vacuoles may be present.

Proerythroblasts (0·5–5 per cent). Size 12–20 μm in diameter. Large round or oval nucleus with coarse reticular pattern of chromatin containing 3–5 prominent nucleoli. Thin rim of deep blue cytoplasm which is homogeneous except for a perinuclear clear zone.

Early or Basophilic Normoblasts (2–20 per cent). Size 12–13 μm in diameter. Round nucleus, coarse chromatin pattern with demarcation between chromatin and parachromatin and no nucleoli present. Cytoplasm is deep blue.

Intermediate or Polychromatic Normoblasts (2–20 per cent). Size 12–16 μm in diameter. Round nucleus becoming smaller with greater condensation of chromatin. Cytoplasm showing some pink areas adjacent to the nuclear membrane.

Late or Acidophilic (Orthochromic) Normoblasts (2–10 per cent). Size 8–12 μm. Nuclear chromatin becomes condensed and pyknotic and may show fragmentation. Cytoplasm is slate-pink or pink in colour (depending upon the reduction of ribonucleic acid and the formation of haemoglobin).

Megakaryocytes (0·1–0·5 per cent). Size varies from 30 to 150 μm in diameter. Nucleus is polypoid varying from 4 to 16 lobes. The nuclear chromatin has coarse strands often with clumps. Cytoplasm is pale blue with azurophilic granules (*Fig. 3.5*).

Monoblasts (occasional cell present in marrow). Size about 14–20 μm in diameter. The nucleus is large with a slight indentation, 'stringy' chromatin and one or two nucleoli. Cytoplasm greyish in colour.

Fig. 3.5.
Megakaryocyte.

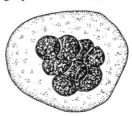

Monocytes (0·05–2 per cent). Size 16–20 μm in diameter. The nucleus is large, oval or indented, with fine chromatin. Cytoplasm is greyish-blue containing very small vacuoles ('ground-glass' appearance) and may be irregular in outline.

Reticulum Cells (0·1–2 per cent). Size 20–30 μm in diameter. The nucleus is round with fine reticular strands, containing 1 or 2 blue nucleoli. The cytoplasm is abundant, pale basophilic, often 'foamy' and may contain a few azure granules.

Osteoblasts (may occur in groups especially in marrow from infants). Oval cells 25–50 μm in length. The nucleus is usually eccentric with coarse chromatin often with clumping and contains 1–3 nucleoli. The cytoplasm is light or dark blue and may contain a few azure granules.

Osteoclasts (may be seen in marrows from infants). Giant cells, sometimes over 100 μm in diameter. There is a polypoid nucleus with individual, nuclei often not touching. There is dense nuclear chromatin with single nucleolus in each nucleus.

ALTERATION IN CELLULARITY AFFECTING ALL ELEMENTS

Hypoplasia—Pancytopenia (*see* Chapter 6)

1. Congenital aplastic anaemia.
2. Chronic acquired.
3. Acute transient.

Hyperplasia

1. Cytopenias due to peripheral destruction including drugs and hypersplenism.
2. Reactive, e.g. tumours or infection.
3. Myeloproliferative disorders.
4. Megaloblastic and some cases of sideroblastic anaemia.

ALTERATION IN MYELOID : ERYTHROID RATIO

The normal M : E ratio 2·5 to 10 : 1.
Alteration in the myeloid : erythroid ratio may be due to:

1. *Myeloid Hyperplasia*

May be subdivided according to the cell types present:

1.1 Myeloblasts and promyelocytes increased in: (i) Acute myeloid leukaemia. (ii) Refractory anaemia with excess blasts and subacute myeloid leukaemia. (iii) Myeloproliferative disorders, especially chronic myeloid leukaemia in accelerated phase. (iv) Occasionally in reactive states, e.g.: infection, especially in childhood. (v) Recovery from some cases of neutropenia.

1.2 Myelocytes, metamyelocytes and neutrophils increased in: (i) Association with peripheral blood neutrophilia. (ii) Peripheral destruction of neutrophils. (iii) Myeloproliferative disorders. (iv) Occasionally in sideroblastic anaemia.

2. *Myeloid Hypoplasia*

2.1 Congenital.
2.2 Acquired, including drugs.

3. *Erythroid Hyperplasia*

3.1 Normoblastic—haemolysis or following blood loss.
            —polycythaemia, primary or secondary.
3.2 Megaloblastic (*see* Chapter 5).

4. *Erythroid Hypoplasia* (*see* Chapter 6)

MORPHOLOGY OF ABNORMAL MARROWS

Megaloblastic Erythropoiesis (*see* Chapter 5)

Iron in Bone Marrow

The Prussian blue reaction stains haemosiderin granules blue; some granules lie free, others within reticulo-endothelial cells. A few granules may be present normally in normoblasts.

Decreased haemosiderin occurs in iron deficiency (*see* Chapter 4).
Increased haemosiderin occurs in:
1. Haemochromatosis.
2. Transfusion haemosiderosis.
3. Pernicious anaemia.
4. Aplastic anaemia.
5. Refractory sideroblastic anaemia.
Sideroblasts are classified into three types:
1. Normal, characterized by granules few in number, small in size and randomly distributed in the cytoplasm.
2. Associated with increased transferrin saturation, characterized by more numerous granules which are larger in size and randomly distributed in the cytoplasm.
3. Not related to increased transferrin saturation:
            3.1 Hereditary sideroblastic anaemias.
            3.2 Acquired sideroblastic anaemias (*see* Chapter 4).

Plasma and 'Myeloma' Cells

An increase in plasma cells is more commonly reactive than malignant. The differential diagnosis of plasmacytosis is discussed in Chapter 18.

Eosinophils

They are increased in:
1. Conditions producing an eosinophilia in the peripheral blood (*see* Chapter 2).
2. Carcinomatosis involving the bone marrow.
3. Eosinophilic granuloma of bone.
They are decreased in conditions associated with eosinopenia (*see* Chapter 2).

Basophils

Increased numbers are found around lymphoid aggregates in the bone marrow; otherwise the number of marrow basophils appear to reflect the peripheral basophil count. Mast cells are increased in the marrow in pancytopenia, acute lymphoblastic leukaemia, chronic lymphocytic leukaemia, with secondary carcinoma infiltration, and in the urticaria pigmentosa—systemic mastocytosis syndrome.

Lymphoblasts

They appear in the marrow in:
1. Acute lymphoblastic leukaemia.
2. Lymphoblastic lymphomas.
3. Chronic lymphatic leukaemia, though the majority of cells are mature lymphocytes.

Lymphocytes

Increased numbers occur physiologically in the newborn and first few months of life (up to 50 per cent of nucleated cells may be lymphocytes during first few weeks of life). Pathological increase occurs in:
1. Peripheral blood lymphocytosis (*see* Chapter 2).
2. Chronic lymphocytic leukaemia.
3. Lymphocytic lymphomas. In lymphomatous infiltration of the marrow, the lymphocytes are predominantly peritrabecular in their distribution.
4. Infectious mononucleosis.
5. Macroglobulinaemia.
6. Cold agglutinin disease.
7. Aplastic anaemia (often relative).
8. Occasionally in myelofibrosis.

Monocytes

Increased in conditions associated with a monocytosis in the peripheral blood (*see* Chapter 2).

Abnormal Macrophages (Foam Cells)

Storage Diseases
1. *Gaucher's disease* is inherited as an autosomal recessive disorder. It is common in Ashkenazi Jews with infantile, juvenile and adult forms due to a

deficiency of β-glucocerebrosidase, characterized by hepatosplenomegaly, skin pigmentation, pingueculae and bone destruction later associated with pancytopenia. Macrophages 20–80 μm in diameter with pale blue cytoplasm and containing wavy fibrils are found in the bone marrow. The cytoplasm stains with PAS and Sudan black B.

2. *Niemann–Pick's disease* is inherited as an autosomal recessive disorder usually occurring in infants (85 per cent) or young children (15 per cent); commoner in Ashkenazi Jews. It is characterized by enlargement of liver, spleen, lymph glands and mental retardation (some have a 'cherry-red' macula). There is jaundice, feeding difficulties, cachexia and death commonly due to bronchopneumonia. The cytoplasm of the macrophages is filled with droplets containing sphingomyelin presenting a honeycomb appearance and staining with Sudan black B.

3. *Gangliosidoses* are of two types, both autosomal recessive:

> 3.1 GM1 type: generalized gangliosidosis affecting brain and viscera, due to deficiency of β-galactosidase.
> 3.2 GM2 type: Tay–Sachs' disease, amaurotic familial idiocy due to hexosaminidase A deficiency.

4. *Fabry's disease* (angiokeratoma corporis diffusum) a sex-linked recessive disorder due to deposition of abnormal glycolipid (due to α-galactosidase deficiency) in nervous system, myocardium vascular smooth muscle and characterized by pain in limbs, punctate telangiectasias around scrotum, umbilicus, thighs and buttocks, proteinuria and oedema. Deposits in organs and histiocytes stain with PAS and Indian black B.

5. *Cholesteryl ester hydrolase and triglyceride lipase deficiency.* Two types of these autosomal recessive disorders are recognized:

> 5.1 Wolman's disease. Infants fail to thrive, have gastrointestinal symptoms and hepatosplenomegaly. Non-polar lipids are found in marrow histiocytes.
> 5.2 Cholesteryl ester storage disease. There is a relatively benign course with massive hepatomegaly with or without splenomegaly. Ceroid pigment and lipid accumulate in macrophages.

6. *Hyperlipoproteinaemia.* Types I to V are recognized by the electrophoretic lipoprotein pattern. Each type may be primary or secondary to other diseases. Foam cells may be found in the bone marrow in all types. Tangier disease is characterized in the homozygote form by absence of high-density lipoproteins and the deposition of cholesteryl esters in reticulo-endothelial cells and the Schwann cells of the peripheral nerves.

7. *Von Gierke's glycogen storage disease* is due to glucose-6-phosphatase deficiency inherited as an autosomal recessive with hepatic and renal enlargement, hypoglycaemia, hyperlipidaemia, anaemia and retarded growth. Glycogen granules are present in macrophages. A mild bleeding diathesis associated with a prolonged bleeding time may occur. There is deficient PF3 activity and abnormal platelet aggregation, probably related to hyperlipidaemia.

Sea-blue Histiocytes. Lipid-containing histiocytes with cytoplasm staining 'sea-blue' are 20–60 μm in diameter with a single eccentric nucleus which has coarse chromatin structure. Granules stain with PAS and Sudan black B. They may be classified into:

1. Primary disorder inherited as autosomal recessive characterized by spleno-

megaly and sometimes hepatomegaly and often mild secondary thrombocytopenia. Occasionally macular disorders, neurological complications and pulmonary infiltrates may occur in more progressive forms of the disease.

2. Acquired disorder may be associated with the following disorders: rheumatoid arthritis, chronic granulomatous disease, sarcoidosis, chronic myeloid leukaemia, polycythaemia rubra vera, sickle-cell disease, thalassaemia, immune thrombocytopenic purpura and some of the lipid storage diseases.

Whipple's Disease. Macrophages containing rod-like cytoplasmic inclusions which are PAS-positive occur in the liver, spleen, lymph nodes and bone marrow. Clinically characterized by arthralgia, abdominal pain and impaired intestinal adsorption.

Hermansky–Pudlak Syndrome. Pigmented macrophages are found in the bone marrow. The syndrome is due to an autosomal recessive disorder characterized by albinism and a prolonged bleeding time due to 5 HT and nucleotide deficiency in platelets.

Histiocytosis X Spectrum (*see* Chapter 13)

Megakaryocytes

Increased in:
1. Platelet destruction, e.g. immune thrombocytopenic purpura, hypersplenism.
2. Reactive marrows, e.g. infection, bleeding.
3. Myeloproliferative disorders, especially primary thrombocythaemia and myelofibrosis.

Decreased in:
1. Congenital hypomegakaryocytic syndromes (*see* Chapter 20).
2. Marrow hypoplasia (including paroxysmal nocturnal haemoglobinuria).
3. Marrow infiltration.
4. Severe infections, especially rickettsial and viral.
5. Drugs, including gold, sulphonamides, chlorpropamide, chlorthiazide, butazolidine, alcohol and steroids.
6. Megaloblastic anaemia.
7. Some cases of cirrhosis.

Malignant Cells present in Bone-marrow Aspirates and Sections

Malignant cells in aspirates are characterized by:
1. Different morphology from normal marrow elements.
2. High nuclear : cytoplasmic ratio.
3. Cells appearing in clumps or trails.
4. Nuclear moulding often present.
5. Very large nucleoli common.

Definitive diagnostic feature of certain neoplasms include:
1. Melanin pigment.
2. Voluminous honeycomb cytoplasm staining with PAS, found in hypernephroma cells.
3. Mucin (stained with muci-carmine) cytoplasmic inclusions in adenocarcinoma.

Common primary tumours that metastasize to bone marrow include breast, lung, kidney, prostate, thyroid, large bowel and, in young children, neuro-blastoma. Generalized neuroblastoma infiltration may resemble an acute lym-phoblastic leukaemic marrow. Sarcomas also may metastasize to the bone marrow.

Although lymphoma infiltration may be diagnosed on marrow aspirates, biopsy sections increase the chance of a positive diagnosis and improve accuracy of diagnosing the type of lymphoma. The same advantages apply to diagnosis of secondary deposits.

Parasites in Bone Marrow

Leishmania donovani protozoa may be diagnosed in bone-marrow aspirates. Culture of an aspirate on special media may establish the diagnosis when few parasites are present in the bone marrow.

Parasites which occur in the peripheral blood associated with malaria, trypano-somiasis, relapsing fever and bartonellosis may be seen in marrow aspirates.

Selected Further Reading

Begemann H. and Rastetter J. (1979) *Atlas of Clinical Haematology,* 3rd ed. Berlin, Springer-Verlag.
Dacie J. V. and Lewis S. M. (1975) *Practical Haematology,* 5th ed. Edinburgh, Churchill Livingstone.

4

Iron Metabolism and Associated Disorders

IRON-DEFICIENCY ANAEMIA

Definition

Iron deficiency occurs when the total body iron is reduced below the level which is 'normal' for the individual's age and sex. Iron depletion refers to the diminution in iron stores and is often accompanied by a low serum iron and a raised transferrin level. Iron depletion without a reduction in the haemoglobin level is designated 'iron deficiency without anaemia' or 'latent iron deficiency'.

When the transferrin saturation falls below 15 per cent, iron-deficient erythropoiesis occurs, the red cells having a low MCV associated with a reduced MCH value and in more severe states also a lowering of the MCHC.

Incidence

Iron deficiency is the commonest cause of anaemia. The incidence of the disorder varies according to the age, sex and social status. Women of the child-bearing age are most commonly affected. In the UK it has been estimated that 8 per cent of women and 0·5 per cent of men have an iron-deficient type of anaemia. An urban survey showed that 20 per cent of the population were iron depleted.

IRON METABOLISM (Fig. 4.1)

Dietary Iron

Contains 10–15 mg/day. Most iron in food is in the form of organic complexes. The ferric compounds are liberated from the complexes by acid digestion in the stomach and must then be converted to ferrous forms by reducing substances such as vitamin C and protein sulphydryl groups prior to absorption. Phosphates and phytic acid in the diet reduce iron absorption by forming insoluble complexes.

It is generally considered that ferrous (Fe^{2+}) ions enter the intestinal mucosal cells, are oxidized to ferric (Fe^{3+}) ions and bind with apoferritin to form ferritin. The ferric ions are transferred across the inner cell membrane where they bind to transferrin. The degree of unsaturated transferrin governs the amount of transfer from the mucosal cells and thus regulates iron absorption, but this 'mucosal block' is poorly understood.

In health, 10 per cent of the dietary iron (1·0–1·5 mg of element iron) is absorbed each day, but this may increase to 30 per cent in iron depletion. The mucosal cells ultimately exfoliate into the gut lumen and contain unutilized ferritin. The plasma contains 3–4 mg of iron; the concentration of this ferric ion attached to transferrin

Fig. 4.1. Iron metabolism.

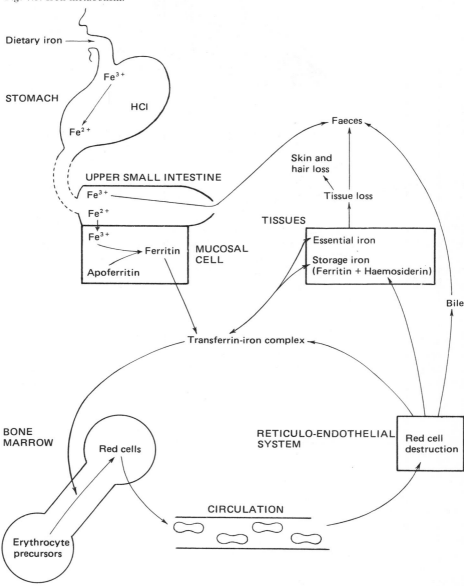

is 13–32 µmol/l (7–80 µg/dl). Males have higher iron levels than females; the level shows diurnal variation (higher in the morning), rises in pregnancy and may fall just before menstruation.

The mol wt of transferrin is 88 000; each molecule of transferrin binds two ferric atoms. The concentration of plasma transferrin is 1·2–3·0 g/dl which is capable of binding 250–400 µg/dl of iron (approximately 44–80 µmol/l). This value is referred to as the total iron-binding capacity of serum. In health, about one-third of transferrin is saturated. The amount of transferrin not bound is referred to as the unsaturated or latent iron-binding capacity. Transferrin transports iron to and from the bone marrow and tissues and is raised in infancy, pregnancy, and by oral contraceptives. Tissue iron may be divided into:

1. Non-essential or 'available' storage iron.
2. Essential and 'non-available' iron.

Storage Iron

In the bone marrow, the reticulo-endothelial system and other body tissues this comprises some 750–2000 mg. It is stored as ferritin and haemosiderin, present in approximately equal amounts. One-third of tissue iron is in the bone marrow, one-third in the liver and the remaining third in the spleen and other tissues.

Ferritin has a variable molecular structure. Apoferritin is made up of about 25 subunits to produce a molecule (mol. wt approximately 460 000) which is capable of binding some 5000 iron atoms. Ferritin does not stain with potassium ferrocyanide, but gives tissue sections a pale blue background hue. The serum ferritin is probably the best simple method of assessing iron stores. Haemosiderin is probably formed by partial denaturation of ferritin. At the same time, some additional 30 per cent of iron is bound to the molecules which become aggregated as insoluble particles appearing as golden brown granules and stain blue with the potassium ferrocyanide reaction.

Essential Tissue Iron

Amounting to about 300 mg, is contained mainly in myoglobin and in certain enzymes such as cytochromes, peroxidases and catalases (these enzymes containing some 40 mg of elemental iron).

Haemoglobin Iron

Some 2–3 g of elemental iron are contained in haemoglobin. Most of the iron from effete red cells is recycled for further haemoglobin synthesis.

Iron Balance

To remain in iron balance it is essential that sufficient iron must be absorbed from the food to meet iron requirements. Iron stores in an infant at term are sufficient for the requirements of the first 4 months of life. From 4 to 12 months 200 mg are required. This means that by the age of 6 months the diet should contain about 6 mg of elemental iron to allow the absorption of the required 0·6 mg/day. Premature and low birth weight infants have markedly reduced iron stores at birth and are thus very prone to iron deficiency. Milk is a poor source of iron (0·5–1·5 mg/l).

Growth, especially rapid during infancy, and the prepubertal growth spurt make exceptional demands for iron.

Adult males lose about 0·5–1·5 mg/day in sweat, desquamation and urine. Females require an additional 1–2 mg/day to compensate for menstrual loss. Pregnancy demands an extra 400 mg of iron and approximately 0·5 mg are lost per day through lactation.

IRON DEFICIENCY

Aetiology

Inadequate Intake

1. *Nutritional lack*. The amount of iron in the diet is closely related to its calorific value (approximately 6 mg/1000 cal). Hence menstruating women are only in marginal iron balance. About 20 per cent of iron-deficiency anaemia in the UK is associated with nutritional lack.

2. *Impaired absorption* may be due to:

> 2.1 Achlorhydria: although histamine-fast achlorhydria is common in patients with iron deficiency, iron deficiency itself may contribute to the achlorhydria. Hydrochloric acid is important for iron absorption from food, but is not necessary for absorption of iron from ferrous salts.
>
> 2.2 Following gastric surgery: about 50 per cent of patients who have undergone subtotal gastrectomy develop iron deficiency. The cause is due to rapid gastrojejunal transit. Maximum absorption of iron occurs just distal to the pylorus associated with the alkali gradient due to the alkaline pancreatic secretions. Bleeding from anastomotic ulcers may also play a part in the iron deficiency.
>
> 2.3 Coeliac disease: sometimes iron deficiency may be the presenting feature and steatorrhoea is only demonstrable by laboratory investigation.

Blood Loss

1. Menorrhagia is the commonest cause of iron deficiency in women. The normal loss is about 40 ml but up to 80 ml is considered as the upper limit of the normal range. Indications of heavy periods are the passage of clots, periods lasting more than 7 days and the inability to control loss by the use of tampons alone.

2. Blood loss from the alimentary tract may occur from the oesophagus to the rectum and this must be borne in mind when investigating iron deficiency. Right-sided colonic malignancies in particular may have no signs or symptoms.

3. Bleeding from the renal tract.

Other Causes of Iron Loss

1. Intravascular haemolysis resulting in iron loss via the urine in the form of haemosiderin and haemoglobin. (*a*) Paroxysmal nocturnal haemoglobinuria. (*b*) Mechanical red cell fragmentation due to: (i) prosthetic heart valves, usually aortic valve replacements when regurgitation through or around a faulty valve is occurring, (ii) prosthetic patch in the repair of an ostium primum defect when the mitral valve is not fully repaired allowing regurgitation directly on to the patch, (iii) pulmonary vasculitis where the roughened vascular endothelium causes red cell fragmentation.

2. Pulmonary siderosis: repeated alveolar capillary haemorrhages cause an increase of haemosiderin in the pulmonary macrophages which are cleared in the sputum. Although patients may develop cough and dyspnoea due to fibrosis, anaemia is commonly the earliest and only symptom.

3. Rarely in exfoliative dermatitis.

Symptoms

1. General symptoms. In iron deficiency the symptoms of tissue anoxia are the presenting feature in approximately 60 per cent of patients. The onset is insidious with increasing dyspnoea on exertion, palpitations, weakness, fatigue, dizziness and sometimes headache and paraesthesiae. It is common that the haemoglobin has dropped to about 8 g/dl before the patient seeks medical advice.

2. Mouth

    2.1 Angular stomatitis with associated red cracks at the angles of the mouth may in part be associated with a coincidental pyridoxine deficiency. Secondary infection with monilia is common.

    2.2 Atrophic glossitis: the tongue is often pale and smooth, but redness due to inflammation around denuded papillae is not uncommon. The inflammation, associated with a burning sensation, starts on the lateral borders of the tongue, but may eventually spread to involve the whole surface.

3. Pharynx. The Plummer–Vinson syndrome or Paterson–Kelly–Brown syndrome (much more common in women) is due to a postcricoid web with desquamated epithelium building up to produce mucosal folds; sometimes monilial infection is present producing one or more 'cuff-like' strictures. Initial dysphagia is only with solids, but not liquids. Diagnosis is confirmed by barium swallow or endoscopy. The condition improves with iron therapy, but may require dilatation. This condition predisposes to the development of a postcricoid carcinoma.

4. Nails become thin, brittle and fragile and may have longitudinal ridges. A proximal depression, koilonychia (spoon-shaped), may occur.

5. Hair becomes brittle and sparse.

6. Nervous system. Headaches may develop and very rarely in severe iron deficiency cerebral oedema, associated with papilloedema, may occur. Retinal haemorrhage and exudates may occur when the haemoglobin level falls below 5 g/dl. Numbness and tingling (attributed to low tissue iron) and vague neuralgic pain may also occur.

7. Pruritus vulvae may be troublesome.

8. Pica, the abnormal craving for such substances as soil, stones, coal and ice, may occur in children and less commonly in adults.

Radiological Findings

In children persistent iron-deficiency anaemia over long periods is associated with bone changes similar to thalassaemia. The diploic spaces become expanded to give mongoloid facies and the outer tables trimmed and striated to give the 'hair-on-end' radiological finding. Expansion of medullary cavities is easily demonstrated in radiographs of the hands and feet.

The postcricoid web is demonstrated by lateral view with barium swallow. A barium meal may demonstrate flattened mucosa of atrophic gastritis.

Peripheral Blood Picture

Anaemia is characterized by being microcytic (MCV below 80 fl, the degree of microcytosis being proportional to the severity of the anaemia) and morphologically by hypochromia. The small cells have a low MCH (lower limit of normal is 28 μg). The MCHC (lower limit of normal level 32 g/dl) only falls in moderate to severe iron-deficiency anaemia. If, however, the PCV is measured directly by centrifugation rather than calculation from the MCV and the red cell count, the PCV is higher due to plasma trapping and the MCHC is low in mild iron-deficiency anaemia.

Microscopically the red cells show microcytosis, hypochromia, ovalocytosis with very narrow elliptocytes called 'pencil' cells, and target cells in severe cases. Anisocytosis and poikilocytosis reflect the abnormal erythropoiesis. Mild polychromasia (associated with a reticulocyte count of some 2–5 per cent) occur, especially with haemorrhage. The leucocyte count is usually normal, but granulocytopenia occurs in longstanding cases. The platelet count also is usually normal, but may be raised with bleeding.

Bone Marrow

Increased cellularity due to erythroid hyperplasia is common. When blood loss is occurring erythropoiesis is micro-normoblastic, intermediate and late normoblasts predominating. Ineffective erythropoiesis is manifested by multinuclearity, nuclear fragmentation, and some pyknotic nuclei. Ragged edges of a reduced cytoplasm are common.

Myelopoiesis appears normal. Megakaryocytes are normal. Iron stain shows absence of iron particles.

Biochemical Findings

Serum iron below the lower limits of the normal range (10–30 μmol/l). Low levels also occur in congenital atransferrinaemia, chronic diseases and after rapid utilization following effective treatment of megaloblastic anaemia with vitamin B_{12} or folate. Total iron binding capacity is high (normal range 40–70 μmol/l). Raised levels are also found with raised serum or body iron levels, haemolytic anaemia, liver disease and with oestrogen ingestion. The ratio of serum iron to the total iron binding capacity is much more useful than either value alone and is less than 10 per cent in iron-deficiency anaemia. In chronic disease the ratio is usually 20 per cent or above (*Fig. 4.2*).

Ferritin levels below 10 μg/dl are characteristic of iron deficiency and levels between 10 and 20 μg/dl are suggestive but not diagnostic. Where inflammation and iron deficiency coexist, normal ferritin levels may occur.

Diagnosis

The diagnosis is often suggested from the history and examination and is confirmed by the typical peripheral blood appearance, the biochemical changes and the demonstration of iron depletion in the bone marrow.

The cause of iron deficiency *must* always be established.

Differential Diagnosis

Other forms of microcytic hypochromic anaemias include:
1. Thalassaemia.

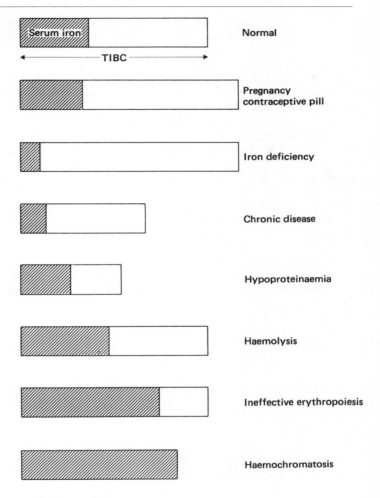

Fig. 4.2. Serum iron and TIBC in various disorders.

2. Some other haemoglobinopathies.
3. Sideroblastic anaemias, hereditary and acquired.
4. Chronic disease (*see* Chapter 12).
5. Inherited sex-linked hypochromic anaemia.

An iron-deficient type of anaemia with systemic iron overload occurs in congenital atransferrinaemia.

Treatment

Oral Iron. Preparations are required to:
1. Restore the haemoglobin level.
2. Replenish the body stores.

An effective preparation should:

2.1 Contain 50–100 mg elemental iron per tablet.

2.2 Contain elemental iron which is releasable and in a suitably absorbable form.

2.3 Be associated with a low incidence of side effects when compared with other similar pharmacological preparations.
2.4 Be cheap.

Ferrous sulphate, 200 mg tablets, containing 63 mg of elemental iron, meets these requirements. The dose should be 1 tablet t.d.s. Side effects include a metallic taste in the mouth, nausea, vomiting, abdominal pain and sometimes diarrhoea or even constipation. Very occasionally, constitutional symptoms similar to those encountered with parenteral iron may occur.

When the side effects are mild, a reduction of the dose to one tablet a day may result in loss of untoward symptoms; the dosage can then be gradually increased often without the return of adverse symptoms. Occasionally an alternative preparation, such as ferrous gluconate 300 mg tablets containing 37 mg of elemental iron or ferrous fumarate 200 mg tablets containing 66 mg of elemental iron, may be tolerated when ferrous sulphate is unacceptable. Ferrous fumarate in a syrup (containing 45 mg/5 ml) is available if a liquid preparation is required. A liquid preparation of sodium iron edetate (containing 55 mg iron in 10 ml) does not contain sucrose and may be given to diabetics.

Parenteral Iron. This is required if:

1. Oral iron preparations cannot be tolerated.
2. Persistent blood loss causes a negative iron balance, despite oral therapy.
3. Gastrointestinal disease (such as ulcerative colitis) exists which would be adversely affected by oral iron.

Intramuscular Iron. Iron dextran (Imferon) is a stable complex of ferrous hydroxide and dextran, Iron-sorbitol-citric acid complex (Jectofer) is more rapidly absorbed, the maximum iron level being attained in 2 hours. Staining of the skin can be avoided by a 'zig-zag' injection. Systemic reactions include: vomiting, headache, arthralgia, urticaria, bronchospasm and occasionally anaphylactic shock. Reactions are especially prone to occur if the unsaturated transferrin level is low; hence parenteral iron must not be given concomitantly with oral iron.

Intravenous Iron. This is dangerous and is rarely given. Saccharated oxide of iron (Ferrivenin) is available in 5-ml ampoules containing 100 mg of iron. It is essential that a test dose of 20 mg of iron is given on the first day. The maximum single dose should not exceed 200 mg.

A total dose of iron infusion may be given using iron-dextran in order to correct iron deficiency by a single treatment. It is important that the following facts are observed:

1. Iron deficiency is definitely present.
2. The patient does not have an allergic tendency.
3. Medical supervision during the initial phase of the infusion and the facilities to deal with anaphylactic reaction are to hand. The iron-dextran (up to a maximum dose of 2·5 g) is added to a litre of saline or dextrose; the risk of thrombophlebitis is less with saline than dextrose, but the latter is indicated if heart failure is incipient.

Dosage Calculation of Parenteral Iron

1. Iron-sorbitol, 200 mg, is required to increase the haemoglobin level by 1 g/dl in women and about 250 mg is required in men; in addition, 500 mg are required to help replenish tissue stores.
2. Iron-dextran, 150 mg, is required to raise the haemoglobin level by 1 g/dl, an additional 500 mg is required to help replenish the tissue stores.

Untoward side effects occurring during a total iron infusion include anaphylactic shock which is most likely to occur soon after the commencement of the infusion. The infusion must be immediately stopped and 200 mg of hydrocortisone, together with 10 mg chlorpheniramine maleate, given intravenously. Subcutaneous adrenaline may also be required. Minor side effects include flushing, sweating, nausea, fever, myalgia and lymphadenopathy.

IRON OVERLOAD

Generalized

Excessive parenchymal iron associated with tissue damage is referred to as haemochromatosis and excessive reticulo-endothelial iron without tissue damage as haemosiderosis. In general, haemochromatosis follows excessive absorption of iron from the gut when the plasma iron and transferrin saturation are raised and haemosiderosis follows excessive parenteral iron administration in the presence of a normal iron and transferrin saturation. There is great overlap between these pathological entities.

Aetiology

1. Idiopathic haemochromatosis, an inherited condition of uncertain inheritance which is probably heterogeneous. Over one-third of patients have an affected relative—often with subclinical disease. There is a close association with one or both specific haplotypes namely A3, B7 and A3, B14. The mechanism of increased iron absorption is undefined. Clinical disease rarely presents before 20 years and is most common in middle age after the accumulation of 15–50 g of iron. It is five times more common in men.

2. Haemolysis associated with ineffective erythropoiesis, especially thalassaemia major, thalassaemia intermedia or sideroblastic anaemia. The mechanism is not known.

3. Liver disease, especially alcoholic cirrhosis, and after portacaval anastomoses.

4. Repeated blood transfusions or parental iron administration.

5. Rarely with excessive oral intake. This is seen in the Bantu who brew beer in iron pots. The volume of alcohol consumed may be highly significant.

Clinical Features. There is increased pigmentation of the skin, cirrhosis of the liver (with an increased risk of developing hepatoma), congestive cardiomyopathy and endocrine failure, particularly diabetes, testicular atrophy and occasionally hypopituitarism. Arthropathy may occur and chondrocalcinosis may be seen on radiography.

Diagnosis

1. The plasma iron is raised with a transferrin saturation of 80–100 per cent. This may be found in ineffective erythropoiesis and does not alone indicate iron overload.

2. The serum ferritin is markedly raised.

3. The 24-hour urinary iron excretion in response to intravenous desferrioxamine (10 mg/kg) is usually greater than 10 mg (normal < 2 mg).

4. Liver biopsy enables the amount of iron to be measured, its distribution to be assessed and the presence of cirrhosis to be detected.

5. Accurate estimations of total body iron can be made using nuclear magnetic resonance techniques.

Management

1. Weekly phlebotomies of 500 ml for 2–3 years will eventually restore iron levels to normal. Only then will the serum iron fall and phlebotomies be less frequently required.

Desferrioxamine given subcutaneously by an infusion pump will increase urinary iron excretion.

3. Testosterone may be given for hypogonadism.
4. Intemperance should be discouraged.
5. Diabetes is managed in the normal way.
6. Immediate relatives should be screened for occult haemochromatosis.

Early treatment is indicated.

Localized

Localized iron deposition in tissues occurs in pulmonary haemosiderosis, paroxysmal nocturnal haemoglobinuria (kidneys) and in rheumatoid arthritis (joints).

SIDEROBLASTIC ANAEMIAS

Definition

A variety of dyserythropoietic disorders in which iron-containing granules occur around the nuclei of some normoblasts (ring sideroblasts) (*Fig. 4.3*).

Fig. 4.3. Ring sideroblasts stained with Prussian blue.

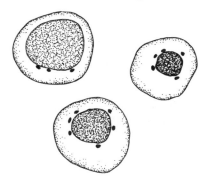

Classification

Hereditary forms are usually inherited as a sex-linked recessive disorder with partial penetrance, though occasionally transmitted autosomally.

Acquired Forms

1. Primary; both sexes are equally affected, highest incidence is in middle-aged and elderly subjects, probably several types of biochemical abnormalities exist.

2. Secondary; may be subdivided according to aetiology into those associated with:

> 2.1 Drugs (such as isoniazid, cycloserine, pyrazinamide and chloramphenicol), chemicals (especially lead) and alcohol.
> 2.2 Associated with malnutrition (dietary or due to malabsorption).

2.3 Associated with other disorders of the marrow. (i) Acute myeloid leukaemias (especially erythroleukaemia); (ii) the chronic myeloproliferative disorders; (iii) haemolytic dyserythropoietic anaemias.

2.4 Associated with non-haematological disorders. (i) Carcinoma; (ii) uraemia; (iii) thyroid disease; (iv) collagen disorders (such as rheumatoid arthritis and polyarteritis nodosa); (v) porphyria.

HEREDITARY SIDEROBLASTIC ANAEMIAS

Aetiology and Pathology

Iron is deposited in the mitochondria. Several types of biochemical disorders exist including abnormalities of glycine, δ-aminolevulinic acid and porphyrin metabolism. The major cause of the anaemia is severe ineffective erythropoiesis and the mean erythrocyte span varies between 40 days and the normal value of 120 days.

Clinical Features

The onset of moderate to severe anaemia occurs in childhood, adolescence or early adulthood. Females are unaffected in the sex-linked disorder. There is no increased susceptibility to infection or to bleeding.

Laboratory Findings

The anaemia may be normocytic, microcytic or slightly macrocytic in type. Some cells are normochromic and some hypochromic, thus producing the typical 'dimorphic' type of anaemia. The diagnosis is made by the iron stain of the bone marrow aspirate which shows the deposition of iron in the mitochondria (stained by the Prussian blue reaction) appearing as granules in a 'ring' surrounding the nuclei of normoblasts. The granulocytic and megakaryocytic lines are normal. Megaloblastosis and dyserythropoiesis may occur though are less common than in the acquired forms.

The serum iron level is raised and the total iron binding capacity usually saturated though may be reduced as with other chronic diseases. Tissue iron deposition is increased and symptoms of haemochromatosis may develop.

Treatment

Some patients may improve with large doses of pyridoxine, 200 mg a day for adults. Secondary folate deficiency may require supplements. Blood transfusion may become necessary, but the problems of iron overload become exacerbated. Treatment with desferrioxamine has been disappointing.

PRIMARY ACQUIRED SIDEROBLASTIC ANAEMIA

Aetiology and Pathology

The severity of the anaemia is chiefly due to ineffective erythropoiesis. Red cell survival is usually normal, only occasionally reduced. As in other types of sideroblastic anaemia iron is deposited in the mitochondria of normoblasts, impairing their function and resulting in premature destruction of the cells. The basic biochemical lesions vary and are ill-understood. There is some evidence that a somatic mutation producing a dominant, yet metabolically ineffective clone, may be responsible for some of the disorders in this group.

Clinical Features

The symptoms of anaemia have an insidious onset; usually the haemoglobin reaches a plateau of about 7 g/dl. There may be increased pigmentation of exposed skin. Hepatic and/or splenic enlargement is not unusual.

Laboratory Findings

These resemble those already described under the congenital sideroblastic section.

Treatment

Pyridoxine, 200 mg per day, causes a complete or partial remission in one-third of patients. Occasionally patients refractory to treatment with pyridoxine respond to pyridoxal 5-phosphate. A coexisting secondary folate deficiency requires supplements (5 mg o.d.). Occasionally ascorbic acid (25 mg b.d.) may improve the haemoglobin level. Blood transfusions may be required for severe anaemia, but increase risks of iron overload; desferrioxamine may be required.

SECONDARY ACQUIRED SIDEROBLASTIC ANAEMIAS

Aetiology and Pathology

The causes have already been enumerated under 'Classification'. Often the sideroblastic changes only contribute in a minor way to the anaemia.

Isoniazid, cycloserine and pyrazinamide inhibit pyridoxal 5-phosphate (*Fig. 4.4*).

Chloramphenicol inhibits protein synthesis by mitochondria. Lead inhibits δ-aminolevulinic acid synthetase and haem synthetase.

Alcohol inhibits pyridoxal kinase.

Clinical Features

The main features often are those of the primary disorder; the possibility of sideroblastic dyserythropoiesis should be considered, especially if the severity of the anaemia is inappropriate.

Fig. 4.4. Haem synthesis pathway.

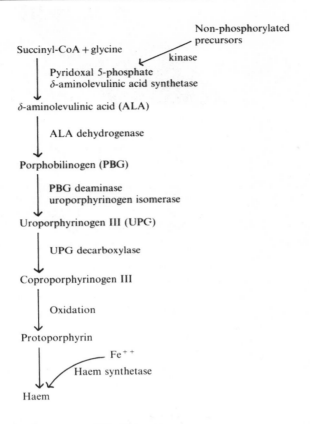

Succinyl-CoA + glycine
Non-phosphorylated precursors
kinase

Pyridoxal 5-phosphate
δ-aminolevulinic acid synthetase

δ-aminolevulinic acid (ALA)

ALA dehydrogenase

Porphobilinogen (PBG)

PBG deaminase
uroporphyrinogen isomerase

Uroporphyrinogen III (UPG)

UPG decarboxylase

Coproporphyrinogen III

Oxidation

Protoporphyrin

Fe^{++}
Haem synthetase

Haem

Laboratory Findings

The findings are of the underlying disorder plus those described.

Treatment

Always directed at the primary disease. Antituberculous drugs should be changed if the sideroblastic changes are not improved by pyridoxine. Chelating agents are required, together with pyridoxine, in lead poisoning. Cessation of alcohol, together with pyridoxine and folate administration is accompanied usually by a rapid response in cases due to alcoholism.

Selected Further Reading

Finch C. A. (ed.) (1982) Clinical aspects of iron deficiency and excess. *Semin. Hematol.* **XIX**, 1.
Jacobs A. (ed). (1982) Disorders of iron metabolism. *Clin. Haematol.* **11**, 2.

Chapter 5 Megaloblastic Anaemia

GENERAL FEATURES

The megaloblastic anaemias are a group of disorders characterized by a common morphological and functional abnormality in the peripheral blood and bone marrow, due to abnormalities in DNA synthesis. The term 'megaloblast' denotes any maturation stage of the nucleated red cell involved in megaloblastic change whilst 'megaloblastic change' refers to morphological and functional changes in erythrocytes, granulocytes and platelet precursors.

In megaloblastic red cell precursors the cells at all stages of development appear larger than corresponding normoblasts and this is most apparent in the later stages. The cytoplasm appears to mature at a more rapid rate than the nucleus and condensation of the nucleus is delayed. The nuclear chromatin appears stippled or finely reticular and is described as 'open', 'sieve-like' or 'lace-like'. Megaloblastic granulocyte precursors are most distinctive at the metamyelocyte stage when nuclear : cytoplasmic asynchrony results in the so-called 'giant metamyelocyte' with a large ragged horseshoe nucleus and voluminous basophilic cytoplasm.

BIOCHEMICAL BASIS OF MEGALOBLASTIC CHANGE

The precise biochemical mechanisms of megaloblastic change are uncertain, but certain facts are apparent; there is impaired conversion of deoxyuridine to deoxythymidine and RNA in megaloblasts is much increased whilst DNA is only slightly increased. The RNA : DNA ratio rises because DNA replication is blocked whilst synthesis of cytoplasmic RNA and protein proceeds unabated. There are four deoxyribonucleoside triphosphates and reduced supply of one or other of these during the 'S' phase of the cell cycle inhibits the elongation of a newly initiated DNA fragment.

Other features of the haematology of megaloblastic change, such as ineffective erythropoiesis, cellular death in the marrow and chromosome anomalies, probably occur secondary to the primary DNA defect.

CLINICAL FEATURES

The general features of megaloblastic anaemia have an insidious onset and are often well compensated. Anorexia is common and glossitis may be florid (especially in B_{12} deficiency). In severe cases, there may be a low grade pyrexia; infections due to neutropenia, and bleeding due to thrombocytopenia, occur. Subfertility is described. Optic atrophy, peripheral neuropathy, subacute degeneration of the cord and dementia are well recognized in B_{12} deficiency (sometimes without severe megaloblastic change), but have also been described in folate deficiency.

On examination, there is pallor and often slight icterus reflecting the haemolytic element of ineffective erythropiesis. The tongue is often raw resembling a 'beef steak'. Slight splenomegaly occurs in a minority of patients and neurological lesions may be present. Vitiligo and goitres may be present in pernicious anaemia.

LABORATORY FEATURES

Peripheral Blood

There are abnormalities of all elements.

Red Cells. The red cells are typically macrocytic with an MCV in excess of 100 fl. The haemoglobin is usually low and the red cell count is more markedly reduced. Macrocytosis may be the initial feature of megaloblastic change. Macro-ovalocytes are often present with profound anisocytosis and poikilocytosis. Inclusions such as stippling, Howell–Jolly bodies and Cabot rings are seen in the more severe cases. The absolute reticulocyte count is usually reduced. Nucleated red cells can appear when the haematocrit is extremely low and these tend to be megaloblasts.

White Cells. Leucopenia, often with a relative lymphocytosis, appears as the anaemia worsens. There is a neutrophil 'right shift' with the number of neutrophil lobes rising. The presence of 5- and 6-lobed neutrophils is characteristic. These changes in the neutrophil may be the very first signs of megaloblastosis.

Platelets. No obvious macroscopic morphological changes are seen on the blood film. Thrombocytopenia develops as the anaemia gets more severe.

Marrow

The marrow findings have been described. If iron deficiency coexists the classic features in the blood may be masked, but megaloblastic change in the marrow persists.

Other Blood Tests

Ineffective erythropoiesis and haemolysis gives rise to a raised unconjugated bilirubin, increased urine urobilinogen, decreased haptoglobins and very high levels of lactate dehydrogenase. The serum iron is often high with rapid iron clearance and poor incorporation into circulating red cells. Ineffective leucopoiesis may cause a rise in serum muramidase.

CLASSIFICATION OF MEGALOBLASTIC ANAEMIA

1. B_{12} deficiency.
2. Folate deficiency.
3. B_{12} and folate refractory megaloblastic anaemias.

VITAMIN B_{12} DEFICIENCY

Sources of Vitamin B_{12}

It is synthesized primarily by micro-organisms, but the human source is food of animal origin, e.g. liver, meat, eggs, milk. B_{12} is not found in plant tissues, though contamination with bacteria and algae may provide some B_{12}.

Some bacteria that cannot synthesize vitamin B_{12} and require an exogenous source of it are the basis of B_{12} assays (*Lactobacillus leishmaniae*).

Absorption and Daily Requirement of Vitamin B_{12}

From the average Western diet of 5–30 µg, 1–5 µg is absorbed. The minimum daily requirement is approximately 1 µg. A minute fraction of ingested B_{12} is absorbed rapidly and passively but the majority of absorbed B_{12} is actively taken up in the terminal ileum as a B_{12}–intrinsic factor complex. The intrinsic factor is secreted by the gastric fundal parietal cells. It serves to protect B_{12} from proteolytic digestion and to attach the B_{12} complex to specific receptors on the intestinal microvilli, this latter process requiring the presence of free calcium ions and a neutral pH. Following attachment to the receptor the vitamin enters the mucosal cell leaving the intrinsic factor behind. The B_{12} then enters the blood attached to trans-cobalamin II which seems to be derived from the ileal enterocyte. This complex is rapidly cleared from the blood by the liver. The total body stores of 2000–3000 µg in the adult (about half in liver and a significant amount in kidneys) are sufficient for 3–4 years if no further B_{12} is absorbed. The normal serum B_{12} level is 150–950 pg/ml, and can be measured either in a bioassay or in a radioim-munoassay. Raised levels are seen in myeloproliferative diseases, liver disease and renal disease.

Metabolic Functions of Vitamin B_{12}

Cobalamin is a co-factor in the methylation of homocysteine to methionine.

Homocysteine + methyltetrahydrofolate $\longrightarrow$ Methionine + tetrahydrofolate

Cobalamin deficiency thus leads to low levels of methionine. Methionine is converted to a methyl derivative and the majority of this compound is oxidized to formate.

Formate is necessary in many reactions including:
1. Purine synthesis.
2. Conversion of deoxyuridine to thymidine.

3. Formation of folate polyglutamate which is the folate coenzyme.

Methionine is also needed to produce 5-adenosylmethionine which is probably an important 'methyl donor' in the nervous system.

It is apparent that B_{12} deficiency will result in a rise in 5-methyltetrahydrofolate and serum folate levels. Folate polyglutamate which is the predominant red cell folate will be reduced.

Aetiology of B_{12} Deficiency

1. Nutritional Deficiency. This occurs with a persistent diet of less than 1–2 μg B_{12}/day. It is seen in vegans, dietary faddists and chronic alcoholics. There is often accompanying folate deficiency. It can be corrected with oral B_{12} 2–10 μg/day.

2. Malabsorption

2.1 Gastric Disease

2.1.1 Intrinsic factor deficiency occurs: pernicious anaemia (*see later*), juvenile pernicious anaemia, atrophic gastritis and after gastrectomy. Iron-deficiency anaemia is the commonest form of anaemia following partial gastrectomy and the less common megaloblastic change may be masked. Five per cent of patients develop overt B_{12} deficiency after gastrectomy, but about 20 per cent of patients will develop low serum B_{12} levels. Folate deficiency is the cause of megaloblastic anaemia after partial gastrectomy in about 20 per cent of cases. Severe B_{12} deficiency is inevitable after total gastrectomy without supplements, if the patient survives long enough. The altered intestinal pH and intestinal hurry also may contribute to the malabsorption. Juvenile pernicious anaemia is a rare autosomal recessive disorder in which there is failure to make the glycoprotein intrinsic factor. The affected children are well until the second year of life when they become weak, lose weight and develop diarrhoea. On examination, there is pallor, hepatosplenomegaly and the typical neurological features of B_{12} deficiency.

2.1.2 Zollinger–Ellison Syndrome. There may be B_{12} malabsorption, probably due to the low ileal pH.

2.2 Terminal Ileal Disease

2.2.1 Ileal Resections. The majority of patients with more than 60 cm ileum resected malabsorb B_{12}.

2.2.2 Crohn's Disease and Ulcerative Colitis involving the Ileum. Megaloblastic anaemia occurs in 20–40 per cent of patients. Bacterial colonization may contribute. The anaemia of Crohn's disease is of mixed aetiology, including also folate deficiency, iron deficiency and the anaemia of chronic disease.

2.2.3 Tropical Sprue. Megaloblastic change due to folate of B_{12} deficiency is usually seen before treatment. Folate deficiency tends to appear first. Even after apparent clinical recovery the B_{12} absorption often remains abnormal.

2.2.4 Congenital selective B_{12} *malabsorption*—the Imerslund–Gräsbeck syndrome is a rare autosomal recessive condition. The defect in B_{12} absorption is not understood. There is associated proteinuria and renal biopsy may be normal or show a glomerulonephritis. Renal function is usually normal. The clinical disorder tends to wax and wane and diagnosis may be delayed.

2.3 Competitive Parasites

2.3.1 Bacterial overgrowth of the gut is seen in disorders of intestinal motility such as in blind loops, Crohn's disease and scleroderma. The bacteria compete for the ingested B_{12}.

2.3.2 Diphyllobothrium latum—about 3 per cent of those infested with the Scandinavian fish tapeworm become anaemic. Although the main cause of B_{12} depletion is by competition, the levels of intrinsic factor are also reported to be low.

2.4 Pancreatic Failure. The B_{12} malabsorption is probably secondary to the low pH and calcium ion concentration.

2.5 Drug-induced Small Bowel Malabsorption

2.5.1 Biguanides. Phenformin and metformin cause malabsorption by unknown mechanisms which may also be related to damage of the brush border enterocytes by abnormal intestinal flora.

2.5.2 Para-aminosalicylic acid (PAS) causes reduced B_{12} absorption and an abnormal Schilling test. Intrinsic factor secretion is unaffected and there may be some abnormality in the gut wall.

2.5.3 Colchicine and neomycin both affect the enterocyte and impair B_{12} absorption.

2.5.4 Potassium supplements may diminish B_{12} absorption by causing a fall in gut luminal pH.

3. Increased Requirement for Vitamin B_{12}. Reserves of B_{12} are usually considerable, but occasionally B_{12} reserves are exhausted in pregnancy, hyperthyroidism and massive erythropoiesis.

4. Disorders of Vitamin B_{12} Storage and Transport—Transcobalamin II Deficiency. Transcobalamin (TC) II is synthesized by the intestinal enterocyte and possibly the liver and transports vitamin B_{12} in the circulation. A small number of infants with severe magaloblastic anaemia, diarrhoea and vomiting are found to have TC II deficiency. These children have normal serum B_{12} levels, complete absence of TC II on measurement of serum proteins, and failure to absorb oral B_{12} with or without intrinsic factor (IF). IF is present in gastric juice in normal amounts. Massive doses of B_{12}, such as 1000 µg weekly or more, may be necessary to bypass the transport mechanism and allow some B_{12} to diffuse directly into cells.

Pernicious Anaemia

Pernicious anaemia (PA) is a disorder of megaloblastic change usually with anaemia and sometimes with neurological abnormalities associated with vitamin B_{12} deficiency secondary to failure of the IF secretory apparatus. There are

120/1 000 000 cases per year in the UK. Males and females are equally affected and it mainly occurs in the elderly.

Aetiology. PA appears to have some degree of genetic determination:

1. There is a high incidence in Scandinavia and Northern Europe.
2. There is a higher incidence of blood group A in PA patients and their relatives.
3. There is an increased incidence in relatives of patients.

Clinical Pathology. There is a central failure of immune control of unknown cause associated with auto-antibodies in gastric juice and serum, and severe atrophic gastritis.

Stomach. There is marked reduction in the volume of gastric juice to about 15–20 ml/h (NR 50–150), and histamine-fast achlorhydria is present. This may antedate PA by many years. IF secretion is virtually absent. The wall of the stomach is atrophic particularly in the fundal two-thirds. All coats of the wall are affected. The gastric glands have only mucus-producing cells and there is infiltration with lymphocytes and plasma cells and metaplasia of intestinal epithelium.

Serum Antibodies. Antibodies to IF at the B_{12}-combining site occur in the serum of 55–60 per cent of PA patients; this antibody is usually IgG but may be IgA. Antibody to IF at the non-B_{12}-combining site occurs in about 35 per cent of patients; usually those who have antibody to the B_{12} combining site. Parietal cell antibodies are seen in over 90 per cent of PA patients. Thyroid auto-antibodies are seen in 50 per cent of cases.

Gastric Juice Antibodies. Free IF antibody is found in 35 per cent of PA and if immune complexes are dissociated, bound antibody is found in a further 25 per cent.

Clinical Features. The duration of symptoms is often extremely long and can be well over a year. Symptoms referable to the gastrointestinal tract are not uncommon—of these, episodic diarrhoea is the most frequent.

The patients often have a modest pyrexia, fair hair and blue eyes and a lemon-yellow colour due to a combination of the anaemia and the mild icterus from the modest haemolytic element. The spleen is palpable in 10–20 per cent of cases.

Laboratory Investigations and Diagnosis. There is a macrocytic blood picture, usually with anaemia and a megaloblastic bone marrow.

The Schilling Test. The serum B_{12} is low and malabsorption of oral vitamin B_{12} can be demonstrated in a Schilling Test Part I. The fasting patient is given radioactive B_{12} (0·5 µg) in water to drink after voiding the bladder. A flushing dose of 1 mg of non-radioactive B_{12} is given intramuscularly to block vitamin B_{12}-binding sites in the plasma and liver and enhance excretion of any absorbed radioactive B_{12}. Normal subjects excrete 10 per cent or more of the administered radioactivity in the first 24 hours. If excretion is low a Part II Schilling Test is performed. The Part I test is repeated with the addition of 60 mg of porcine intrinsic factor given orally with the radioactive B_{12}. If poor excretion in Part I was due to IF deficiency, then the excretion will be higher in Part II. A creatinine clearance should be performed on both occasions to check that the urine collections were complete and that there is no renal failure (*Fig. 5.1*).

The Dicopac Test. The Dicopac* test uses two different isotope-labelled vitamin B_{12} preparations. The free cyanocobalamin is labelled with [58]Co and the IF-bound cyanocobalamin is labelled with [57]Co. Both isotope preparations are

* Radiochemical Centre, Amersham.

Fig. 5.1. Schilling test.
Vitamin B_{12} excretion
in urine.

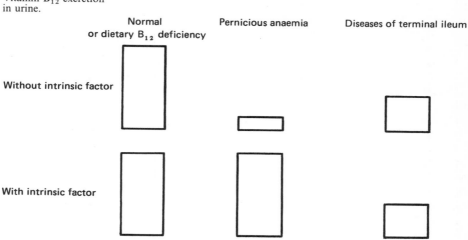

administered at the same time so that the Part I and Part II of the Schilling test can be performed concurrently. During the counting procedure the substantial difference in the energy of the gamma emissions between ^{57}Co and ^{58}Co allow separate quantitation of the isotopes by the use of a pulse height analyser.

Methylmalonic acid excretion in the urine is raised in B_{12} deficiency, but is rarely measured.

Circulating parietal cell antibodies are found in over 90 per cent of cases, but are found in 15–20 per cent of normals over 60 years of age.

Circulating IF antibodies are found in over 50 per cent of patients.

The patients also have histamine-fast achlorhydria associated with severe atrophic gastritis. The serum gastrin is raised.

The Deoxyuridine Suppression Test. A test has been devised in which a suspension of marrow cells is incubated with deoxyuridine which converts it into thymidine and incorporates it into DNA. Deoxyuridine suppresses radioactive thymidine incorporation into DNA and in normoblastic marrow less than 10 per cent of thymidine is utilized. However, in megaloblastic anaemia due to B_{12} or folate deficiency there is a block in deoxyuridylate conversion to thymidylate. Tritium-labelled thymidine is added to the test suspension and if there is further requirement for thymidine it is taken from the radioactive element. Hence, the more normal the marrow the less the incorporation of radioactivity (NR < 10 per cent). In B_{12} or folate deficiency less deoxyuridine is utilized and relatively more of the radioactive thymidine is incorporated. In B_{12} deficiency the abnormal result can be ameliorated by B_{12}, folic acid, folinic acid and tetrahydrofolate but in folate deficiency there is no correction by B_{12}. The test gives a normal (i.e. non-megaloblastic) result in refractory macrocytic anaemia not due to B_{12} or folate deficiency.

Differential Diagnosis. Other causes of megaloblastic anaemia and particularly other causes of B_{12} deficiency. Other concomitant 'autoimmune diseases' should be excluded, e.g. immune thyroid and adrenal disease. Other clinical associations include: diabetes mellitus, vitiligo, hypoparathyroidism, mucocutaneous candidiasis, ovarian failure, myasthenia gravis, hypogammaglobulinaemia, rheumatoid arthritis and Sjögren's syndrome and myeloproliferative disorders.

Course. The haematological disorder is completely corrected by B_{12} adminis-tration, whilst the neurological lesion may be fully or only partial remediable. Recovery may continue for up to 1 year. Carcinoma of the stomach occurs in patients with PA about 4–8 times as frequently as in other persons of the PA age group. The tumour is more likely to be in the body or fundus of the stomach and only one-third occur in the pylorus and antral end.

Treatment of B_{12} deficiency

1. Treat cause if possible.
2. Vitamin B_{12} is given by parenteral injection except in cases of dietary deficiency when oral supplements are suitable. Hydroxocobalamin is retained by the body far more efficiently than cyanocobalamin although both will produce a good haematological response in PA. A reticulocyte response is seen by the third day and peaks about 6–7 days. Levels of 10 per cent are often seen. The bone marrow is frequently normoblastic within 48 hours. It is often helpful to load the new patient with around 6 injections of 1000 µg of hydroxocobalamin in the first few weeks of treatment. Thereafter, hydroxocobalamin 500–1000 µg at 2-monthly intervals, 1000 µg at 3-monthly intervals or 8×1000 µg in 2-3 weeks every year, have all proved satisfactory. Hypokalaemia may develop when severe vitamin B_{12} deficiency is initially treated; this is particularly hazardous if diuretics are also given. If folate is given in B_{12} deficiency there may be a partial haematological remission, but the neurological condition may deteriorate further.
3. Blood transfusion should be avoided, where possible, since the circulation can easily be overloaded in very anaemic patients. However, with a haemoglobin of 3–4 g/dl or less it is sometimes unavoidable and in these circumstances small volumes of blood (< 2 units of packed red cells) should be given slowly with diuretic cover. Exchange transfusion, during which small volumes of blood are removed from the other arm, may be appropriate during this transfusion.

FOLIC-ACID DEFICIENCY MEGALOBLASTIC ANAEMIA

Folic Acid

Folic acid is the parent compound of a large group of compounds known as the folates. Folic acid is pteroyl-glutamic acid and many folates have multiple glutamic acid residues and are known as polyglutamates. It is the tetrahydrofolates which are the active folates in enzyme reactions and the two-stage reduction of folate to the tetrahydro derivatives is catalysed by a single NADPH-linked enzyme dihydrofolate reductase.

Folate Sources and Requirements

Folate is found in a wide variety of vegetables and fruits, as well as in liver and kidney. Excess cooking can destroy much of the folate in foodstuffs. The minimum daily requirement is around 50 µg of folic acid. The average folate stores are 5–10 mg of which one-third is in the liver. This is sufficient to last about 4 months if dietary intake ceases.

Metabolic Functions of Folates

Folate is an acceptor/donor of one carbon units in the synthesis of purine and pyrimidine bases. Thymidine synthesis is particularly dependent on folate and in folic-acid deficiency this results in impaired DNA synthesis and megaloblastic change.

Folate Absorption and Metabolism

Folate is absorbed in the small bowel, particularly the upper jejunum, and the polyglutamates in the diet are hydrolysed in the small gut to monoglutamate. Folate is carried in the plasma by a protein of two components one of mol. wt. 200 000 and the other around 50 000. There may also be a membrane-derived intracellular folate-binding protein acting as an important regulator of folate uptake into the cell. The protein resembles β-lactoglobulin—the folate-binding protein of cow's milk.

Clinical Features of Folic-acid Deficiency

The clinical features are similar to other forms of megaloblastic anaemia, but usually without significant neurological abnormalities.

Aetiology of Folate Deficiency

1. Nutritional deficiency is seen in the elderly, premature infants, especially if milk-fed, chronic alcoholics (also impaired hepatic storage of folate), those living alone and the mentally subnormal.

Whereas nutritional B_{12} deficiency usually occurs as a pure deficiency, nutritional folate deficiency is often part of a widespread deficiency of many vitamins and is often easily diagnosed from the history.

2. Malabsorption

2.1 Partial gastrectomy. Although B_{12} deficiency is the classic cause of postgastrectomy megaloblastic anaemia folate deficiency does occur in 20–50 per cent of patients caused at least in part by decreased dietary intake.

2.2 Coeliac disease. Iron deficiency usually occurs also and macrocytosis may be masked.

2.3 Tropical sprue.

2.4 Jejunal resections.

2.5 Extensive Crohn's disease.

2.6 Whipple's disease.

2.7 Scleroderma.

2.8 Infiltration of the gut with lymphoma.

2.9 Drugs (e.g. phenytoin) interfere with folate absorption at the brush border.

3. Increased folate requirements are seen in:

3.1 Pregnancy (5–10 fold increase in requirements).

3.2 Lactation.

3.3 Prematurity.

3.4 Prepubertal growth spurt.

3.5   Haematological disorders, such as chronic haemolysis and myeloproliferative disorders.

3.6   Malignant diseases, e.g. lymphoma.

3.7   Severe inflammatory disorders including exfoliative dermatitis.

3.8   Repeated dialysis.

3.9   Homocysteinuria.

4. Defective utilization of folate is seen with:

4.1   Antifolate drugs, e.g. methotrexate, trimethoprim (including high dose co-trimoxazole).

4.2   Anticonvulsant drugs, such as diphenylhydantoin, phenobarbitone and primidone. The mechanism is uncertain, and some interference with absorption of polyglutamates also occurs.

4.3   Other drugs including glutethimide, isoniazid, cycloserine and oral contraceptives.

4.4   Alcohol.

4.5   Vitamin C deficiency which probably permits increased oxidation of tetrahydrofolate.

5. Folate Deficiency Associated with Inborn Errors. Congenital deficiency of various enzymes concerned with folate metabolism can occur. The patient has a normal B_{12}, poor response to oral folate and may have elevated urinary formiminoglutamic acid or megaloblastic anaemia in infancy. Amongst the enzymes which may be congenitally deficient are:

5.1   Dihydrofolate reductase.

5.2   Glutamate formiminotransferase.

5.3   Methyl tetrahydrofolate homocysteine methyltransferase.

Laboratory Features

There is a low serum folate, low red cell folate and raised folate-binding proteins. Serum folate levels reflect recent dietary intake whereas red cell folate levels reflect the folate status at the time of their formation. Folate can be measured by a microbiological assay or by a radioactive isotope technique. Serum B_{12} and urinary methylmalonate are normal.

Treatment of Folate Deficiency

In deficiency states 5–15 mg of folate are given orally every day for about 4 months after exclusion of B_{12} deficiency. Long-term folate therapy may be necessary in chronic haemolytic diseases and other causes of increased folate requirement. Oral supplements are usually adequate even in malabsorption syndromes.

Prophylactic folate is often given to pregnant women, premature babies, in chronic haemolytic anaemias and to those receiving dialysis. After high-dose methotrexate therapy the acute effects of folate deficiency can be ameliorated by folinic acid rescue.

B_{12} AND FOLATE REFRACTORY ANAEMIAS

A small group of rare poorly understood disorders including:

1. Pyridoxine-responsive megaloblastic anaemia.

2. Thiamine-responsive megaloblastic anaemia.

3. Refractory anaemia and preleukaemia. Unexplained refractory megaloblastic anaemia may be associated with an increasing number of myeloblasts and later in the disease the patient may become frankly leukaemic.

4. Erythemic myelosis is a leukaemic disorder associated with severe DNA abnormalities in erythropoiesis. It is associated with severe megaloblastic change and progression to frank leukaemia which may be mixed erythroid and myeloid.

5. Anti-DNA drugs (i) 6-Mercaptopurine and 6-thioguanine interfere with purine synthesis and inhibit RNA and DNA synthesis early and late in the purine nucleotide interconversion steps. (ii) Cytosine arabinoside causes megaloblastic change due to inhibition of DNA polymerase. Its effects are reversible by deoxycytidine. (iii) 5-Fluorouracil inhibits pyrimidine synthesis by blocking the methylation of deoxyuridylate to deoxythymidilate. (iv) Hydroxyurea interferes with DNA synthesis at many sites and chelates iron in ribonucleoside diphosphate reductase.

6. Hereditary orotic aciduria. This is a genetic disorder of two main types: (i) Deficiency of orotidylic decarboxylase and pyrophosphorylase with excretion of orotic acid in the urine. (ii) Deficiency of orotic decarboxylase only and excretion of orotic acid and orotidase. Clinical picture is of severe megaloblastic anaemia in a young child, often with discoloration of the auricular cartilage, failing to respond to B_{12} and folate. Orotic acid administration may produce improvement.

7. Lesch–Nyhan syndrome. This is a sex-linked enzyme deficiency due to reduction or absence of hypoxanthine-guanine-phosphoribosyl transferase. There is self-mutilation associated with hyperuricaemia and hyperuricosuria. Treatment is with adenine.

Selected Further Reading

Chanarin I. (1979) *The Megaloblastic Anaemias,* 2nd ed. Edinburgh, Blackwell Scientific Publications.
Hoffbrand A. V. (ed.) (1976) Megaloblastic anaemias. *Clin. Haematol.* **5**, 3.

Chapter 6

Aplastic Anaemia and Bone Marrow Failure

The aplastic and hypoplastic anaemias are a group of disorders characterized by a decrease in haemopoietic bone marrow accompanied by selective cytopenias or pancytopenia.

The aplastic anaemias (AA) can be classified as follows:

1. Congenital
- 1.1 Non-familial
- 1.2 Fanconi's anaemia
- 1.3 Other familial disorders

2. Chronic Acquired
- 2.1 Idiopathic
- 2.2 Drugs
- 2.3 Chemicals
- 2.4 Irradiation
- 2.5 Associated with infections, particularly viral hepatitis
- 2.6 Associated with autoimmune disease
- 2.7 Associated with pregnancy
- 2.8 Associated with PNH

3. Acute Transient As (2) above plus many viral, bacterial and fungal infections.

PATHOGENESIS

1. Congenital

The congenital or constitutional aplastic anaemias account for 20–30 per cent of childhood aplastic anaemias and can be classified as:

1.1 Congenital, but not familial.

1.2 Familial and usually associated with physical abnormalities. This is known as Fanconi's anaemia and is an autosomal recessive condition.

1.3 Other familial bone marrow failure syndromes including that associated with pancreatic insufficiency, neonatal thrombocytopenia, amegakaryocytosis with absent radii and dyskeratosis congenita. There are various inheritance patterns.

The commonest of these disorders is Fanconi's anaemia. The mechanism is uncertain, but a chromosomal instability is frequently found with chromatid exchanges, breaks and endoreduplication. This abnormality is most pronounced in blood lymphocytes, but is also found in marrow cells and fibroblasts.

2. Chronic Acquired

2.1 Idiopathic Aplastic Anaemia (IAA) is by far the commonest type of aplastic anaemia and is thought to be due to a numerical or functional deficiency of stem cells rather than to a deficient microenvironment. This view is based on the fact that progenitor cells (CFU-GM and BFU-E) are usually low or absent and that bone marrow transplantation from an identical twin, without preparative therapy, can be curative. It should be noted, however, that marrow regeneration often takes longer after transplantation in aplasia than it does in acute leukaemia. It is commonly thought that some cases of idiopathic aplastic anaemia are immune mediated. IAA may be associated with other autoimmune disorders and serum inhibitors and abnormal suppressor cells have been reported in some patients, although technical difficulties and lack of reproducibility between centres make this data difficult to interpret. There is no widely accepted test to indicate which patients might benefit from immunosuppression, and response to intensive immunosuppressive therapy including cytotoxic drugs does not necessarily imply an immunological basis for the disease.

2.2 Drug-related Aplastic Anaemia may develop in three ways:

2.2.1 Direct cytotoxic action, e.g. cytotoxic drugs.

2.2.2 Dose-related marrow suppression, e.g. chloramphenicol, diphenylhydantoin, chlorpromazine, thiouracil, methicillin. Chloramphenicol dose-related abnormalities begin with vacuolation of marrow erythroblasts and may be related to suppression of ferrochelatase and inhibition of mitochondrial protein synthesis. Chloramphenicol aplasia may also be idiosyncratic.

2.2.3 Idiosyncratic or hypersensitivity aplasia, e.g. chloramphenicol, chlorpromazine, quinine, phenylbutazone, gold, barbiturates, colchicine, hydantoin, oral anticoagulants, streptomycin, sulphonyl ureas, thiazides and thiouracils.

The mechanism is in most cases unknown. This type of aplasia almost invariably occurs in the first few months of treatment. In chloramphenicol idiosyncratic aplasia there is evidence of genetic predisposition and effect on DNA synthesis. Chloramphenicol, quinine and some other drugs can be shown to affect CFU-GM in vitro in affected individuals.

2.3 Chemicals and Toxins. Benzene and related compounds—lindane, DDT, toluene. Benzene can cause a whole variety of haematological abnormalities, but most commonly pancytopenia associated with hypoplasia. Hypoplasia commonly occurs soon after exposure though this is not invariable.

2.4 Irradiation. With sufficient dose of irradiation bone marrow aplasia will certainly ensue. Indeed this is the rationale for the irradiation of 10 Gy or thereabouts to leukaemic recipients prior to bone marrow transplantation. The erythroid series is more sensitive to irradiation than the granulocytic and megakaryocytic series, but this tends to be masked by the long red cell survival.

2.5 Associated with Viral Hepatitis. Males are more commonly affected; 75 per cent are under 20 years. Hypoplasia usually occurs within 2 months of the diagnosis of hepatitis and is often very severe and intractable.

2.6 Pregnancy Associated. Several types of aplastic anaemia occur in pregnancy, but there is evidence that in a few instances marrow hypoplasia originates in pregnancy and remits at delivery only to relapse in later pregnancies. In some cases termination of the pregnancy is associated with improvement in marrow cellularity.

2.7 Associated with PNH (*see* Chapter 11).

CLINICAL FEATURES OF ACQUIRED APLASTIC ANAEMIA

Most of the clinical and laboratory features are similar regardless of the underlying cause. The onset is usually insidious and the patient ultimately presents with the clinical features of anaemia secondary to red cell failure, bleeding secondary to thrombocytopenia or infection secondary to neutropenia. Occasionally the onset is much more rapid and it is these patients who often have an extremely poor prognosis.

On examination, there are signs of anaemia and often purpura with haemorrhage into the gums and retinae, inflammatory lesions on the skin, mouth and anus. Modest splenomegaly occurs in approximately 10 per cent of cases in the late stages of the disease.

LABORATORY FEATURES

1. Anaemia is usually normocytic but may be macrocytic. The Hb is variable, but may be as low as 3–4 g/dl at presentation.

2. There is an absolute reticulocytopenia; usually $<40 \times 10^9/l$ (<1 per cent) though occasional nucleated red cells may be found in the peripheral blood.

3. Absolute granulocytopenia is always present and in severe cases is $<0.5 \times 10^9/l$.

4. Monocytopenia is usually present.

5. Lymphocytes usually decreased, but much less so than granulocytes.

6. Platelets usually $<20 \times 10^9/l$.

Severe aplastic anaemia is defined as having reticulocytes $<20 \times 10^9/l$, granulocytes $<0.5 \times 10^9/l$ and platelets $<20 \times 10^9/l$.

7. Bone marrow aspirate almost devoid of haemopoietic cells, but with mononuclear lymphocytoid cells, reticulum cells, mast cells and plasma cells. A few early myeloid cells are often seen, but megakaryocytes are virtually absent.

8. Bone marrow biopsy is hypoplastic, fat spaces predominate though small foci of hypercellular marrow may be seen. A bone marrow biopsy should ideally be taken from more than one site (*Fig. 6.1*).

9. Serum iron is often elevated, but plasma iron turnover may well be normal. Bone marrow may contain much iron, but rarely is it in the nucleated red cells.

10. Plasma erythropoietin is usually considerably elevated.

11. Often modestly raised HbF levels, especially during recovery phases.

Fig. 6.1. Trephine biopsies (low power). *a*, Normal marrow showing cellular elements and fat spaces. *b*, Hypoplastic marrow with increased fat spaces. *c*, Myelofibrosis showing whorls of reticulin and reduced cellularity.

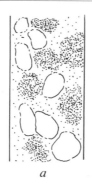 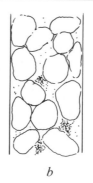 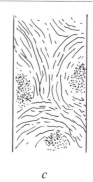

a   *b*   *c*

TREATMENT OF APLASTIC ANAEMIA

Management of Infections

Infection is the commonest form of death in aplastic anaemia and early recognition and treatment with potent broad-spectrum bactericidal antibiotics is essential. Risk of infection rises when the neutrophil count is $< 1 \times 10^9/l$ and is particularly likely if the neutrophil count falls below $0 \cdot 2 \times 10^9/l$. Many centres give co-trimoxazole prophylactically when the neutrophil count is low. Aggressive anti-biotic therapy should be started if a significant fever ($> 38\,°C$) persists for more than 12 hours or if a fever is associated with any clinical deterioration, in the absence of another cause such as blood product administration. A throat swab, swabs from the site of venous catheter insertions, sputum specimen if available, MSU, stool specimen and several blood cultures should be sent to bacteriology, but treatment should not await these results. Special culture media should be used if patients have been receiving prophylactic antibiotics. If a central line is in use at least one set of cultures should be taken from the line. A chest radiograph should be taken even if the chest is clinically clear. Ten ml of serum should be saved for possible viral antibody titres at a later date.

A broad-spectrum antibiotic regime must be chosen to suit local and individual needs. An aminoglycoside should be given in adequate doses, e.g. gentamicin 160 mg i.v. stat then 120 mg i.v. 8-hourly in adults for 24 hours with later dosage adjustment according to serum gentamicin levels. A penicillin is usually also given. Benzyl penicillin 2 megaunits i.v. bolus and then 1 megaunit i.v. 6-hourly in adults is useful for many chest infections, but if a pseudomonas infection is thought likely then a broad-spectrum penicillin with anti-pseudomonas activity should be given. Carbenicillin 20–30 g i.v./day in divided doses is commonly used, but azlocillin 5 g 8-hourly is equally effective and involves less sodium load. If the fever does not respond within 48 hours and no organism has been identified or if a mouth or anal lesion is present at the onset, metronidazole 400 mg 8-hourly should be given to provide cover against anaerobic organisms. If fever persists or local lesions develop in the severely neutropenic patient, despite adequate antibiotics, then granulocytes are usually given if available. Continued failure to respond is a desperate situation. Fungal infections, pneumocystis and viral infections should be sought and therapy with amphotericin, high dose co-trimoxazole or acyclovir (if proven DNA virus infection) considered. Amphotericin almost invariably impairs renal function and close monitoring of gentamicin levels is necessary. Second-line antibacterial agents include cephuroxime (useful for penicillin hypersensitivity) and chloramphenicol. Methylprednisone 1 g i.v. may be useful in the management of septicaemic shock. Antibiotics are ideally continued until the symptoms and fever have resolved and the neutrophil count is $>0.5 \times 10^9/l$ though this latter criteria cannot always be achieved.

The importance of good nursing and particularly mouth care with nystatin, amphotericin, or ketaconazole, mouth lozenges must be emphasized. Protective isolation may be useful in the nursing of the severely neutropenic and some centres use skin and gut decontamination, particularly if intensive immunosuppression or transplantation is anticipated. Close co-operation with the microbiology department is essential and where there are local problems with specific resistant organism, different antibiotics to those described above may be necessary.

Blood Product Support

1. Red Cell Transfusions. Blood transfusions are given as required, but sensitization to red cell, white cell, platelet and plasma antigens can occur and should be minimized by extended red cell phenotyping and the use of leucocyte-depleted blood were possible.

2. Platelet Support. This is much more difficult than red cell support. The infusion of 1×10^{11} platelets/m^2 should produce an increment of about $12 \times 10^9/l$ in a non-sensitized recipient. Antibodies will develop to HLA and platelet specific antigens if random platelets are repeatedly transfused, but bleeding is a significant risk if platelet levels are not kept above $10 \times 10^9/l$.

3. Granulocyte Support. It is not technically possible to consistently and prophylactically achieve useful levels of circulating granulocytes. No attempt is made therefore to supplement granulocytes until severe infection not responding to multiple parenteral antibiotics supervenes. The role of tissue typing in granulocyte transfusion is not fully established.

Therapy to Stimulate the Marrow in Aplastic Anaemia

1. Conventional Doses of Glucocorticoids. Glucocorticoids have been given for a considerable number of years in an attempt to stimulate haematopoiesis in aplasia. Their effectiveness in this situation is far from proven, but low-dose prednisone may mitigate against the effects of thrombocytopenia, by a vascular stabilization.

2. Androgens. A variety of androgenic steroids have been tried to stimulate the marrow in aplastic anaemia. This treatment is occasionally thought to be successful, but may need to be continued for 3–6 months or much longer before any noticeable effect is seen. The androgen is often given in combination with a glucocorticoid. Amongst the androgens used are testosterone, fluoxymesterone and, less frequently, oxymethalone. Oxymethalone is only one-fifth as virilizing as the testosterone derivates and because of this can be given at a dosage of 4–5 mg/kg/day compared with 1–2 mg/kg/day for testosterone derivates. Many of the androgenic steroids cause significant hepatic complications.

3. Folic Acid. As in many dyserythropoietic disorders, folic acid is often given in hypoplasia or aplasia, perhaps starting at 5 mg t.d.s. in the adult and going on to a maintenance dosage of 5 mg daily. There is no proof of genuine benefit.

4. Immunosuppressives. An immune basis to aplastic anaemia is often suspected. For this reason, immunosuppressive drugs have been tried with reports of success. The use of these agents where there is already leucopenia and thrombocytopenia is not without risk. The following agents are amongst those used: high-dose methylprednisone (initially 20 mg/kg/day), chlorambucil, cyclophosphamide, azathioprine and antilymphocyte serum (ALS). Horse or rabbit ALS are given by repeated i.v. infusions, usually in combination with high-dose steroids. Results similar to those achieved by bone marrow transplantation have been reported. Monoclonal anti-T cell antisera are becoming available for clinical use as immunosuppressants. Immunosuppression with ALS has in some centres been followed by i.v. infusion of mismatched haplotype identical bone marrow from a parent or sibling in the hope of tiding the patient over as a temporary split haematopoietic chimera until autologous recovery of marrow takes place. Autologous recovery has been reported following standard haplotype identical marrow grafts.

BONE MARROW TRANSPLANTATION FOR APLASTIC ANAEMIA

Results of supportive therapy only in the treatment of AA have been extremely poor (up to 75 per cent of patients dead at 2 years) and were not improving. This provided the rationale for bone marrow transplantation.

Eligibility for Transplantation

Severe aplastic anaemia <40 years with compatible donor.

Preparation of the Recipient

An agent, usually cyclophosphamide at 200 mg/kg in divided doses over 4 days, is given to immunosuppress the recipient in order that the graft can be accepted. It is essential to maintain a high urinary output during this procedure. 2-Mercaptoethane sulphonate is also effective in reducing the urothelial toxicity of cyclophosphamide. Total nodal irradiation is used in some centres to reduce rejection. Cyclosporin A also appears to be effective in reducing graft rejection.

Tissue Typing

A 4/4 match at the HLA A+B loci is usually required with a negative mixed lymphocyte culture between recipient and potential donor, thus usually limiting potential donors to an identical twin or 1 in 4 siblings. Parents or siblings with a single locus mismatch (A, B or D) also may be considered as donors.

Technique of Marrow Grafting

The donor is given a general anaesthetic and 500–800 ml of marrow are aspirated from the posterior and anterior iliac crests and sternum to produce a recipient dose of around 2–4×10^8 nucleated marrow cells/kg of recipient. The marrow is taken into heparin and tissue culture medium and infused i.v. into the recipient.

Immunosuppression

Methotrexate or cyclosporin A are given to minimize graft versus host disease. Manipulation of the bone marrow with monoclonal or polyclonal antisera to remove mature immunocompetent cells may also be appropriate.

Support

Platelet infusions are given to keep the platelet count above $20 \times 10^9/l$ and antibiotics and granulocyte transfusions are given as necessary. All blood products are irradiated before being given to the recipient to prevent any undesired grafting.

Results

Forty to fifty per cent of patients transplanted for severe AA are long-term survivors at 1–5 years and these results in a prospective, but uncontrolled trial were significantly better than those from conventional therapy with androgens, steroids, etc. Recent studies using cyclosporin A are even more encouraging.

Problems of Bone Marrow Transplantation in Aplastic Anaemia

Graft Failure and Graft Rejection. Failure of the graft occurs in < 10 per cent of cases, but in AA a significant number of patients successfully take the graft, and then reject it. This is reduced by use of cyclosporin A

Graft Versus Host Disease (GVHD). Graft versus host disease is a poorly understood immunological reaction of donor lymphoid cells against host tissues. The acute form comes on 1–4 weeks after transplantation in 50–70 per cent of cases and manifests itself as a maculopapular rash, especially on the hands and feet, hepatocellular liver damage and diarrhoea. These problems may be minimized by the prophylactic use of methotrexate or cyclosporin A; the incidence of GVHD is not very different with these two regimes but the mortality from GVHD is less in those given Cyclosporin A. Florid GVHD is alarming but may respond to high-dose methylprednisone. Chronic GVHD coming on several months after transplantation manifests as sclerodermatous skin changes and obstructive liver disease. When severe it is usually refractory to treatment.

Interstitial Pneumonia. This is a late problem occurring after bone marrow transplantation in up to half the patients in some series. It is sometimes proven to be associated with cytomegalovirus or pneumocystis, but TBI (especially fast dose rate) and graft versus host disease may be implicated.

Infections. Initially bacterial, but after granulocyte recovery, opportunistic fungal and viral infections predominate.

FANCONI'S ANAEMIA

Clinical Features

It usually presents in boys between 4 and 7 years and girls between 6 and 10 years. It is slightly more common in boys and may present much later. Inheritance autosomal recessive. There is insidious onset of anaemia and bruising with no enlargement of lymph nodes, liver or spleen. There is increased pigmentation in 75 per cent of cases and skeletal abnormalities including absent radii and thumbs and abnormalities of the long bones and hips, in two-thirds. Microsomy, microcephaly, renal anomalies, hypogonadism and strabismus are commonly found. There is an increased incidence of congenital heart disease.

Laboratory Features

Characteristically there is pancytopenia with macrocytic red cells and markedly reduced reticulocytes. In the early stages there is an increase in HbF and antigen on the red cells. Red and white cell precursors are not seen in the blood. The ESR is very high. A bone marrow aspirate and biopsy are both hypoplastic with morphological changes in erythroblasts resembling megaloblastic change, but with normal B_{12} and folate levels. A chromosome instability can be demonstrated, in most cases, but is not essential for the diagnosis. These chromosome changes resemble those found in acute luekaemia and in this syndrome there is an increased incidence of acute leukaemia. Radiography of the long bones frequently shows retarded bone age. An IVU should be done in all suspected cases.

A diagnosis of Fanconi's anaemia can be made if there is aplastic anaemia with the classic physical features, or aplastic anaemia with typical chromosomal abnormalities or with relatives with a more classic disease.

Treatment

Is that for other forms of aplastic anaemia. Bone marrow transplantation may be effective, but great care must be taken in selecting sibling donors who may have incipient disease.

Prognosis

Ultimately fatal, unless treated by a successful graft; 5–10 per cent of cases terminate in acute leukaemia.

PURE RED CELL APLASIA (PRCA)

This is a heterogeneous disorder in which there is an isolated depletion of the erythroid series.

1. Acute PRCA

There is acute self-limiting erythroid hypoplasia.

a. It is most commonly seen in the chronic haemolytic anaemias, such as hereditary spherocytosis and paroxysmal nocturnal haemoglobinuria, in which situations it is commonly referred to as an 'aplastic crisis'. In most instances there is only moderate erythroid hypoplasia but anaemia rapidly develops because of the shortened red cell survival. This condition is usually a complication of viral infections.

b. Some drugs have been reported to cause acute PRCA including diphenyl-hydantoin, chlorpropamide and chloramphenicol.

c. Acute PRCA is occasionally seen without a history of haemolytic anaemia or drug ingestion. It usually follows an infective episode.

2. Chronic PRCA

2.1 Congenital (Diamond–Blackfan Syndrome)

Aetiology. This is a congenital disorder which in at least some cases is genetically inherited. The mode of inheritance is uncertain. Associated minor congenital defects are seen in about 25 per cent of cases; these include strabismus, inverted nipples and webbing of the neck. More rarely, major abnormalities such as musculoskeletal abnormalities, hydronephrosis and heart defects occur. The disorder is probably a primary stem cell defect. Claims of a T cell-mediated immune suppression have not been substantiated. In some patients there is increased urinary excretion of anthranilic acid after an oral tryptophan load but this is not invariable and the significance of this finding is not clear.

Clinical. Anaemia usually develops within the first few weeks of life producing pallor, dyspnoea and congestive heart failure. The haemoglobin may be less than 10 g/dl at birth. Hepatosplenomegaly is common and is secondary to the heart failure. There is no haemorrhagic tendency or susceptibility to infections in the early stages. Occasionally the diagnosis is not made until the child is several years old. Ultimately multiple transfusions lead to iron overload and portal hypertension; hypersplenism may then cause leucopenia and thrombocytopenia. In the late stages there is an increased risk of overwhelming sepsis.

Laboratory Features. There is normocytic anaemia with severe reticulocytopenia. The bone marrow is normocellular with a great increase in the M : E ratio with a normal granulocyte and megakaryocyte cell series. The few nucleated erythroid cells seen are usually proerythroblasts which may show mild megaloblastic change. Cases have been described in which there are normal numbers of normoblasts with marked dyserythropoiesis, but such cases should probably be considered as 'congenital dyserythropoietic anaemias'.

The HbF is usually raised even when the patient is repeatedly transfused.

Treatment. Transfusions are given as required to maintain an acceptable Hb level. Iron chelators must also be given. Approximately one-third of otherwise untreated patients have spontaneous remissions though these are often temporary. Prednisone may induce a complete or partial remission in up to one-half of cases; 1–2 mg/kg should be given for at least 6 weeks; a reticulocytosis heralds a response. Whether there has been a response or not, this high steroid dose must then be reduced to minimize side effects, particularly growth retardation. Responders usually require some maintenance therapy, and not infrequently relapse. Splenectomy should not be performed.

Prognosis. Non-responders inevitably develop transfusion siderosis. Overwhelming sepsis is the commonest cause of death in these patients, especially if the spleen has been removed.

2.2 Acquired.

Aetiology. This is a disorder primarily affecting middle-aged adults, though childhood cases do occur. Between one-third and one-half of cases are associated with a thymoma which in most instances (80 per cent) is a benign tumour. Myasthenia gravis may also be present. The mechanism in acquired PRCA with and without a thymoma is thought to be immunological. There is an association with other auto-immune diseases (e.g. SLE), antibodies to erythropoietin and erythroid progenitor and precursor cells have been demonstrated, and in some cases there is a proliferation of T cells with a 'suppressor phenotype'.

Laboratory Findings. The anaemia is usually normocytic but may be macrocytic. Unlike the congenital variety some suppression of leucocytes frequently occurs, especially in the later stages. Abnormalities of immunoglobulins including hypogammaglobulinaemia and paraproteins are not infrequent.

Treatment. Primary treatment is by transfusion.

Thymomas should be sought and removed if found, though complete recoveries are not the rule.

A trial of high-dose steroid therapy and other immuno-suppressive drugs should be given. Anti-lymphocyte globulin is effective in some cases. Where relevant autoantibodies are present, plasmapheresis may have a part in a combined modality approach.

Selected Further Reading

Geary C. G. (ed.) (1979) *Aplastic Anaemia.* London, Baillière Tindall.

Storb R. et al. (1978) One hundred and ten patients with aplastic anaemia treated by bone marrow transplantation in Seattle. *Transplant Proc.* **10**, 135

Thomas E. D. (1975) Bone marrow transplantation. *New Engl. J. Med.* **292**, 832.

7

General Features of Haemolytic Anaemia

CLINICAL

1. Symptoms of anaemia, such as breathlessness on exertion, tiredness, palpitations, headache and faintness, are more common if the haemolysis is of sudden onset. Patients may have symptoms of general debility and malaise and also symptoms related to the underlying cause.

2. Pallor, due to vasoconstriction of skin capillaries.

3. Jaundice, usually mild and may fluctuate. The absence of jaundice does not exclude haemolytic anaemia. Urine darkens on standing due to oxidation of urobilinogen to urobilin.

4. Splenomegaly, degree depending on underlying cause.

5. Pigment gallstones—increased incidence.

6. Leg ulcers may occur, especially with congenital haemolytic anaemias, such as thalassaemia major and sickle-cell disease; occasionally in hereditary spherocytosis.

LABORATORY

1. Evidence of Increased Haemoglobin Breakdown (*Fig. 7.1*)

a. Raised serum bilirubin (normal value less than 17 mmol/l, 1 mg/100 ml); usually only mild elevation of unconjugated pigment which gives the raised indirect van den Bergh reaction. Pigment gallstones may occasionally cause obstructive jaundice.

b. Raised urine urobilinogen—produces red colour with Ehrlich's reagent. Urobilinogen can be distinguished from porphobilinogen by shaking the coloured solution with n-butanol. If the colouring is due to urobilinogen it is extracted into the butanol (upper layer). With porphobilinogen the colour remains in the lower layer.

c. Haptoglobin levels are reduced or absent. Marked reduction occurs with intravascular haemolysis, but a reduced level may occur with extravascular haemolysis. These α_2-glycoproteins bind free haemoglobin to form complexes which are rapidly removed by the reticulo-endothelial system. Haptoglobin level returns to normal approximately 1 week after cessation of haemolysis.

d. Plasma haemoglobin level rises with intravascular haemolysis (normal less than 10 mg/l).

e. Haemoglobinuria occurs when the amount of haemoglobin released exceeds the binding ability of haptoglobin.

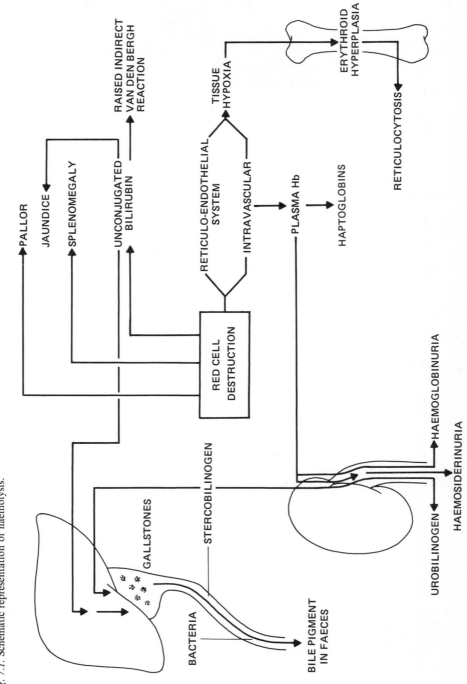

Fig. 7.1. Schematic representation of haemolysis.

f. Haemosiderinuria occurs in chronic haemolysis in association with haemoglobinuria. The pigment is taken up by tubules and iron may later be released into the urine as haemosiderin granules.

g. Methaemalbuminaemia is present in the plasma when there is marked intravascular haemolysis; the haem moiety of free haemoglobin is oxidized to methaem which has a greater affinity for albumin than globin.

2. Evidence of Increased Red Cell Production

a. Reticulocytosis, due to increased production and partly due to earlier release from the marrow. Reticulocytes have an MCV of approximately 110 fl. Normoblasts may occur in the peripheral blood with severe haemolysis.

b. Erythroid hyperplasia may produce frontal bossing, radiological evidence of marrow expansion which predisposes to bone pain and pathological fracture. The myeloid : erythroid ratio is less than 1 : 1.

3. Red Cell Morphological Abnormalities

Inborn errors responsible for abnormal shapes include: hereditary spherocytosis, hereditary elliptocytosis and sickle-cell disease. Spherocytosis occurs in hereditary spherocytosis and in a variety of acquired haemolytic anaemias and is not of specific diagnostic value. Red cell fragmentation occurs in microangiopathic haemolytic anaemia; fragmentation associated with irregular contraction of cells occurs in some drug-induced haemolytic anaemias. Target cells occur in thalassaemic syndromes, haemoglobin C disease and sometimes in sickle-cell disease. Siderocytes occur in some haemolytic anaemias and are even more numerous when splenectomy has been performed and haemolysis continues.

4. Demonstration of Reduced Red Cell Survival

Red cells labelled with ^{51}Cr have a normal $T_{\frac{1}{2}}$ of 25–35 days. Haemolytic anaemias are associated with $T_{\frac{1}{2}}$ of less than 15 days (shortened $T_{\frac{1}{2}}$ greater than this are associated with a haemolytic state). (*See* Chapter 28.)

GENERAL APPROACH TO THE INVESTIGATION OF HAEMOLYTIC ANAEMIA

1. Clinical History

A careful history often will determine whether a haemolytic anaemia is congenital or acquired, though it must be remembered that many congenital haemolytic anaemias do not become manifest until adult life. Recent viral infections (especially pneumonia or glandular fever), evidence of lymphoma, chronic lymphatic leukaemia, systemic lupus erythematosus, rheumatoid arthritis, polyarteritis nodosa or sarcoid, are particularly relevant.

A careful history of drug ingestion is essential, especially methyldopa, mephenamic acid or high-dose penicillin.

Fig. 7.2. The direct antiglobulin test.

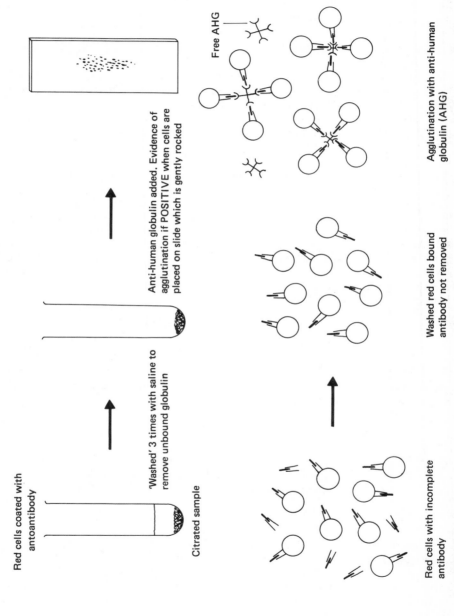

Red cells coated with antoantibody

'Washed' 3 times with saline to remove unbound globulin

Citrated sample

Anti-human globulin added. Evidence of agglutination if POSITIVE when cells are placed on slide which is gently rocked

Free AHG

Agglutination with anti-human globulin (AHG)

Washed red cells bound antibody not removed

Red cells with incomplete antibody

A positive family history often is obtained in patients suffering from haemo-globinopathies or red cell enzyme defects. Troublesome leg ulcers, symptoms suggestive of sickle crises, problems with pregnancies or the history of splenectomy in relatives are relevant.

2. Examination of the Peripheral Film

a. Red cells: the morphology of the red cells frequently suggests the cause of haemolysis.

b. White cells: atypical mononuclear cells, neutrophilia or evidence of chronic lymphatic leukaemia should be sought.

c. Platelets: a reduction, together with fragmented cells, is found in disseminated intravascular haemolysis.

3. Direct Antiglobulin Test (Coombs' Test)

Having determined that haemolysis is occurring, it is essential to determine whether or not the haemolysis is immune mediated by the direct antiglobulin test (DAT) (*Fig. 7.2*).

Further investigations are dictated by the history, clinical findings and results of the DAT.

Selected Further Reading

Dacie J. V. (1981) *The Haemolytic Anaemias,* Vol. 1, 3rd ed. Edinburgh, Churchill Livingstone.

Chapter 8 / Hereditary Haemolytic Anaemias

I. MEMBRANE DEFECTS

Hereditary Spherocytosis

Definition. An inherited defect of the membrane cytoskeleton causes the red cells to be rounder, more rigid and fragile, have increased osmotic fragility and be more prone to splenic sequestration.

Aetiology and Pathology. Inherited as an autosomal dominant with incomplete penetrance affecting 1 in 5000 of the population. In 25 per cent there is no family history and is presumably due to a spontaneous mutation. The membrane cytoskeletal abnormality has not been precisely defined. It is associated with increased sodium influx and increased ATP utilization for the compensatory increased pumping out of sodium ions. Intracellular glycolysis may be increased twentyfold.

The spherocytes enter the pulp cords of the spleen and their shape delays entry, via the slit-like apertures of the walls, into the splenic sinuses. The splenic cords are therefore congested.

Clinical Features. Symptoms vary in severity. In mild, well-compensated disease there is no anaemia. However, the anaemia may be moderate to severe. Because of the shortened red cell survival marrow depression (as may occur with intercurrent infection) exacerbates the anaemia to produce the so-called 'aplastic crisis'; folic acid depletion due to compensatory increased erythropoiesis may also be a contributing factor. 'Haemolytic crises', which are less common than 'aplastic crises', are associated with increased splenic red cell destruction. The spleen almost always is palpable; it is not tender except during the haemolytic crisis.

In the more severe cases jaundice may be present at birth and persist after the first week; kernicterus can occur in the neonatal period. The usual bilirubin level is between 20 and 70 µmol/l (1·2–4 mg/100 ml).

Radiographic Findings. Skeletal changes are rare but sometimes 'tower skull' and thickening of the frontal and parietal bones occur.

Laboratory Findings

Blood. The haemoglobin level is usually between 8 and 12 g/dl, but lower levels occur during crises. The red cells are usually normocytic, but occasionally microcytosis is present. If there is a marked reticulocytosis, macrocytosis occurs.

The mean cell average thickness (MCAT) is increased (from the upper limit of 2 µm to as high as 3·5 µm). The increase in the MCAT is associated with increased fragility in hypotonic saline. Some patients have only a small proportion of cells susceptible to hypotonia which are demonstrable as a 'tail' in the fragility curve. In some other patients the increased osmotic fragility may only be demonstrated after 24 hours incubation of the red cells at 37 °C prior to the fragility test. The autohaemolysis test is positive and the degree of haemolysis is reduced or even corrected by the addition of glucose, which helps generate the ATP required in increased amounts. The reticulocyte count is usually between 5 and 20 per cent, very high levels occur during the haemolytic crisis. ^{51}Cr studies show a shortened red cell survival with increased uptake of counts over the spleen.

Bone Marrow. There is erythroid hyperplasia, the myeloid : erythroid ratio usually being between 2 : 1 and 1 : 2. Megaloblastic change occurs if there is concomitant folate deficiency.

Urine. There is an excess of urobilinogen in the urine, but no bile pigment (unless there is the complication of obstructive jaundice due to stones or hepatitis).

Diagnosis. This is based on clinical and laboratory findings and usually a family study.

Differential Diagnosis. If the disorder presents in the neonatal period it must be differentiated from haemolytic disease of the newborn, G-6-PD deficiency and α-thalassaemia. In later life the disorder must be distinguished from autoimmune haemolytic anaemia, and thus the negative Direct Antiglobulin Test is extremely important.

Treatment. Blood transfusion may be required for aplastic crisis in the first 2 years of life. Folic acid supplements may be required during childhood and also especially during pregnancy if splenectomy has not been performed previously. Splenectomy increases red cell survival to some 80 per cent of normal, abolishes the crises and prevents pigment stone formation. Because of the associated risk of infection in splenectomized patients, the operation is usually postponed until after puberty. Prophylactic maintenance penicillin should be given. Polyvalent pneumococcal vaccine may be of limited value.

In older children and adults an ultrasound should be performed prior to splenectomy so that, if required, consideration may be given to cholecystectomy being performed at the same time as splenectomy.

Hereditary Elliptocytosis

Definition. An inherited disorder of the red cell membrane characterized by oval red cells. The abnormality does not become manifest morphologically before the reticulocyte stage of maturation.

Aetiology and Pathology. Inherited as an autosomal disorder (with variable penetrance) affecting about 1 in 25 000 of the population. Two types of inheritance occur: (1) Non-Rh-linked, associated with a high incidence of severe anaemia in the homozygote. (2) Rh-linked, usually associated with a milder disorder. There is no correlation between the degree of elliptocytosis and the severity of the anaemia. The percentage of elliptocytes varies from 50 to 90 per cent. The cause of elliptocytosis is unknown, but is probably due to a protein rather than a lipid abnormality of the membrane.

Clinical Features. Most of the patients have no symptoms; in about 12 per cent there is either a compensated haemolytic state or haemolytic anaemia which may be associated with splenomegaly, leg ulcers and occasionally skeletal changes.

Laboratory Investigations. The peripheral film is characteristic with usually over 50 per cent of the red cells being elliptocytes, though occasionally only a slight excess above the accepted upper limit of 15 per cent elliptocytes is found. The red cells are normocytic or microcytic. The osmotic fragility and autohaemolysis tests are normal.

Diagnosis and Differential Diagnosis. The diagnosis is made from the peripheral film morphology and family studies. Differentiation must be made from other conditions where elliptocytosis occurs: iron deficiency, thalassaemia, megaloblastic anaemias and the anaemias associated with chronic disease.

Prognosis and Treatment. Often the disorder is asymptomatic and longevity is not affected. Anaemia and associated symptoms, if present, are usually corrected by splenectomy.

Hereditary Stomatocytosis

Definition. The red cells have a slit-like central pallor. There are many variants of this inherited disorder, some of which may be associated with anaemia. It is not certain whether additional inherited red cell abnormalities contribute to the severe forms of this disease.

Classification. Many varieties of the disorder have been reported, some due to autosomal recessive, others due to autosomal dominant inheritance.

Aetiology and Pathology. The red cells of some patients show a marked increase of sodium levels with markedly reduced potassium levels. In other patients the sodium and potassium levels are normal and these patients show increased red cell glucose consumption in vitro, suggesting compensation for increased cation permeability. Many patients have an increased red cell osmotic fragility.

Clinical Features. Symptoms are very variable in this heterogeneous group of disorders. Many patients are symptom-free, others are anaemic and jaundiced from birth. Splenomegaly is common in these latter patients.

Laboratory Investigations. The peripheral film shows stomatocytosis, usually between 10 and 50 per cent of the red cells being affected. Anaemia, if present, is associated with a reticulocytosis and hyperbilirubinaemia.

Differential Diagnosis. Stomatocytosis may occur in thalassaemia, some red cell enzyme defects, viral infections, lead poisoning, some drugs such as quinidine and chlorpromazine, some malignancies, liver disease and alcoholism.

Treatment. Splenectomy may be beneficial if haemolysis is severe.

Hereditary Acanthocytosis

Definition. Acanthocytes have thorn-like projections which vary in length and width and are irregularly distributed over the surface of the red cells.

Aetiology and Pathology. The condition is inherited as an autosomal recessive in a syndrome associated with malabsorption, diffuse nervous system involvement and an atypical retinitis pigmentosa due to abetalipoproteinaemia.

Clinical Features. Symptoms usually present within the first 2 years of life with steatorrhoea. Only fat absorption is impaired (cf. coeliac disease), therefore vitamin B_{12} and folate levels are normal. Neurological symptoms include weakness, ataxia and nystagmus. The atypical retinitis pigmentosa with macular atrophy often results in blindness. Anaemia, if present, is only mild. Death usually occurs during childhood.

Laboratory Investigations. The diagnosis is confirmed by the absence of betalipoprotein in the plasma and by the diagnostic appearance of the small intestine obtained by biopsy.

Differential Diagnosis. Acquired acanthocytosis occurs in uraemia, cirrhosis, microangiopathic haemolytic anaemia, myxoedema, pyruvate kinase deficiency and in association with some neoplasms.

Hereditary Pyropoikilocytosis

Definition. A congenital haemolytic anaemia associated with in vivo red cell fragmentation and marked in vitro fragmentation of red cells at 45 °C.
Aetiology and Pathology. Inherited as an autosomal recessive. There is an increased ratio of cholesterol to membrane protein and cell deformity is decreased.
Clinical Features. There is anaemia, usually between 7 and 9 g/dl, jaundice and splenomegaly.
Treatment. Patients respond well to splenectomy.

II. RED CELL ENZYME DEFECTS

The enzyme systems of the red cell are almost exclusively involved in oxygen and to a lesser extent carbon dioxide transport. ATP is required to maintain the biconcave disc shape and flexibility of the cell wall (enables the cell to travel readily through small capillaries and facilitates the diffusion of gases within the cell) and is essential for ion transport across the cell membrane. ATP is produced by the metabolism of glucose to lactate by the glycolytic (Embden–Meyerhof) pathway, two mols of ATP being produced for every mol of glucose metabolized (*Fig. 8.1*). 2,3-Diphosphoglycerate (2,3-DPG) is synthesized by an offshoot of this pathway and modulates haemoglobin oxygen affinity. NADH is also produced by the glycolytic pathway and maintains haem iron in the ferrous state. NADPH is produced by the hexose monophosphate shunt; this is necessary for glutathione reduction which prevents denaturation (oxidation of SH groups) of haemoglobin. There is no tricarboxylic acid cycle, protein or nucleic acid synthesis in the mature red cell. Erythrocyte enzyme defects are usually due to production of an abnormal enzyme, often with a shortened life span, rather than the absence of the enzyme protein. An enzyme deficiency may be suggested by the history (e.g. haemolysis following drug ingestion) but in the investigation of the congenital non-spherocytic haemolytic anaemias a pragmatic approach is necessary. With the exception of glucose-6-phosphate dehydrogenase (G-6-PD) deficiency (estimated 100 000 000 affected individuals) symptomatic enzymopathies are rare and it is wise to very carefully exclude more common causes of haemolysis such as immune haemolysis. G-6-PD and pyruvate kinase are the first enzymes to be assayed as they are the most common deficiencies. Measurement of 2,3-DPG is often helpful; the level is usually raised in anaemia but the level is often higher than expected in enzymopathies distal to the 2,3-DPG pathway (e.g. pyruvate kinase deficiency) and lower in proximal enzymopathies (e.g. phosphofructokinase deficiency). The importance of appropriate control specimens and full family studies in the investigation of enzymopathies must be emphasized.

Glucose-6-Phosphate Dehydrogenase Deficiency

Definition. Glucose-6-phosphate dehydrogenase (G-6-PD) catalyses the first stage of the hexose monophosphate shunt:

$$\text{G-6-P} + \text{NADP} \xrightarrow{\text{G-6-PD}} \text{6-PG} + \text{NADPH}$$

Fig. 8.1. Glucose metabolism.

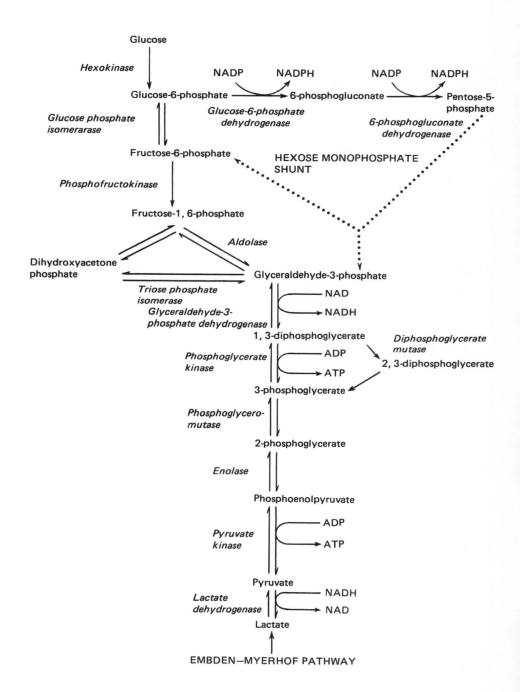

The active enzyme is a dimer or tetramer of monomeric subunits which have a molecular weight of about 50 000. The normal enzyme is designated B +. The inheritance of the enzyme is sex-linked. Low levels of G-6-PD lead to low levels of reduced glutathione at times of oxidant stress with consequent precipitation of haemoglobin, oxidation of membrane SH groups and membrane lipid peroxidation.

Classification. Variants of G-6-PD deficiency may be classified by the electrophoretic findings. A very large number of variants (over 100) occur due to alterations in the amino acid sequence in the enzyme. The 'normal' enzyme, designated B +, is present in Caucasian subjects and about 60 per cent of Negroes. The African A + variant (incidence about 25 per cent of Negroes) has a more rapid electrophoretic mobility than B, but only slightly reduced enzyme activity. The African A − variant (incidence 5–15 per cent) is quantitatively normal, but the enzyme is unstable and declines as the red cell ages. The Mediterranean and Oriental types of G-6-PD deficiency have very low or absent levels of enzyme activity. Female heterozygotes have a dimorphic population of red cells with respect to G-6-PD levels (Lyon hypothesis). The overall level tends to be over 50 per cent of normal as the normal red cells in the heterozygote survive preferentially. The males are either affected or normal.

Pathology and Clinical Features

1. Neonatal jaundice may occur with most variants, but is most common with the Mediterranean and Oriental varieties. Female heterozygotes of this type occasionally haemolyse in the newborn period. Dye-containing compounds, used to sterilize the umbilical cord, and the administration of vitamin K have been precipitating factors.

2. Chronic congenital haemolytic anaemia has been found in over 30 variants. About 60 per cent of this clinical type have been reported in Northern Europeans. The anaemia is usually mild, the haemoglobin being below 10 g/dl in about one-fifth of patients.

3. Stress-induced haemolytic episodes are caused by infections, particularly viral hepatitis, diabetic acidosis and other acute illnesses.

4. Stress and drug-induced haemolysis is more severe in the Mediterranean and Oriental varieties. The Negro type is self-limiting as the reticulocytes released from the marrow at this time have normal G-6-PD levels. The intravascular haemolysis may be so acute as to cause prostration and occasionally death.

Drugs which may cause haemolysis with G-6-PD variants are shown in *Table 8.1.* Favism is characterized by severe acute haemolysis (associated with jaundice and haemoglobinuria) occurring in persons sensitive to uncooked or lightly cooked fava beans or in some patients the inhalation of the fava pollen. Children between 2 and 5 are most commonly affected. The disorder is relatively rare in adults. Favism is mostly confined to the G-6-PD Mediterranean variant.

Laboratory Findings. There is anaemia and reticulocytosis at the time of haemolysis. The red cells show anisocytosis and frequent Heinz bodies. The red cells have normal osmotic fragility and show type I autohaemolysis. The neutrophil count is frequently raised. Screening tests for G-6-PD deficiency and enzyme assay are described in Chapter 28. Young cells have a higher G-6-PD activity than older cells, hence the increase in young cells after a haemolytic episode may mask the diagnosis. In heterozygous females, as one X chromosome per cell is non-functioning (Lyon hypothesis), there will be two populations of red cells which differ in their enzyme activity.

Table 8.1 Some drugs known to cause haemolysis in G-6-PD deficiency

Aspirin

Sulphonamides
Phenazopyridine
Nitrofurantoin
Nalidixic acid
Chloramphenicol

Quinine
Chloroquine
Primaquine

Dapsone
Para-aminosalicylic acid
Vitamin K
Vitamin C
Probenecid
Diazoxide
Benzocaine

Treatment. Patients should avoid drugs and agents which precipitate haemolysis. Infections should be treated promptly. In neonates exchange transfusion may be required for severe jaundice. In children and adults transfusion may be required for several haemolytic episodes. Care must be taken not to transfuse blood from a G-6-PD-deficient donor!

Pyruvate Kinase Deficiency

Definition. Pyruvate kinase (PK) deficiency is associated with gross impairment of ATP generation in the Embden–Meyerhof pathway, hence potassium and water are lost through the red cell membrane and the cell becomes sequestrated by the reticuloendothelial system.

Aetiology and Pathology. Inherited as an autosomal recessive and characterized by a moderate to severe haemolytic anaemia. Variants of the disorder have been associated with haemolysis in the heterozygous state. Most patients are of Northern European origin. The inability to generate ATP and to convert NAD to NADH leads to a shortened red cell life span. The 2,3-DPG levels are raised, hence a 'shift to the right' in the haemoglobin oxygen dissociation curve occurs. PK deficiency may be due to a quantitative reduction or due to a mutant enzyme having abnormal kinetic properties.

Clinical Features. There is a considerable variation in the severity of this congenital non-spherocytic anaemia (Hb usually between 4 and 10 g/dl). Exacerbations of the anaemia may be precipitated by infection or other stress. Symptoms tend to be less severe than the haemoglobin level would indicate due to the improved oxygen delivery to the tissue caused by the shift of the haemoglobin oxygen dissociation curve. Severe cases may require frequent transfusions from birth. The level of the jaundice and the degree of splenomegaly vary with the severity of the anaemia. Pigment gallstones may be a complication.

Laboratory Findings. The anaemia is associated with a reticulocytosis. The peripheral film shows polychromasia with some macrocytosis, some of the red cells have an irregular outline. The red cells have slightly increased osmotic fragility. The autohaemolysis test is usually positive with poor correction by glucose (type II). Diagnosis is confirmed by the PK enzyme assay.

Treatment. Exchange transfusion may be required during the neonatal period. Splenectomy often improves the haemoglobin level and reduces transfusion requirements. Folic acid supplements may be required.

Other Red Cell Enzyme Defects

The following enzyme defects are associated with haemolytic anaemia.
6-Phosphogluconate Dehydrogenase (6-PGD). 6-PGD is the second enzyme in the hexose monophase shunt and converts 6-phosphogluconate to pentose-5-phosphate.

6-PGD deficiency is a very rare cause of haemolytic anaemia which is inherited as an autosomal recessive. Dietary factors appear to affect the enzyme level and may relate to exacerbations of the disorder. A high carbohydrate diet appears to impair synthesis of the enzyme. Drugs which produce haemolysis in 6-PGD deficiency should be avoided.

Defects in Embden–Meyerhof Pathway

Hexokinase, an autosomal recessive disorder. The anaemia improves after splenectomy.

Glucose phosphate isomerase (phosphohexose isomerase), an autosomal recessive disorder. The anaemia improves after splenectomy. Progressive neurological degeneration may occur in some patients.

Phosphofructokinase (phosphohexokinase), an autosomal recessive disorder. Three clinical types are recognized. Type I in which there is severe deficiency of the muscle enzyme, but only slight red cell enzyme impairment. Type II in which the muscle enzyme activity is normal and the red cell enzyme activity is only moderately decreased. Type III in which the muscle enzyme activity is normal, the red cell enzyme activity is, however, severely deficient.

Aldolase, an autosomal recessive disorder. The anaemia may improve after splenectomy. Neurological disorders occur in some patients.

Triosephosphate isomerase, an autosomal recessive disorder. The anaemia is mild and well compensated, but severe progressive neurological disease occurs in childhood. Cardiac arrhythmias may occur.

Phosphoglycerate kinase, a sex-linked recessive disorder which is associated with a severe haemolytic anaemia in males. Females are only mildly affected and two red cell populations may be demonstrated (as with G-6-PD deficiency). Neurological symptoms have occurred in a few patients.

Diphosphoglycerate mutase, an autosomal recessive disorder. There may be a mild haemolytic state. The urine contains mesobilifuchsin.

Enolase deficiency, an autosomal recessive disorder. There is a chronic haemolytic anaemia exacerbated by drugs having an oxidant action.

Defects of Glutathione Metabolism

Glutathione reductase, an autosomal dominant disorder. Haemolytic anaemia is precipitated by drugs having an oxidant action. Thrombocytopenia has occasionally been reported. Neurological symptoms occur in some patients.

γ-Glutamyl cysteine synthetase, an autosomal recessive disorder. There is a well compensated haemolytic anaemia.

Glutathione synthetase, an autosomal recessive disorder. There is a well compensated haemolytic anaemia, exacerbated by drugs having an oxidant action.

Glutathione peroxidase, an autosomal recessive disorder. Acute haemolytic episodes occur after exposure to drugs having an oxidant action.

Laboratory Investigations. Enzyme defects affecting the Embden–Meyerhof pathway produce the blood picture of a non-spherocytic haemolytic anaemia with no denaturation of haemoglobin.

Enzyme defects affecting glutathione metabolism produce a variable degree of anaemia; haemolytic episodes precipitated by drugs having an oxidant action are associated with morphological changes of stippling, Heinz body formation, sometimes spherocytosis and always polychromasia. Dietary deficiency of riboflavin may exacerbate these changes.

III. DEFECTS OF HAEMOGLOBIN SYNTHESIS

Thalassaemic Syndromes

See Chapter 9.

Abnormal Haemoglobins

See Chapter 10.

Selected Further Reading

Beutler E. (1978) *Haemolytic Anaemia in Disorders of Red Cell Metabolism.* New York, Plenum.
Dacie J. V. (1981) *The Haemolytic Anaemias*, Vol. I, 3rd ed. Edinburgh, Churchill Livingstone.
Huehns E. R. (1976) Disorders of carbohydrate metabolism in the red blood corpuscle. *Clin. Endocrinol. Metab.* **5**, 651–674.

Chapter 9

Haemoglobin and the Thalassaemia Syndromes

STRUCTURE OF HAEMOGLOBIN

Haemoglobin consists of two moieties. Haem is of constant structure throughout the animal kingdom; it consists of 4 pyrrole groups linked by methene (—CH=) bridges to form a porphyrin ring (*Fig. 9.1*).

Fig 9.1. The porphyrin ring of haem.

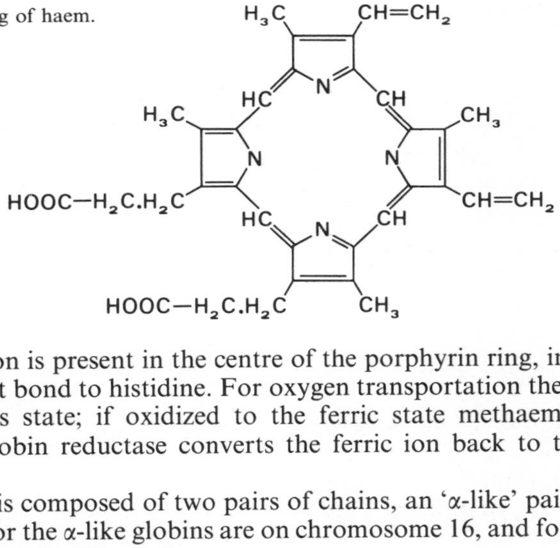

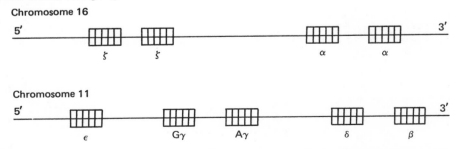

One molecule of iron is present in the centre of the porphyrin ring, in a pocket, attached by a covalent bond to histidine. For oxygen transportation the iron must remain in the ferrous state; if oxidized to the ferric state methaemoglobin is formed. Methaemoglobin reductase converts the ferric ion back to the ferrous state.

The globin moiety is composed of two pairs of chains, an 'α-like' pair and a 'β-like' pair. The genes for the α-like globins are on chromosome 16, and for the β-like globins on chromosome 11 (*Fig. 9.2*).

Fig. 9.2. Genetic coding of globin chains.

Chromosome 16

5′   ζ   ζ   α   α   3′

Chromosome 11

5′   ε   Gγ   Aγ   δ   β   3′

Different globin genes are expressed at different stages of development, with transition from the 5′ gene→3′ genes. The major haemoglobins at the different developmental stages are shown below.

Embryonic Haemoglobins

Hb Gower 1	$\zeta_2\varepsilon_2$	50%	possibly
Hb Gower 2	$\alpha_2\varepsilon_2$	25%	higher at
Hb Portland	$\zeta_2\gamma_2$	5%	earlier stages.

Fetal Haemoglobins

HbF	$\alpha_2\gamma_2$	90%
HbA	$\alpha_2\beta_2$	10%

Adult Haemoglobins

HbA	$\alpha_2\beta_2$	97%
HbA$_2$	$\alpha_2\delta_2$	2%
HbF	$\alpha_2\gamma_2$	1%

The different haemoglobins can often be demonstrated by electrophoresis (*Fig. 9.3*).

Fig. 9.3. Haemoglobin electrophoresis.

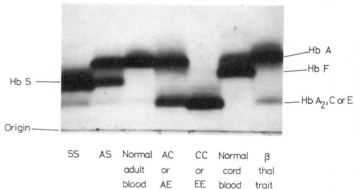

Note that the γ chain consists of two components γ^G and γ^A, the difference being the presence of glycine or an alanine residue at position 136. The switch from HbF→HbA synthesis occurs at birth and is related to the period of gestation and not the act of parturition. The mechanism is unknown. Minor (post translation) variants of HbA$_1$ occur, the most important being the glycosylated variant HbA$_{1c}$ which can be used as an indicator of diabetic control.

THALASSAEMIA SYNDROMES

These are inherited disorders in which the rates of synthesis of one or more globin chains are reduced, resulting in unbalanced globin chain production, ineffective erythropoiesis, haemolysis and variable anaemia.

Genetic Mechanisms

These have been extensively studied as the thalassaemias provide an excellent model for the understanding of gene regulation. The following investigative tools

have been employed:
1. DNA cleavage with a variety of bacterial restriction endonucleases.
2. Separation of DNA fragments by gel electrophoresis.
3. Identification of the DNA fragments containing the appropriate genes by using radioactive-labelled complementary DNA to hybridize with its complementary sequence. The cDNA probes are made from isolated mRNA (reticulocytes) using viral reverse transcriptases.
4. Isolated DNA fragments can be inserted into bacteriophages and then cloned in bacteria to provide large amounts of pure genes which can then be sequenced.

These techniques have shown that normal genes contain intervening sequences that do not code for protein. Initially the whole gene sequence is translated to form heterogeneous nuclear RNA (HnRNA), and the intervening sequences are then removed by enzymatic cleavage and splicing to give cytoplasmic mRNA. This is the template for protein synthesis (*Fig. 9.4*).

Fig. 9.4. Diagram of globin chain synthesis.

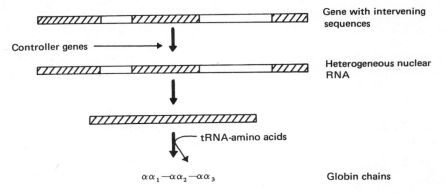

The defect in thalassaemia is in the DNA sequence, but this defect could be manifest at any of the stages of protein synthesis. Defects have been found at all levels except for the 'controller genes' which are not at present amenable to investigation, e.g.: (i) deleted globin genes account for most α-thalassaemias, and hereditary presence of fetal haemoglobin; (ii) partial β gene deletion preventing transcription to HnRNA occurs in some β^0-thalassaemias; (iii) abnormalities of cleavage or splicing sites in the intervening sequences account for some cases of $\beta^+ + \beta^0$-thalassaemia by preventing HnRNA processing to cytoplasmic mRNA; (iv) point mutations in the original structural gene may prevent transcription of the mRNA (e.g. by insertion of a stop sequence) and has been described in β^0-thalassaemia.

In the β^0-thalassaemias no β chains are produced. In the β^+-thalassaemias some β chains are present. All cases of β^+-thalassaemia so far investigated have correspondingly low levels of β mRNA.

The thalassaemias are complicated by the presence in some cases of Hb Constant Spring, a variation of the normal α globin. There is a mutation in the normal terminating codon of the chain so that the chain is elongated by an additional 31 amino acid residues. This structural variant is synthesized at low rates (i.e. thalassaemia). A single Hb Constant Spring gene causes very mild or silent thalassaemia with an abnormal band on starch gel electrophoresis at pH 8·5 (runs just behind HbA_2),

α-THALASSAEMIA SYNDROMES

Mainly due to α gene deletions, Hb Constant Spring genes, and their interactions. As more α genes are affected (4 in total) the thalassaemia increases in severity. α-thalassaemias are mainly found in the Orient, Africa and the Middle East.

Clinical Forms of α-Thalassaemia

Silent α-Thalassaemia. Mildest form which has no detectable evidence of the disorder except that at birth Hb Bart's (a tetramer of γ-chains–$γ_4$) is present to a concentration of 1–2 per cent (normal level less than 0·5 per cent). Subsequently, the red cells appear morphologically normal, but there may be a slight reduction in the MCV and MCH values. (This form is usually due to a 'single gene' disorder and is commonly referred to as a 'silent' thalassaemia.)

The α-Thalassaemic Trait. This trait is asymptomatic and is characterized by a concentration of about 5 per cent Hb Bart's at birth with subsequent red cell morphological abnormalities of hypochromia, target cell, poikilocytosis and the occasional inclusions. HbH ($β_4$) is unstable and easily denatured and is responsible for red cell inclusions (most easily demonstrated by cresyl blue supravital stain). The trait often involves 'two genes'.

Haemoglobin H disease is characterized by the presence of 5–20 per cent HbH and small amounts of Hb Bart's. The HbA_2 level is reduced. It is important that if iron deficiency exists it must be corrected before a definitive diagnosis can be made. Iron deficiency results in a reduction in haem synthesis hence there is no relative excess of β chains conjugated with haem forming HbH. The disease is associated with haemolysis (the $^{51}CrT_{\frac{1}{2}}$ varies from 5 to 20 days, but red cell survival findings may be spurious due to ^{51}Cr transfer from HbH to HbA molecules). Haemoglobin levels may be normal though levels around 9g/dl are common. Patients are especially susceptible to infection; the reason is unknown. Acute infections are often associated with a marked drop in the haemoglobin level. Low haemoglobin levels may be found during pregnancy. Haemoglobin H disease may be due to the involvement of 'three genes'.

Hb Bart's hydrops fetalis syndrome results from a total absence of α-chain synthesis, hence no HbA, HbA_2 or HbF is produced. About 80 per cent Hb Bart's, with small amounts of HbH and Hb Portland 1 $ζ_2γ_2$, is present. The syndrome is usually due to involvement of all α genes.

Hydrops fetalis associated with Hb Bart's is fatal and is associated with miscarriage of a non-viable fetus during late pregnancy. Toxaemia during pregnancy is commonly found. The haemoglobin level is usually 4–10 g/dl. Hb Bart's has a high oxygen affinity which contributes to tissue anoxia. The fetus is pale and oedematous, jaundice is mild or even absent, and the degree of liver enlargement is greater than splenic enlargement (cf. immune haemolysis hydrops fetalis). It has been postulated that hepatic sinusoidal erythropoiesis produces portal hypertension leading to reduced flow in the umbilical vein and placental oedema with consequent reduction of placental transfer of proteins and other nutriments.

Management

No treatment is required for the thalassaemia traits. Haemoglobin H disease management consists of:

1. The support of red cell production—folic acid supplements (5 mg p.o. daily) should be given continuously and are essential during pregnancy, as is a good protein diet.

2. Vigorous treatment of any cause of stress to erythropoiesis, such as infection.

3. Avoidance of iron overload. Erythropoietic hyperplasia may be associated with slightly increased iron absorption, but haemochromatosis does *not* occur (cf. β-thalassaemia). No oral iron supplements should be given unless deficiency has been proven biochemically.

4. If a patient also has G-6-PD deficiency or is a carrier of an unstable haemoglobin, drugs with an oxidant action must be avoided.

α-*Thalassaemia Associated with* β-*chain Variants*

1. Sickle-cell trait. The reduced availability of α chains leads to a lower percentage of HbS as α chains interact preferentially with β chains compared to β^s chains.

2. Sickle-cell disease. Individuals with concomitant homozygous HbS and α-thalassaemia have small and poorly haemoglobinized cells with a lower mean cell HbS. In Saudi Arabia, where α-thalassaemia is common, individuals with sickle-cell disease have a high HbF and this reduces the severity of the clinical condition.

3. HbC trait associated with an α thal trait has a lower concentration of HbC than without the 'interaction'.

4. HbE trait individuals usually have some 40 per cent HbE demonstrable; the double heterozygotes with an α thal trait have between 15 and 30 per cent HbE.

β-*THALASSAEMIA SYNDROMES*

Classification

These may be classified as:

1. True β-thalassaemias which may be β^0 or β^+ (*see* Genetic mechanisms, p. 77).

2. Other β-thalassaemias including the Hb Lepore syndromes, and hereditary persistence of fetal haemoglobin.

These are found mainly in the Mediterranean populations, the Middle East, India, Pakistan and S.E. Asia. They occur sporadically in all racial groups.

Clinical Forms of β-*Thalassaemia and Associated Laboratory Findings*

There is a spectrum in this disorder varying from mild impairment of β-chain synthesis to complete absence. Genetically, thalassaemia minor refers to the heterozygous state and thalassaemia major to the homozygous state. Clinically, thalassaemia minor and major have referred to the clinical severity, intermedia being used to indicate symptoms of intermediate severity and minima to indicate absence of clinical symptoms but a detectable laboratory anomaly.

β-Thalassaemia Minima. Mildest heterozygote. The so-called silent β-thalassaemia gene can only be detected by demonstrating diminished β globin chain synthesis. There are normal values for A_2 and HbF. The red cell indices may show a slight reduction in the MCV and MCH values. It is essential that iron deficiency be excluded before laboratory tests be undertaken, for iron deficiency may be associated with normal HbA_2 levels in thalassaemic trait; only when the iron deficiency is corrected will the raised HbA_2 occur.

β-Thalassaemia Minor. To divide this group of heterozygotes into $β^0$ and $β^+$ variants, family studies must be performed. The HbA_2 level is increased to 4–6 per cent (normal 1·5–3 per cent) and there is no, or only slight elevation of HbF (2–5 per cent). Usually there is no anaemia. Even if present, the haemoglobin level is only reduced by some 2 g/dl if the individual remains healthy, but with pregnancy, malnutrition or infections, haemoglobin levels can drop dramatically. It is always important not to overlook an associated disease if a previous asymptomatic thalassaemic presents with anaemia.

β-Thalassaemia Intermedia. This is a heterogeneous group of disorders including:
1. Homozygotes for mild $β^+$-thalassaemia.
2. Homozygotes for β-thalassaemia of the high fetal haemoglobin type.
3. Homozygotes for $δβ$-thalassaemia.
4. Heterozygotes for β and $δβ$-thalassaemia.
5. Carriers of two β-thalassaemic genes and an α-thalassaemic gene.

Often the diagnosis is not made until 4 or 5 years of age and then it is normally as a result of intercurrent infection precipitating transitory deterioration. Signs of anaemia, jaundice and splenomegaly with an appropriate ethnic origin suggest the diagnosis, which is confirmed by haematological examination. Growth is not retarded. In later life pigment gallstones, osteoporosis with a predisposition to renal calculi and haemochromatosis may occur. Pregnancy may occasionally be associated with marked anaemia, requiring transfusion. Ulceration of the legs, usually over the distal end of the tibiae, is a troublesome and common feature.

Thalassaemia Major. This is due to homozygous severe $β^+$-thalassaemia or $β^0$-thalassaemia. The amount of HbF does not correlate well with the severity of the anaemia. As the disorder affects the β-globin chain the newborn child is healthy. Symptoms associated with anaemia develop after the first 2 months of life: poor appetite, failure to thrive, genu valgum, proximal muscle weakness and delay in walking are common features. Physical retardation becomes more apparent with age though there is normal mental development. Without regular transfusions, death usually occurs during childhood; the few who survive into teenage are sexually underdeveloped. Expansion of the marrow cavity creates characteristic protuberance of facial bones producing 'mongoloid' facies, and often severe dental malocclusion. A high cardiac output associated with severe anaemia causes left ventricular hypertrophy. Dysrhythmias are common and congestive heart failure (of which haemosiderosis may be a contributory cause) frequently develops. Splenomegaly is usually sufficiently great to produce abdominal swelling. The degree of hepatomegaly is variable. Leg ulcers are common.

Radiology

The radiological findings are not specific for thalassaemia, but reflect an expanded marrow cavity. The skull shows thickening of the cranial bones due to expansion of the diploe. Fine spicules traverse the diploe giving a 'hair-on-end' appearance to the vault of the skull. Another site where marrow cavity expansion is especially manifest is the phalanges. Apart from other haemolytic anaemias, such as hereditary spherocytosis, similar radiological findings occur in congenital syphilis.

Peripheral Blood Appearances

The classic findings in all forms of β-thalassaemia are that the red cells are microcytic, the MCH is reduced, and the MCHC may be reduced. Target cells, poikilocytes, schistocytes, stippled cells, normal haemoglobinized cells, polychromasia, normoblasts (especially with the more severe forms of the disease) and even macrocytes may be present despite the overall marked microcytosis. If the patient has undergone splenectomy, the number of schistocytes is reduced but the other red cell abnormalities become more florid. Polychromasia reflects the number of reticulocytes which, when corrected for the degree of anaemia, are raised in thalassaemia intermedia but not in thalassaemia major.

Management

For accurate diagnosis and prognosis family studies may be required. Principles of management applicable to the management of HbH disease also apply to β-thalassaemia. Management of thalassaemia major requires additional consideration.
1. Blood transfusion. Previously transfusions were administered only for the symptomatic relief of severe anaemia but the quality of life was poor. Present transfusion regimes maintain a high haemoglobin level, suppress erythropoiesis and permit normal growth. However, desferrioxamine must be given to reduce transfusion siderosis producing cardiac complications and diabetes mellitus.
Desferrioxamine is administered by slow subcutaneous injection using an automatic syringe pump; the optimal dose (which varies from 0·5 to 2 g per day, given over 8 hours), being determined by measurement of iron balance.
The simultaneous administration of oral vitamin C to improve iron excretion is debatable as it also increases iron absorption.
2. Splenectomy is indicated if (a) there has been a progressive increase in the frequency of transfusion unassociated with any detectable, atypical antibody; (b) development of neutropenia or thrombocytopenia attributable to hypersplenism occurs. Following splenectomy there is an increased risk of infection, particularly pneumococcal. Prophylaxis with penicillin and polyvalent pneumococcal vaccine reduces the risk.

THALASSAEMIA SYNDROMES AFFECTING δ CHAINS

There is depression of δ as well as β chains, hence there is no increase of HbA_2 in the trait.

δβ-*Thalassaemia*

This results from a partial deletion of the $\delta + \beta$ genes. Heterozygotes have similar haematological findings to β-thalassaemia except that HbA_2 level is not raised and the HbF level varies from 5 to 15 per cent. Homozygotes have been reported to have only HbF.

Lepore Thalassaemia

The Lepore chain is a hybrid composed of part of a δ and part of a β chain—at least three variants of δ and β combinations have been recognized. The Lepore gene is responsible for absence of β chain synthesis and only a low production of $\delta\beta$ chains unable to match the number of α chains. Hence the Lepore trait is haematologically similar to β-thalassaemia trait except that 5–15 per cent of the Hb Lepore is present, the remainder being HbA and homozygous Lepore is associated with a thalassaemia major-like clinical condition except for the presence of 10–20 per cent of Hb Lepore and the remainder HbF.

Hereditary Persistence of Fetal Haemoglobin (HPFH)

This is a heterogeneous group of disorders. The Negro type of HPFH results from a major deletion involving the $\delta + \beta$ genes (larger than in $\delta\beta$-thalassaemia). The mechanism of continued γ chain expression is not known, but the defective $\delta + \beta$ chain synthesis is almost totally compensated for. The HbF is distributed evenly throughout the red cells in the Negro and Greek forms of HPFH, but is unevenly distributed in the Swiss type.

In the Negro type of HPFH the heterozygote has about 25 per cent of HbF and homozygote 100 per cent HbF. The Greek type has slightly lower levels of HbF.

Reactivation of HbF Synthesis in Adults

Reactivation of HbF occurs physiologically when there is a sudden increase in erythropoietic activity, such as in pregnancy, and after recovery from hypoplasia. The HbF level is usually at the upper limit of the accepted normal range.

Raised HbF (above 10 per cent) occurs in:

1. Juvenile chronic myeloid leukaemia, the level often increases with the duration of the disease.
2. Juvenile myelomonocytic leukaemia.
3. In some cases of adult acute leukaemia (lymphoid, myeloid and monocytic).
4. Chronic myeloid leukaemia.
5. Myelofibrosis.
6. Myeloma.
7. Acquired aplastic anaemia.
8. Paroxysmal nocturnal haemoglobinuria.

In most of these conditions there is an abnormal haemopoietic clone. Very rarely raised HbF levels have been reported in carcinoma of the bronchus, hepatoma, thyrotoxicosis and testicular tumours.

Haemoglobin S/β-Thalassaemia

Genetic Classification. The clinical effects of heterozygosity for HbS and β-thalassaemia are very variable depending upon whether the thalassaemia gene is $β^+$ or $β^0$. In HbS/$β^+$ up to 30 per cent HbA may be present, the remainder being HbS, apart from some 5 per cent HbF and 5 per cent HbA_2; in HbS/$β^0$ no HbA is detectable. Ethnically the HbS/$β^+$-thalassaemia is more common in Negroes and HbS/$β^0$-thalassaemia is more common in those of Southern European origin.

Clinical Forms and associated Laboratory Findings. In Negroes there may be only mild anaemia and little disability. Splenomegaly predisposes to splenic infarction and a few patients develop hypersplenism.

In Southern Mediterranean races, anaemia is often severe, growth retarded, sickle crises frequent, and death before puberty common.

Interaction between β-Thalassaemia and other β Chain Variants

With other β chain variants such as D, C and E, the majority of the haemoglobin found is that of the Hb variant whereas with the simple abnormal Hb trait, the majority of the haemoglobin is HbA. The ratio of abnormal haemoglobin to HbA is determined (as with HbS) by the type of thalassaemia gene. With $β^0$-thalassaemia heterozygotes, family studies may be required to determine the genetic status which may appear identical, both clinically and in the laboratory, with the homozygous form of the abnormal haemoglobin.

ANTENATAL DIAGNOSIS OF THALASSAEMIA

Pregnant women should be screened at the earliest opportunity for thalassaemia trait (low MCV and MCH). If thalassaemia is suspected, the husband should also be screened and haemoglobin electrophoresis of both future parents be performed.

If both parents are found to have thalassaemia trait antenatal diagnosis can be offered in the early part of the second trimester with a view to abortion if the fetus is found to have β-thalassaemia major. The diagnosis is made by globin chain synthesis studies of fetal blood obtained at fetoscopy in a specialist centre. The ethical problems must be discussed fully prior to fetoscopy.

Selected Further Reading

Nathan D. G. (1979) Progress in thalassaemia research. *Nature* **280**, 275.
Weatherall D. J. and Clegg J. B. (1981) *The Thalassaemic Syndromes*, 3rd ed. Oxford, Blackwell.

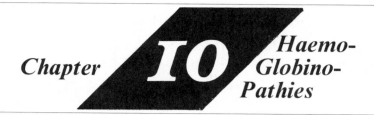

Chapter 10 Haemo-Globino-Pathies

A haemoglobinopathy is an inherited structural abnormality of the globin chains. Mutations in the gene sequence cause a variant amino acid to be substituted for the normal component in the amino acid sequence comprising that globin chain. Although only a single variant (e.g. HbS) occurs in most patients with haemoglobinopathies, occasionally two (e.g. HbC Harlem) or three variants occur. Additional amino acids (e.g. Hb Constant Spring) and hybrids of β and δ chains (Hb Lepore) have been considered in Chapter 9.

SICKLE-CELL DISORDERS

The normal glutamine amino acid at the sixth position of the β chain is replaced by valine in sickle haemoglobin. Deoxygenated HbS, in sufficient concentrations, aggregates into long fibrils presumably because the valine residues in the deoxy configuration can form polar contacts with adjacent molecules (*Fig. 10.1*). These fibrils distort the red cell to form the characteristic sickle cell. With oxygenation the process is initially reversible but eventually the cell membranes become damaged and 'irreversibly sickled cells' are formed which are then soon cleared from the circulation. The likelihood of sickling is increased by exposing the cells to excessive hypoxia and by acidosis. The presence of other haemoglobins such as HbA or HbF reduces the concentration of HbS and makes sickling less likely. The major problems caused by sickling are haemolysis and vascular occlusions by sickled cells. The homozygous condition (HbS/S) is referred to as sickle-cell anaemia, the heterozygous state (Hb A/S) is referred to as sickle-cell trait.

Sickle-cell Trait

Clinical Features. The trait is not associated with anaemia and is usually asymptomatic. The importance of diagnosis is to avoid anoxia, such as may occur with anaesthetics or flying in an unpressurized aircraft. Infections, especially respiratory, dehydration and other causes of sluggish venous and capillary circulation (where blood is deoxygenated) and acidosis can occasionally give rise to a sickling vaso-occlusive crisis (*see below*).

The beneficial effect of the sickle-cell trait in areas where *Plasmodium falciparum* infection is endemic appears to be restricted to young children. Probably infected red cells become preferentially sickled and are hence sequestered in the spleen and liver where reticulo-endothelial cells destroy the parasites.

Life expectancy is not reduced and many athletes, known to have the trait, compete successfully in strenuous sports.

Laboratory Investigations. The haemoglobin level, the red cell indices and the peripheral film examination are normal. The screening test (described in Chapter

Fig. 10.1. Diagrammatic representation of sickle fibril formation.

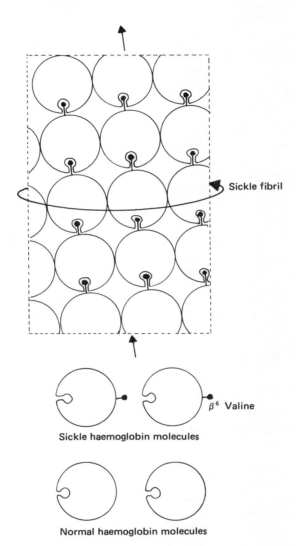

Sickle fibril

β^6 Valine

Sickle haemoglobin molecules

Normal haemoglobin molecules

28) is positive. Electrophoresis demonstrates the presence of HbS usually in concentrations between 35 and 50 per cent (*see Fig. 9.3*, p. 76). Concomitant iron deficiency may reduce the relative concentration of the HbS.

Sickle-cell Disease

Clinical Features
Onset. The symptoms usually develop during the second 6 months of life as haemoglobin F protects against sickling during intrauterine life and the neonatal period. As more β^s chains are synthesized so the concentration of HbS rises until adult levels are present by the sixth month.

Some patients present in later childhood and occasionally the first crisis does not occur until adulthood.

Anaemia may be due to:

1. So-called aplastic crises, which are associated with a rapid drop in the haemoglobin level; because of the short red cell survival the effect of relative hypoplasia becomes manifest rapidly. Infections, especially viral, cause such marrow depression. Recovery associated with a marked reticulocytosis occurs after about 1 week.

2. Acute splenic sequestration crisis which occurs in young children is a major cause of death in the young.

3. Haemolytic crises; these are rare and in many cases have been demonstrated to be due to G-6-PD deficiency in which haemolysis has been precipitated by drugs.

4. Folate deficiency frequently occurs in children and pregnant women.

Vaso-occlusive crises are characterized by pain. In children splenic infarcts are common with left hypochondrial pain often associated with referred pain to the left shoulder. Frequent infarctions lead to splenic fibrosis and atrophy (auto-splenectomy), thus splenic infarction is rare in adults. Pain of infarction commonly occurs in the bones of the limbs, back and abdomen, chest and near joints. Infarction of bone may be followed by periosteal reaction which may be difficult to separate from osteomyelitis during the initial days of a crisis. Infection (commonly malaria in tropical countries and chest infections in temperate climate) often precipitate vaso-occlusive crisis. The infarction pain, which varies from mild rheumatic type pain to agonizing pain requiring powerful analgesics, is accompanied by constitutional symptoms which vary greatly in severity: fever, anorexia, prostration and sometimes mental symptoms such as somnolence and temporary psychotic behaviour occur.

Dactylitis due to medullary infarction may be a presenting symptom in infancy, with a painful swelling of the dorsum of the hands and feet (the 'hand-foot' syndrome).

Aseptic femoral head necrosis is a common complication producing marked disability; less common is necrosis of the humeral head.

Osteomyelitis is a common complication, especially due to infection with salmonellae. It may prove to be very difficult to differentiate between infarction and osteomyelitis; rigors, positive blood cultures and evidence of suppuration substantiate the diagnosis.

Ankle ulceration is a distressing and chronic complication which may also occur with other congenital haemolytic anaemias such as thalassaemia. The aetiology appears to be a combination of hypoxia and poor circulation.

Cholelithiasis occurs with increasing frequency with age; about 50 per cent of the patients in late middle age have gallstones, though less than 10 per cent of the patients develop symptoms.

Retinopathy visual impairment may occur due to arteriolar occlusion, arterio-venous anastomoses and vascular proliferation. The latter is described as 'sea-fan' appearance which may be complicated by vitreous haemorrhage or retinal detachment.

Genito-urinary system. Haematuria is a common manifestation due to ischaemia papillary necrosis, but it is essential that other potential causes are investigated. Many patients are unable to produce a concentrated urine due to an acquired tubular reabsorption defect. Priapism is usually due to massive sickling in the corpora cavernosa.

Lung complications. Acute 'pulmonary episodes' are the most common complication of sickle disease. The aetiology is due to pulmonary vascular occlusion from in-situ sickling and microemboli or infection. It is probable that often the cause is multifactorial. The lower lobes are most commonly affected. Chronic pulmonary insufficiency and pulmonary hypertension may be a late complication of recurrent 'pulmonary episodes'.

Laboratory Investigations. A normochromic, normocytic anaemia with a haemoglobin of 8–11 g/dl is present. The peripheral film shows evidence of abnormal erythropoiesis, anisocytosis, poikilocytosis and 'sickle cells'. Older children and adults may have findings in the peripheral film which reflect autosplenectomy, with target cells, Howell–Jolly bodies and ovalocytes.

The sickle screening test is positive and haemoglobin electrophoresis shows HbS, no HbA, but a varying amount of HbF (*see Fig. 9.3*, p. 76).

Intrauterine diagnosis of the homozygous state can be made by aspiration of a fetal blood sample under fetoscopic control and termination of such cases may be considered in some centres.

Radiological Findings. Skeletal radiographs show rarefaction with a broad diploic zone in the skull and with thickening of the frontal and parietal bones. In infants the long bones show evidence of marrow hyperplasia with increased diameter, decreased medullary density (ground-glass appearance) and often increased coarse patterning of the cortex. These changes are often conspicuous in the metacarpals. Bone sclerosis due to infarction occurs, associated with periosteal reaction and sometimes narrowing of the medullary cavity.

Prevention of Crisis
  1. Avoid dehydration.
  2. Avoid cold.
  3. Avoid hypoxia.
  4. Treat infections early.
  5. Avoid acidosis.
  6. Avoid hypotension.
  7. Hypertransfusion can be given to suppress the bone marrow; within 2 weeks 70 per cent of the circulating haemoglobin will be transfused HbA. Such regimes are often used prior to major surgery, and in the management of major complications.
  8. In acute surgical emergencies exchange transfusion or hyperbaric oxygen can be used to reduce sickling.

Treatment of Sickle Crisis
  1. Hydration is essential.
  2. The patient must be kept warm to improve the circulation.
  3. If the patient is acidotic i.v. bicarbonate is indicated.
  4. Suspected infections must be treated.
  5. Non-narcotic analgesics should be given freely.
  6. Blood transfusion is of help in the management of patients:
      a. requiring surgical procedures;
      b. in severe crisis;
      c. with priapism;
      d. with severe anaemia.
Anti-sickling agents such as urea, potassium cyanate and piracetam have proved to be either not suitable or ineffective in vivo. Recently it has been suggested that

fresh frozen plasma may ameliorate crisis possibly by alteration of prostacyclin metabolism. Crises nearly always symptomatically resolve within about 5 days.
Management of Pregnancy. Transfusion should be given to maintain the haemoglobin above 7 g/dl. Oral folic acid supplements are essential. Avoid prolonged labour and, if there is delay in the second stage, forceps delivery or Caesarean section is indicated. Anoxia, cooling, acidosis and dehydration must be avoided. Sickle crisis during the puerperium are common and initial presentation of symptoms may occur with sickle traits at this time.

Other Sickling Disorders

Sickle Disorders with Hereditary Persistence of Fetal Haemoglobin (S/HPFH). In the HbS/HPFH double heterozygote virtually no normal β chains are synthesized but the high levels of HbF reduce the risks of sickling.
Clinical Features. The disorder is relatively mild; crisis occurring in about 25 per cent of the patients. The spleen is palpable in about 40 per cent.
Laboratory Investigations. The haemoglobin level is normal. The approximate levels of the different haemoglobins are HbS 80 per cent, HbF 20 per cent, HbA nil, HbA_2 level variable (may be normal or reduced). The peripheral film shows poikilocytosis, hypochromia and target cells. The ^{51}Cr red cell survival is normal.
Sickle/α-Thalassaemia. The inheritance of α-thalassaemia genes mitigates against the severity of sickle-cell disease.

Reduced α chain synthesis leads to lower intracorpuscular levels of HbS. This genetic combination is particularly common in Saudi Arabia.
Sickle/β-Thalassaemia
Definition. The disorder is the double heterozygous state for sickle and β-thalassaemia genes. If the thalassaemia gene is β^0 the condition is more severe than the β^+ gene.
Clinical Features
Mediterranean type, usually a severe disorder with marked anaemia, retarded growth and frequently death in childhood. The *hand-foot* syndrome is a common manifestation and infarcts are common.
Negro type—most Negroes have a milder form of the disorder, some with little disability and mild anaemia. Splenomegaly occurs in about 60 per cent. Those with HbA present have the milder disorder; those patients with no haemoglobin A may have symptoms similar to sickle disease, though usually of less severity.
Laboratory Investigations. Peripheral blood films show target cells, stippling and polychromasia. Electrophoresis reveals HbS 60–90 per cent, HbF 10–30 per cent, HbA 0–30 per cent.
Treatment. Generally management is similar to sickle disease. Splenectomy should be performed if isotope studies demonstrate hypersplenism.
Sickle Haemoglobin C
Definition. Inheritance of the β^s gene from one parent and the β^c gene from the other results in the red cells containing approximately 50 per cent HbS and 50 per cent HbC.
Clinical Features. There is a great variation in the incidence and severity of the symptoms. The symptoms usually occur less frequently and are less severe than in sickle disease except:
   1. Ocular complications, especially retinal thrombosis and detachment.
   2. Aseptic femoral head necrosis, which is often bilateral.

3. Acute 'pulmonary episodes'.
4. Haematuria.
There is splenomegaly in about 60 per cent of patients.
Laboratory Investigations. Anaemia is mild to moderate (Hb above 8 g/dl).
The peripheral film shows target cells with occasional pointed and folded cells, the 'paper hat' appearance.

HAEMOGLOBIN C TRAIT AND DISEASE

In some parts of West Africa, especially North Ghana, up to 20 per cent of the population have this abnormal haemoglobin. The trait is without symptoms and the haemoglobin level is normal; there is no evidence of haemolysis and no splenomegaly. The homozygous haemoglobin C disease may be asymptomatic, but occasionally is associated with fleeting abdominal pain, and splenomegaly is common and may be massive. Ocular lesions occur frequently. Mild anaemia is common; cholelithiasis may occur.
Laboratory Investigations. In the trait, electrophoresis demonstrates 50 per cent HbA and 50 per cent HbC. The peripheral film may show the occasional target cell, but may be normal.
In the disease, electrophoresis demonstrates only HbC. The haemoglobin level is usually between 8 and 12 g/dl, the red cells being normochromic or macrocytic; occasionally microcytosis and hypochromia occur. Whatever the indices there are very numerous target cells and the osmotic fragility is reduced. The reticulocyte count is usually 4–6 per cent. The ^{51}Cr $T_{\frac{1}{2}}$ is often reduced to 8–10 days.

HAEMOGLOBIN D TRAIT AND DISEASE

Definition. HbD migrates, at pH 8·6, at the same rate as HbS but is of normal solubility. It can be separated from HbS by starch-gel electrophoresis at pH 6·2. There are several variants, the most common variant being HbD Punjab.
Clinical Features. Although most common in persons from North-West India the abnormality may be found in English, Portuguese and French patients. The heterozygotes are asymptomatic, the homozygotes have a mild anaemia.

HAEMOGLOBIN E TRAIT AND DISEASE

Definition. HbE is due to replacement of glutamine by lysine in position 26 of the β-chain.
Clinical Features. Most common in persons from South-East Asia. The trait is symptomless; the disease is associated with a mild haemolytic anaemia.
Laboratory Investigations. Electrophoresis of haemoglobin reveals 30–45 per cent HbE in the trait and mainly HbE in the disease (*see Fig. 9.3*, p. 76). The peripheral film shows microcytosis, some polychromasia and some target cells.

HAEMOGLOBIN M

Definition. Inherited as an autosomal condition producing cyanosis due to methaemoglobinaemia.

Aetiology. A haem moiety is carried in a pocket of each α and β chain. The 'proximal' histidine holds the haem securely to the α and β chain and the 'distal' histidine protects the ferrous iron from oxidation. Amino-acid substitutions of the four histidine sites occur producing haemoglobin M.

Clinical Features. Cyanosis is present from birth in α chain variants, whereas cyanosis develops between 6 and 9 months in the β chain varieties. The β chain abnormalities may be associated with mild anaemia and jaundice. Sulphonamide therapy may exacerbate the anaemia. The course is benign and uneventful but the diagnosis is important to prevent subsequent unnecessary investigations.

Laboratory Investigations. In an α chain disorder the haemoglobin level usually is normal. A compensatory erythrocytosis does not usually occur as the oxygen affinity is reduced. In the β chain disorder the oxygen affinity is often high but because of mild haemolysis, erythrocytosis is rare. Methaemoglobin may be seen on a starch gel and quantified by difference spectroscopy. HbM is identified by specific absorption spectra (*see* Chapter 28).

Differential Diagnosis

Congenital methaemoglobinaemia, which is inherited as an autosomal recessive, is due to NADH-reductase deficiency and is diagnosed by enzyme assay on a haemolysate. Treatment is not required, but cosmetically the condition can be managed by 500 mg ascorbic acid daily. NADPH-reductase deficiency is not associated with cyanosis.

Toxic methaemoglobinaemia may be due to:

1. Compounds such as marking ink or coloured crayons.
2. Nitrobenzene present in furniture and shoe polish.
3. Nitrates—especially likely in high concentrations in reservoir and well water after droughts.
4. Drugs such as sulphonamides and trinitrin.

The clinical history reveals the recent onset of cyanosis.

Cyanotic heart disease is associated with cardiac anomalies and clubbing. Arterial Po_2 is low.

UNSTABLE HAEMOGLOBINS

Definition. The unstable haemoglobins can arise from amino-acid substitutions at many sites. The precipitation of the unstable haemoglobin occurs with subsequent conversion to methaemoglobin. The unstable haemoglobins include Zurich, Köln, Leiden, Shepherd's Bush and Chesapeake.

Clinical Features. There is usually a mild compensated haemolytic state; episodes of anaemia follow infection or ingestion of oxidative drugs. With severe variants (e.g. Hb Hammersmith) there is a chronic haemolytic anaemia and cyanosis, due to methaemoglobin.

Diagnosis. Large Heinz bodies may be seen in the peripheral blood, especially after splenectomy. Heinz bodies are generated in vitro by incubation with brilliant cresyl blue. Reticulocytosis reflects the haemolytic state. Unstable haemoglobins are demonstrated by heat or isopropanol precipitation (*see* Chapter 28). Approximately half the haemoglobins may be demonstrated by electrophoresis. Many of the haemoglobins have an altered oxygen affinity.

Treatment
1. Avoid oxidative drugs.
2. Treat infections early.
3. Consider splenectomy for severe haemolysis.
4. Blood transfusion is occasionally necessary.

HIGH AFFINITY HAEMOGLOBINS

This is a group of autosomal dominant disorders associated with a left shift of the oxygen dissociation curve, due to a relative increase in the oxyhaemoglobin stability (*Fig. 10.2*). The various mutations occur in the α or β chains and usually affect either one of the sites of interaction of the four chains (e.g. Hb Chesapeake), the 2,3-DPG binding site (e.g. Hb Rahere), or the haem pocket (e.g. Hb Heathrow).

Fig. 10.2. Haemoglobin oxygen affinity curves.

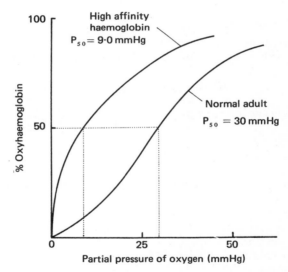

Clinical Features. If the high affinity haemoglobin is stable, polycythaemia occurs; apart from a ruddy complexion the patient is asymptomatic and the diagnosis often an incidental finding. Many high affinity haemoglobins are unstable (especially haem pocket mutations), hence the haemoglobin level is not raised.
Treatment. Treatment for hyperviscosity is rarely required.

Selected Further Reading

Huehns E. R., Hardistry R. M. and Weatherall D. J. (1982) The structure and function of haemoglobin: clinical disorder due to abnormal haemoglobin structure. In: *Blood and its Disorders*, 2nd ed. Oxford, Blackwell Scientific Publications.
Lehmann H. and Huntsman R. G. (1974) *Man's Haemoglobins*. Amsterdam, North-Holland.
Weatherall D. J. (ed.) (1974) Abnormal haemoglobins. *Clin. Haematol.* **3**, 2.

Chapter II

Acquired Haemolytic Anaemias

AUTOIMMUNE HAEMOLYTIC ANAEMIA

This may be classified as:
1. Warm antibody type
    1.1 Idiopathic
    1.2 Secondary
2. Cold antibody type
    2.1 Cold haemagglutinin disease
    2.2 Paroxysmal cold haemoglobinuria
3. Associated with drugs
4. Complicating blood transfusion
5. Immune haemolytic disease of the newborn

Warm Antibody Type

Haemolysis occurs due to auto-antibodies, against the patient's own red cells, most active at 37 °C. The antibody, which is usually IgG, causes coated erythrocytes to be destroyed by the reticulo-endothelial system. Complement activation with intravascular haemolysis is unusual.

Aetiology
1. Idiopathic: more common in females and usually after the age of 40 years. Less common than idiopathic cold antibodies.
2. Secondary type may occur with:
    a. Neoplasms, especially chronic lymphocytic leukaemia, lymphocytic lymphomas and Hodgkin's disease.
    b. Autoimmune disorders such as systemic lupus erythematosus, rheumatoid arthritis, chronic active hepatitis, ulcerative colitis and myasthenia gravis.
    c. Drugs, methyldopa, L-dopa, mefenamic acid.
    Infections, viral or bacterial, may precede the disorder in children and young adults.

Clinical Features. In adults the onset is usually insidious and the course chronic. Sometimes a haemolytic anaemia will antedate manifestations of an underlying disorder by months or even years. Jaundice, mild to moderate in severity, occurs in about 75 per cent of patients; slight to moderate splenomegaly is usual; if marked, pathology of the underlying disorder is a probable contributory factor. Persistent purpura due to associated thrombocytopenia suggests a serious prognosis.

In children and young adults a 'secondary' form of the disorder may have a sudden onset often following a viral infection; it may sometimes occur during pregnancy. The anaemia and jaundice may be accompanied by fever, headache, abdominal and back pains. Oliguria and rarely renal failure occurs. Recovery usually occurs within a few weeks although occasionally the disorder may become chronic.

Laboratory Findings. Anaemia is usually slightly macrocytic, due to the reticulocytosis (usually between 5 and 30 per cent); if secondary folate deficiency exists the macrocytosis is greater. Occasionally normoblasts may be present in the peripheral blood. Spherocytosis often occurs, the degree being correlated with the severity of the anaemia. The osmotic fragility is increased, but the enhancement obtained by incubation is less than with hereditary spherocytosis. The direct antiglobulin test (DAT) is positive. Freshly collected blood may show mild spontaneous agglutination though this is not as marked as when cold agglutinins are present. The white cell count is usually normal in chronic cases, in acute cases there is usually a neutrophilia with a 'left shift'. Thrombocytopenia is rare (Evan's syndrome). The sedimentation rate is markedly raised.

The auto-antibodies are usually IgG, but occasionally IgM or IgA. Some antibodies bind complement but if of Rhesus specificity the IgG antibodies are not complement binding. Sometimes there is a polyclonal excess of globulins but in 50 per cent of patients immunoglobulin deficiency occurs. IgA deficiency is the most common but IgG and IgM levels may be reduced. Very occasionally all immunoglobulin levels are reduced.

Isotope studies demonstrate red cell sequestration in the spleen and to a lesser extent in the liver.

Diagnosis. The findings of a positive DAT with an antibody most active at 37 °C establishes the diagnosis. It is essential to determine whether the disorder is primary or secondary.

Prognosis. In the primary disorder there is no correlation with age of onset, initial severity of the disease, or response to therapy. Spontaneous remissions are common. If the primary disorder is chronic the disorder may last for many years. Despite a normal haemoglobin and reticulocyte count, if the DAT remains positive, the prognosis must be guarded.

If the haemolysis is secondary the prognosis is chiefly related to that of the underlying disorder.

Treatment. In children with the acute form of the disorder recovery may be spontaneous without therapy. The basis of treatment is:

1. Support with blood transfusion, if necessary.
2. Induction of remission with corticosteroids (prednisone, 1 mg/kg). Steroids are tailed off gradually according to the response.
3. Splenectomy if there is no or poor response to corticosteroids.
4. Immunosuppressive therapy, initially with azathioprine (1–2 mg/kg), is indicated if there has been failure of response to corticosteroids and splenectomy, or to corticosteroids alone if splenectomy is contraindicated.
5. Supplement with folic acid.
6. Treatment of underlying disorder if haemolysis is secondary.
7. In infants under 1 year, resistant cases may respond to thymectomy.

Cold Antibody Type

Cold Haemagglutinin Disease (CHAD)
Pathogenesis. Exposure to cold results in agglutination of red cells by an

agglutinating antibody reacting at low temperature (under 30 °C); these are usually IgM antibodies. The red cell agglutinates have increased mechanical fragility.

Aetiology

1. Idiopathic
2. Secondary to:

> 2.1 Neoplasms, particularly lymphocytic lymphoma, chronic lymphocytic leukaemia.
>
> 2.2 Systemic lupus erythematosus.
>
> 2.3 Infections, especially *Mycoplasma pneumoniae*, but also in infectious mononucleosis and some viral infections.

Clinical Features. Idiopathic CHAD usually occurs after 50 years; the sexes are equally affected. The anaemia has an insidious onset and is chronic. The secondary disorders have similar clinical features.

Depending on the thermal amplitude of the auto-antibody two types of manifestations occur:

a. Acute intravascular haemolytic episodes which occur in the cold weather; the haemoglobin level remains within the normal range between attacks.

b. Mild, well compensated haemolytic anaemia. The haemoglobin level falls with exposure to cold, but acute haemolysis does not occur. Exposure to cold is accompanied by cyanosis and Raynaud's phenomenon due to red cell agglutinates.

Postinfectious cold haemolysis is manifested by an acute onset of haemolysis; the sudden fall in haemoglobin is accompanied by jaundice and haemoglobinuria. The haemolysis usually occurs 2–3 weeks after the onset of the illness and subsides within several weeks.

Laboratory Investigations. Even following acute haemolytic episodes the haemoglobin level rarely falls below 7 g/dl. Red cell aggregates are apparent on the blood film (only avoided if blood taken with a warm syringe, kept at 37 °C in EDTA, and smears made on warmed slides). There is polychromasia, spherocytosis and an occasional normoblast may be present. The white cell and platelet counts are usually normal, though with the acute infectious type neutrophilia and occasionally thrombocytopenia may occur.

The bilirubin level reflects the degree of haemolysis. Methaemoglobinaemia and haemoglobinaemia occur with acute episodes. Haemosiderin is frequently found in the urine; haemoglobinuria occurs with acute attacks.

The antibody responsible for CHAD is most commonly anti-I, most active at 4 °C and inactive at 37 °C; the thermal amplitude varies. Anti-I is found after infectious mononucleosis and with some lymphomas. The titre at 4 °C in the idiopathic variety or secondary to neoplasms or autoimmune disorders is high (up to 1 in 1 000 000); that secondary to infection is seldom higher than 1 in 4000. The postinfectious CHAD is due to polyclonal IgM (κ and λ chains), the other forms are due to monoclonal IgM. The direct antiglobulin test is positive and complement (C3d) is demonstrable on the cell surface. In many cases only complement can be demonstrated on the red cells.

Treatment. If the disease is primary and the haemolysis mild and chronic no specific therapy is necessary. During exacerbations cold must be avoided, and environmental temperatures above 25 °C are optimal. Bed rest may be required. If transfusion is given, washed cells are used to avoid administration of complement which exacerbates haemolysis. The blood should be pre-warmed. In severe chronic disease chlorambucil or cyclophosphamide may help. Steroids and splenectomy are seldom beneficial. If the disease is secondary to malignancy or autoimmune disease management of the primary disorder is indicated.

Acute disease secondary to viral infection is often only of 2–3 weeks' duration; no specific therapy other than keeping the patient warm is usually required, though for very severe haemolysis plasmaphoresis may be required.

Paroxysmal Cold Haemoglobinuria

Pathogenesis. A very rare disorder. There is acute intravascular haemolysis precipitated by exposure to cold. The antibody is IgG, usually IgG_3 and is specific for the P blood group system. The haemolysins become fixed to red cells in the cold, the red cells lyse in the presence of complement at $37\,^{\circ}C$.

Aetiology. The condition may be idiopathic or secondary to viral infections (measles, mumps, influenza) or syphilis.

Clinical Features. The degree of 'chilling' necessary to precipitate an attack is variable; an ice-cold drink or immersion of hands in cold water may be sufficient. Rigors, headache, backache and abdominal pain develop after an interval of minutes or hours; urticaria may occur. Haemoglobin in the urine may occur for many hours. Splenic enlargement may occur during an attack.

Diagnosis. The Donath–Landsteiner test for the detection of the bithermal haemolysin is positive (*see* Chapter 28). The direct antiglobulin test is positive only during an acute episode.

Management. Avoidance of exposure to 'chilling'.

Autoimmune Haemolytic Anaemia associated with Drugs

Pathogenesis. This may be classified as:

Type 1: drugs acting as haptens absorbed on the red cell surface, e.g. penicillin and cephalothin.

Type 2: immune-complex absorbed on to the red cell surface (innocent bystanders). The red cells become lysed by this passive absorption of drug-IgM-complex.

Type 3: antibodies to existing red cell antigens especially Rhesus. It has been suggested that suppressor T cells are inhibited (possibly due to a rise in cyclic AMP produced by methyldopa) and uninhibited B cells produce IgG antibodies. Suppression of macrophage activity (also produced by methyldopa) reduces the likelihood of haemolytic anaemia despite antibody-coated red cells.

Clinical Features

a. Drugs absorbed on to the red cell surface. Penicillin requires to be given in very large doses (10 million units/day for over a week). IgM antibodies to penicillin form readily but paradoxically do not cause haemolysis; only with very large doses do IgG antibodies develop which react with penicillin which has become integrated into the red cell membranes. Haemolytic anaemia with cephalothin is rare, but may occur with modest dosage.

b. Immune-complex mediated haemolytic anaemia has been reported with a large number of drugs including quinidine, sulphonamides, some antituberculous drugs and chlorpromazine. The patient becomes sensitized, usually due to previous administration of the drug, then after taking only a small quantity of the drug acute intravascular haemolysis occurs often associated with haemoglobinuria. Renal failure may occur.

c. Drug-induced autoimmune haemolytic anaemia is a well-known complication of methyldopa. Some 20 per cent of patients taking the drug develop a positive direct antiglobulin test, but less than 1 per cent develop haemolytic anaemia. The larger the dose and the greater the duration of medication the higher the incidence of autoimmune antibody production. Mefenamic acid, L-dopa and chlordiazepoxide may also cause this type of haemolysis.

Laboratory Investigations. Acquired haemolytic anaemia occurring during drug ingestion requires testing with:

a. Anti-IgG and anti-C3 sera by the direct antiglobulin test.

b. Testing by the indirect antiglobulin test against normal cells.

c. An eluate prepared from the patient's cells; if it does *not* react with normal cells, this suggests drug-induced haemolysis of type 1 or type 2. Penicillin and cephalothin-induced antibodies do not react with normal cells unless pretreated with the causative drug. Most antibodies due to methyldopa, L-dopa and mefenamic acid are of Rh specificity and will not react with Rh^{null} cells.

It should be remembered that drugs also cause haemolysis in association with red cell enzyme defects (Chapter 8) and unstable haemoglobins (Chapter 10).

Prognosis. Haemolysis ceases within a few days of stopping the drug if haemolysis is due to absorption of drug onto red cell membranes or immune complex medicated. With methyldopa type haemolysis the haemoglobin level ceases to fall within 2 weeks, but the direct antiglobulin test may remain positive for up to 2 years.

Immune Haemolysis complicating Blood Transfusion

See Chapter 27.

Immune Haemolytic Disease of Newborn (HDN)

Pathogenesis. Serious disease is due to anti-D in 90 per cent of patients; other antibodies include anti-c, anti-E, anti-Kell, anti-Duffy, and indeed all blood group antibodies which occur as IgG. Immune anti-A and anti-B (although common) are rare cases of HDN. Of the British population 85 per cent are Rhesus D positive, and this is higher in India and South-East Asia. Of UK marriages 13 per cent are between a D-negative woman and a D-positive male, and 3 in 4 of their children will be D positive. Few mothers are sensitized during the pregnancy until delivery so that only second and subsequent Rhesus-positive children are affected. Not all mothers become sensitized and there is less risk in group O mothers with group A and to a lesser extent group B children. This is presumably due to rapid clearance of the child's red cells from the maternal circulation by naturally-occurring antibodies. Rhesus sensitization can also be caused by Rhesus-positive blood transfusions and other blood products.

Antenatal Diagnosis

Maternal history. History of previous pregnancies, especially if an affected infant was born and blood transfusion is essential.

Maternal serum testing, using a panel of cells which contain antigens involved in HDN, may demonstrate antibodies by the indirect globulin test or by the use of enzyme-treated red cells. There is not a close correlation between antibody titre and the severity of HDN, perhaps because antibody avidity and titre may differ. A rising titre is of serious import. A titre of greater than 1:16 by the direct antiglobulin test at 18 weeks is an indication to perform amniocentesis.

Phenotype testing of the maternal and paternal red cells using specific grouping sera. Knowing the ethnic origin, the probable genotype of the parents can be derived; thus the probability of an affected infant may be determined.

Amniocentesis is performed at 22 weeks or later (depending on past obstetric history and maternal antibody titres). Absorption level of bilirubin is measured at 450 nm.

Fetal blood sampling obtained under fetoscopy from the umbilical cord is occasionally performed so as to determine the fetal phenotype.

Assessment of Severity of HDN at Birth

Cord haemoglobin concentration with levels below 10 g/dl occur in severe cases. However, levels above 15 g/dl do not exclude the possibility of kernicterus.

Cord bilirubin level does not reflect the severity of HDN so closely as the haemoglobin concentration. However, levels above 70 µmol/l (4 mg/100 ml) indicate the need for exchange transfusion.

Cord normoblast count has not proved a useful guide to management.

Treatment

Intrauterine transfusion. In severely affected cases there is a high mortality with births before 34 weeks. Transfusion into the peritoneal cavity of washed red cells (tested for compatibility with the mother's serum) improves the fetal prognosis. Direct transfusion into the umbilical vein under fetoscope control is also possible.

Maternal plasmapheresis requires to be carried out twice a week or more if to be of benefit.

Exchange transfusion, if performed soon after delivery, will remove sensitized cells; reduction of the slightly raised bilirubin level is only of slight value. Subsequent exchange transfusions are performed to keep the bilirubin level well below 270 µmol/l (16 mg/100 ml), above which kernicterus may occur.

Phototherapy by exposure of the neonate to artificial 'day-light spectrum' illumination augments the degradation of bilirubin.

Albumin infusions may be required to treat severe hypoproteinaemia; if extreme, hydrops fetalis occurs. Bilirubin is bound to albumin, thus the risk of kernicterus is reduced.

ACQUIRED NON-IMMUNE HAEMOLYTIC ANAEMIA

This may be classified as:
1. Acquired red cell membrane defects
   - 1.1 Paroxysmal nocturnal haemoglobinuria
   - 1.2 Liver disease
   - 1.3 Vitamin E deficiency
2. Trauma to red cells
   - 2.1 Cardiac prostheses
   - 2.2 March haemoglobinuria
   - 2.3 Burns
3. Microangiopathic haemolytic anaemias
   - 3.1 Haemolytic uraemic syndrome
   - 3.2 Thrombotic thrombocytopenic purpura
   - 3.3 Disseminated intravascular coagulation and others

4. Toxic causes

        4.1 Drugs and chemicals
        4.2 Venoms
        4.3 Infections

5. Hypersplenism

Acquired Red Cell Membrane Defects

Paroxysmal Nocturnal Haemoglobinuria (PNH)

Pathogenesis. There is an abnormal clone of haemopoietic stem cells which produce abnormal red cells, leucocytes and platelets and a predisposition to aplasia. The red cell membranes are abnormally sensitive to complement at reduced pH, this complement activation being by the alternative pathway. The abnormality is associated with low erythrocyte cholinesterase activity, and pitting of the red cell membrane demonstrable on electron microscopy. The defect is more severe in young cells.

Clinical Features. A rare disorder commoner in women. Several clinical entities are recognized.

    1. Classic PNH. There is insidious onset of anaemia; haemoglobinura is present at onset in 25 per cent of the patients. Haemoglobinura is related to sleep (not time of day); stress may also precipitate haemolysis. Jaundice is usually mild. Accompanying symptoms (probably due to venous thromboses) include fever, headache, abdominal and low back pain, which usually lasts about 3 days. Infections, especially of the urinary tract, may occur and haemorrhagic phenomena due to thrombocytopenia are not uncommon. Hepatosplenomegaly is frequent. Gross signs of venous thrombosis are common (*see below*).

    2. Chronic haemolysis without haemoglobinura is a frequent mode of presentation. Iron deficiency develops due to urinary haemosiderin loss. Occasionally the diagnosis is made when iron therapy precipitates haemoglobinuria. Chronic haemolysis may decline or even disappear after many years.

    3. Aplastic anaemia may follow the classic presentation of PNH, or the disorder presents in 12 per cent of patients with marrow aplasia and the PNH red cell defect becomes apparent later.

    4. Thromboses. Venous thromboses are more common than arterial. They often occur in atypical sites. Abdominal pain may be very severe. Hepatic vein thrombosis may cause portal hypertension and hepatic failure. Thromboses have been attributed to intravascular red cell lysis with red cell stroma lipid initiating coagulation, stromal occlusion of small vessels, increased activity of coagulation factors and abnormalities of platelets rendering them very sensitive to the lytic action of complement.

Diagnosis. There is usually anaemia, reticulocytosis, anisocytosis and poikilocytosis. The MCV is usually only slightly decreased and may even be raised, despite the frequent iron deficiency. There may be neutropenia and thrombocytopenia. The NAP score is low unless there is concomitant aplastic anaemia. A positive Ham's test is diagnostic (Chapter 28); the sucrose lysis test is more sensitive, but less specific. Haemosiderinuria is frequently demonstrable even if there is no haemoglobinuria.

Prognosis. This disorder is very chronic and the median survival is 10 years from diagnosis, though many patients live much longer and there are occasional reports of recovery. Death is usually due to venous thrombosis, infection or haemorrhage; occasionally acute leukaemia or myelofibrosis develops.

Treatment. There is no specific therapy. Support therapy includes oral iron supplements and transfusions with washed cells. Iron administration may pre-cipitate acute haemolysis, probably due to the outpouring of the reticulocytes. Androgens are occasionally beneficial for hypoplasia and steroids sometimes reduce the degree of haemolysis. Splenectomy carries a high mortality.

Liver Disease. There is a slightly decreased red cell survival in hepatitis and cirrhosis. In cirrhotic patients an acute excess of alcohol can result in acute haemolysis with abdominal pain and jaundice. There is hyperlipidaemia which may be responsible for the haemolysis by causing alteration of the erythrocyte membrane lipids. This self-limiting condition is known as Zieve's syndrome.

Vitamin E Deficiency. May cause haemolysis in premature infants of 4–8 weeks of age. It is due to deficient artificial milk formulae.

Traumatization of Red Cells

Cardiac Prostheses

Aetiology. The haemolysis of normal red cells in an abnormal environment occurs most commonly with prosthetic aortic valves. Haemolysis may be due to regurgitation around a valve with a fault in placement, regurgitation through the valve, or if the ball becomes swollen due to uptake of lipids and does not ride freely. Haemolysis is more common if both mitral and aortic valve prostheses have been inserted. Patch repair of the endothelial cushion is frequently followed by haemolysis.

Clinical Features. Symptoms are related to the degree of anaemia; often there is a well-compensated haemolytic state. Increased cardiac output with anaemia in-duces a 'vicious circle'.

Laboratory Investigations. The anaemia is associated with a reticulocytosis; schistocytes, microspherocytes and polychromasia are found in the peripheral film. Findings of iron deficiency develop if there is loss of iron due to haemoglobinuria and haemosiderinuria. The haptoglobin level is low. The platelet count may be low due to increased destruction; there is, however, no evidence of disseminated intravascular coagulation (DIC), clotting investigations being normal. Bacterial endocarditis may complicate the disorder and increase the anaemia due to marrow depression. Autoimmune haemolytic anaemia must be excluded.

March Haemoglobinuria

Aetiology. Red cells rupture in the vessels of the soles of the feet of a few, otherwise healthy, individuals. 'Heaviness of stride', inadequate cushioning of feet by footwear on hard surfaces and local increase of temperature have been considered contributory.

Clinical Features. Nausea, abdominal cramps and a burning sensation in the soles of the feet associated with haemoglobinuria following running or other strenuous exercise, such as squash.

Prevention. Patients are advised to wear softer, thicker, resilient insoles.

Burns. Haemolysis may occur due to direct destruction of red cells by heat or by the production of spherocytes with destruction during the subsequent 24 hours.

Microangiopathic Haemolytic Anaemia

This term refers to intravascular haemolysis and fragmentation of the red cells due to disease in small vessels.

Haemolytic Uraemic Syndrome (HUS)

Aetiology. The exact mechanism is uncertain. Damage of renal capillaries due to immune complexes following infection, and disseminated intravascular coagulation with subsequent further renal vascular damage may be responsible for the haemolysis, thrombocytopenia and renal failure in some cases. Various abnormalities of endothelial prostacyclin production have also been demonstrated in both HUS and thrombotic thrombocytopenic purpura. In many patients there is a deficiency of a plasma factor which normally stimulates release of prostacyclin from endothelial cells; this may account for the beneficial effect of fresh frozen plasma. In some cases there are inhibitors of prostacyclin release, and in others the half life of the prostacyclin may be reduced. HUS and thrombotic thrombocytopenic purpura may represent a spectrum of the same disorder.

Clinical Features. Most common between 6 months and 3 years and are rare after 8 years. The classic triad of purpura, haemolytic anaemia and renal failure is frequently preceded by respiratory distress and diarrhoea.

Laboratory Investigations. The anaemia is accompanied by characteristic red cell morphological changes—schistocytes, helmet cells and microcytes. Leucocytosis is common. Thrombocytopenia is usual and fibrin degradation products are increased but only in severe cases is there disseminated intravascular coagulation. The blood urea and creatinine are raised and there is haematuria and proteinuria.

Treatment. This should be directed primarily at the renal failure; early dialysis improves the prognosis. Heparin, steroids, inhibitors of platelet function, fresh frozen plasma and fibrinolytic therapy have all been used, but with only moderate benefit. Mortality is about 30 per cent and is due to renal failure.

Thrombotic Thrombocytopenic Purpura (Moschcowitz's Syndrome)

Aetiology. Unknown, but may be due to autoimmune damage to the arteriolar endothelium which is associated with deposition of hyaline PAS-positive material and fibrin strands within the vessel lumen causing red cell fragmentation and platelet aggregates which occlude the vessels. Abnormalities of endothelial prostacyclin production, possibly due to prostacyclin-stimulating factor deficiency, have recently been postulated. The syndrome may be associated with SLE, rheumatoid arthritis, polyarteritis nodosa and Sjögren's syndrome.

Clinical Features. Incidence, females : males, 3 : 2. Most common before 40 years. The acute fulminant form may be fatal within a few weeks, the chronic form may persist for a few years. Purpura, neurological manifestations (especially paraesthesia and alterations in consciousness), anaemia, abdominal pain and cardiac arrhythmias are most frequent findings. There may be enlargement of the liver and spleen.

Laboratory Findings. The peripheral blood findings are similar to those found in the haemolytic uraemic syndrome; thrombocytopenia is always present. Changes in prostacyclin metabolism have been discussed under HUS. Secondary forms also have the laboratory findings of the primary condition.

Treatment. Steroids (which may be required to be given in high dosage up to 1 g/day of methyl prednisolone) and splenectomy may induce remission. Plasmapheresis may be life-saving as may fresh frozen plasma infusion. Fresh plasma may provide prostacyclin stimulating factor. Heparin, aspirin and dipyridamole and dextran infusions have all been advocated.

Other Types of Microangiopathic Haemolytic Anaemia. In addition to the HUS and thrombotic thrombocytopenia purpura, DIC (*see* Chapter 22), malignant hypertension and eclampsia (associated with arteriolar fibrinoid necrosis as well as DIC) and haemangiomas may be associated with microangiopathic haemolytic anaemia.

Toxic Causes of Haemolytic Anaemia

Drugs and Chemicals. The long list of potential haemolytic substances include water (entering the circulation due to trauma during bladder irrigation and via the lungs in drowning), hyperbaric 100 per cent oxygen (astronauts), copper (haemodialysis using copper tubes), lead (from ingestion of lead paint, especially by children, petrol fumes, lead water pipes and industrial use in printing and battery manufacture). Lead poisoning is associated with basophilic stippling of red cells and sideroblastic marrow changes. Quantitation of urinary levels is essential for diagnosis and monitoring at-risk patients.

Venoms. Spider bites, snake bites (especially cobras) and occasionally insect stings (including bees) may be associated with severe haemolysis.

Infections. Malaria and bartonella are characterized classically by severe haemolysis. Many other infections may be complicated by haemolysis.

Hypersplenism

See Chapter 16.

Chapter 12
The Anaemia of Chronic Disorders

The anaemia of chronic disease is usually mild or moderate and is characterized by:

1. Poor iron utilization, probably due to a failure to release iron from the reticulo-endothelial system to circulating transferrin, the levels of which are also reduced. This disturbance of iron metabolism occurs in most infective or inflammatory injuries.

2. Slightly decreased red cell survival due to extracorpuscular factors rather than an intrinsic red cell defect. The mechanism is not known.

3. Relative erythroid hypoplasia which is apparently due to resistance to erythropoietin and occasionally due to failure of erythropoietin production or release.

In addition to these general features of chronic disease, other factors may contribute to the anaemia depending on the cause of the chronic disease. Some of these factors are considered under the appropriate headings below.

INVESTIGATIONS

The anaemia is most often normocytic and normochromic but may be microcytic and hypochromic.

There is a low serum iron, a low total iron binding capacity, a raised serum ferritin level and increased tissue iron stores.

Bone marrow examination shows normal or reduced erythroid precursors unless there is concomitant severe haemolysis or blood loss in which case there may be erythroid hyperplasia.

The leucocyte count is frequently raised in chronic disease and this is reflected in myeloid hyperplasia in the bone marrow. Specific features of the chronic disease may be apparent in the blood and/or marrow, e.g. malarial parasites, malignant cells (*see* Chapter 3).

SPECIFIC CAUSES OF CHRONIC DISEASE

Infections

1. Infections commonly associated with marked marrow depression include chest infections (especially tuberculosis, chronic suppurative lesions and fungal

infections), brucellosis, subacute bacterial endocarditis, osteomyelitis, pelvic infections, chronic skin lesions (especially discharging sinuses) and chronic renal infection.

2. Infections causing frank haemolysis include malaria, kala-azar, trypanosomiasis and infections around prosthetic heart valves (producing increased turbulence). Acute autoimmune haemolytic anaemia may occur in infectious mononucleosis, infective hepatitis and *Mycoplasma pneumoniae*.

3. Blood loss associated with infection occurs with hookworm infestation (each worm is estimated to extract 0·2 ml daily) and *Schistosoma haematobium*.

If chronic infection coexists with a 'deficiency' type of anaemia (e.g. iron, vitamin B_{12} or folate deficiency) the response to replacement therapy is suboptimal.

Malignancy (Fig. 12.1)

Anaemia may be due to:

1. Nutritional deficiencies due to anorexia, dysphagia, vomiting, diarrhoea or impaired absorption. The requirement for folate is markedly increased especially in lymphomas.

2. Infection; common with carcinoma of bronchus, bladder, skin and uterus.

3. Renal impairment; due to obstruction of ureters in retroperitoneal or pelvic malignancy, disseminated intravascular haemolysis associated with localized or generalized carcinoma or acute leukaemia (especially promyelocytic) or infiltration of renal tissue as may occur with the lymphomas.

4. Marrow infiltration with metastases. Common primary sites are lung, kidney, thyroid, breast, prostate, stomach and skin (melanoma).

5. Sideroblastic erythropoiesis; most common with haematological malignancies.

6. Severe marrow hypoplasia may be due to heavy tumour load, radiotherapy or cytotoxic therapy.

7. Blood loss; common with carcinoma of gastrointestinal tract, carcinoma of cervix or uterus, tumours of the renal tract.

8. Haemolytic anaemia

> 8.1 Autoimmune type occurs most commonly in chronic lymphocytic leukaemia, malignant lymphomas and ovarian tumours.
>
> 8.2 Microangiopathic type especially liable to occur with mucus-secreting tumours such as adenocarcinoma of the breast and adenocarcinoma of the stomach.
>
> 8.3 Hypersplenism in some malignant lymphomas.
>
> 8.4 Increased activity of the reticulo-endothelial system— erythrophagocytosis has been noted around tumour nodules and also in histiocytic medullary reticulosis.

9. Relative anaemia due to increased plasma volume. This may be due to the large vascular volume of some tumours, an enlarged spleen involved by lymphoma, an altered threshold for vasopressin release, or inappropriate antidiuretic hormone (ADH) secretion by some tumours, especially carcinoma of the bronchus.

Peripheral Blood. The findings will depend on specific aspects of the disease. The anaemia is typically normochromic and normocytic though may be hypochromic

Fig. 12.1. Mechanisms
of anaemia in malign-
ant disease.

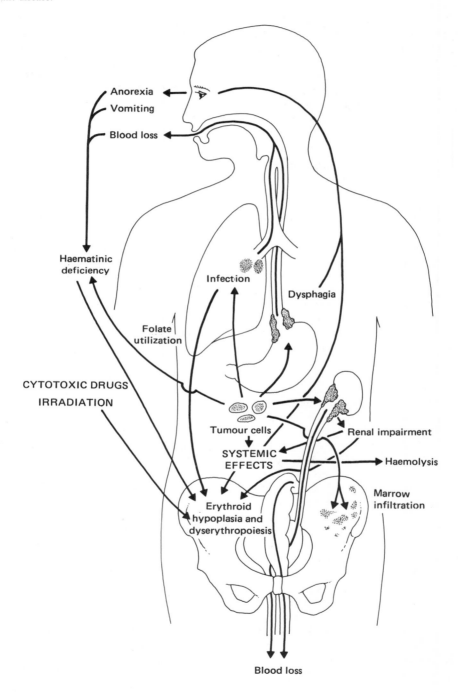

and microcytic. A leuco-erythroblastic blood picture with immature white cells and nucleated red cells in the blood reflects marrow infiltration.

Bone Marrow. The marrow findings will depend upon the principal causes of anaemia associated with the malignancy. Secondary deposits are most frequently demonstrated if a biopsy rather than an aspirate is performed. Sites of bone tenderness are most likely to be involved.

Renal Disease

Factors responsible for anaemia include:
1. Decreased erythropoiesis due to:
    1.1 Reduced erythropoietin levels.
    1.2 Metabolic causes related to retained metabolites. The Hb level falls by approximately 2 g/dl for every 8 mmol rise in urea from 8 mmol/l to 40 mmol/l though the raised urea is not directly responsible. The acidosis causes a right shift in the oxygen dissociation curve, thus minimizing tissue hypoxia. Phosphate retention leads to increased 2,3-DPG levels, also shifting the oxygen dissociation curve to the right.
    1.3 Infection in chronic pyelonephritis and renal tuberculosis.
    1.4 Systemic disorders associated with renal disease such as polyarteritis nodosa, systemic lupus erythematosus and amyloid disease.
2. A shortened red cell survival may be demonstrated by ^{51}Cr labelling in many patients with chronic renal failure. Haemolysis may be pronounced when renal failure is severe and in the microangiopathic haemolytic syndrome.
3. Blood loss. Haematuria may be due to tumours; urinary tract obstructions and calculi; infections such as *Schistosoma haematobium*; and renal parenchymal lesions, including polycystic kidneys and active glomerulonephritis.

Hepatic Disease

The anaemia associated with liver disease may be due to:
1. The primary liver disease itself may produce an anaemia due to decreased production and reduced red cell survival related to impairment of liver function, but there is little correlation with the severity of the hepatic disease. Treatment must be directed at improving hepatic function.
2. Complications of liver disease:
    2.1 Hypersplenism; the anaemia is due to: (i) splenic sequestration of red cells; (ii) reduced cell survival; (iii) expanded plasma volume producing a 'relative' anaemia.
    2.2 Blood loss due to: (i) portal hypertension with oesophageal varices, haemorrhoids and an increased tendency to peptic ulceration; (ii) impaired coagulation due to low levels of vitamin K-dependent Factors II, VII, IX and X, low levels of Factors V and XIII (though low XIII levels are a rare cause of bleeding), disordered synthesis of fibrinogen which fails to polymerize effectively, and disseminated intravascular coagulation which occurs particularly in cirrhosis and

chronic hepatic failure. Thrombocytopenia frequently occurs due to portal hypertension with hypersplenism; qualitative platelet defects also have been reported.

2.3 Haemolysis (i) slight reduction of red cell survival contributes to anaemia in many cases with liver disease; (ii) acanthocytosis may occur and be associated with marked haemolysis; (iii) a positive direct antiglobulin test may occur in chronic active hepatitis; (iv) Zieve's syndrome is the triad of acute haemolysis, hyperlipidaemia, and hepatitis following excessive alcohol intake; alcoholic cirrhosis usually pre-exists.

Peripheral Blood Findings. Liver disease itself causes a moderate anaemia which is often macrocytic. Severe anaemia suggests a complication of the liver disease. Target cells are common, and a mild reticulocytosis may be present. In the absence of hypersplenism or haematinic deficiency the leucocyte count is usually normal though the platelet count is often reduced.

Bone Marrow Findings. The findings may be modified by complications of liver disease. However, the usual findings are slightly increased cellularity due to erythroid hyperplasia. Erythropoiesis is often macronormoblastic. Myelopoiesis is normal; some increase of plasma cells is common. Megakaryocytes may be reduced.

Pancreatic Disease

Chronic pancreatic disease with diminished exocrine function may be associated with malabsorption of vitamin B_{12} without gastric atrophy or ileal disease (*see* Chapter 5). In the Zollinger–Ellison syndrome the lower pH reduces vitamin B_{12} absorption in the ileum.

Adrenal Disease

Addison's disease is associated with a mild to moderate anaemia, normochromic and normocytic in type, due to decreased erythropoiesis. A reduction in plasma volume is common, which masks the anaemia. Treatment may be accompanied initially by a fall in the haemoglobin level due to correction of the plasma volume.

An associated high incidence of antibodies to parietal cells and intrinsic factor exists, so pernicious anaemia may complicate the findings. There is also a high incidence of antibodies to thyroglobulin and thyroid microsomes.

Thyroid Disease

Thyroid hormone affects erythropoietin production due to its metabolic action affecting tissue oxygen consumption. There is probably also a direct metabolic effect on erythropoiesis.

Anaemia occurs occasionally in severe hyperthyroidism. Mild anaemia is common in myxoedema; macrocytosis occurs but is not common unless there is concomitant vitamin B_{12} or folate deficiency. Iron deficiency due to menorrhagia is very common.

Pituitary Hypofunction

Hypopituitarism is characterized by a moderate anaemia (about 10g/dl). It is usually normochromic and normocytic though microcytic and macrocytic types may occur. The anaemia is due to hypofunction of end-organs; it is corrected by replacement therapy.

Rheumatoid Arthritis

The anaemia is normochromic and normocytic or microcytic and hypochromic in type. The anaemia may be multifactorial.

1. The degree of the anaemia is related to activity of the disease as is often reflected by the height of the ESR. There is poor iron utilization in active phases of the disease.

2. The anaemia may be partly due to shortening of the red cell survival, if hypersplenism exists (Still's disease and Felty's syndrome).

3. Blood loss due to ingestion of aspirin and other anti-inflammatory analgesic drugs may contribute to the anaemia.

4. Megaloblastic anaemia may occur and is more commonly due to folic acid deficiency than vitamin B_{12} deficiency; folate deficiency may be due to: (i) nutritional deficiency; (ii) poor folate absorption; (iii) increased demands to cellular proliferation related to the disease; (iv) reduction of folate released from effete red cells.

Systemic Lupus Erythematosus

The commonest form of anaemia is mild to moderate normochromic and normocytic, though the haemoglobin level is lower with coexisting renal disease or ercurrent infection. The direct antiglobulin test is positive in about 15 per cent of patients and autoimmune haemolytic anaemia occurs in about 10 per cent of patients. The anaemia is usually controlled by steroid therapy; initially prednisolone is given in a dose of 60–80 mg per day then gradually reduced after a few weeks.

Polyarteritis Nodosa

Anaemia may result from:

1. Associated renal failure.

2. Intestinal involvement causing blood loss.

3. Increased reticulo-endothelial system avidity for iron (as occurs in rheumatoid arthritis).

4. Haemolytic anaemia.

Cranial Arteritis

There is frequently a mild normochromic and normocytic anaemia which responds to steroid therapy.

Polymyositis and Dermatomyositis

Anaemia, normochromic and normocytic in type, is especially common if there is an underlying malignant neoplasm.

Selected Further Reading

Israëls M. C. G. and Delamore I. W. (ed.) (1972) Haematological aspects of systemic disease. *Clin. Haematol.* **1**, 3.

Chapter **13** Disorders of Granulocytes and Monocytes

PRODUCTION OF GRANULOCYTES AND MONOCYTES

Neutrophils and monocytes arise from a common progenitor cell (CFU-GM). Various regulatory mechanisms have been postulated based on in vitro culture studies (*Fig. 13.1*). CFU-GM divide and differentiate into monocytes and neutrophils under the influence of colony stimulating factors (CSF); local marrow CSF levels are more important than serum levels. Monocytes produce CSF giving a positive feedback loop; stimulated lymphocytes also produce CSF. At high monocyte levels, however, prostaglandin E is produced and this inhibits CFU-GM proliferation and overrides the CSF effect. High neutrophil levels give rise to factors that inhibit CSF production; lactoferrin is possibly one of these factors. Other serum factors increase CSF production and these rise at times of infection. Eosinophils and probably basophils are derived from the same multipotent myeloid stem cell (*see Fig. 3.1*, p. 17) but their proliferation is controlled by separate factors.

Newly-formed granulocytes remain in the marrow for several days and then enter the circulation either to circulate in the blood or to adhere to the vessel walls (marginated pool). These two populations are in dynamic equilibrium. After only 6–7 hours granulocytes leave the circulation and pass into the tissues. Monocytes also enter the tissues to become macrophages, which probably still have proliferative potential.

Fig. 13.1. Possible control mechanisms of granulopoiesis.

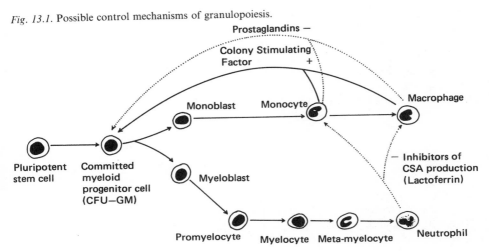

FUNCTION OF NEUTROPHILS

Neutrophils are principally involved in the elimination of micro-organisms (*Fig. 13.2*). The neutrophils generally do not recognize the microbes themselves but depend on them being coated with specialized proteins for which there are receptors on the neutrophil membrane (opsonization). The major opsonins are C3b and IgG. The killing of the ingested micro-organisms is a complex process.

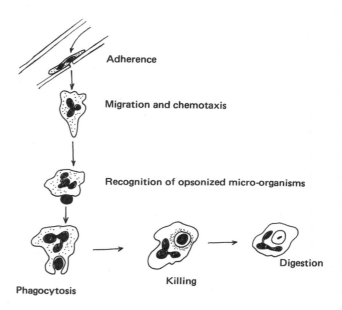

Fig. 13.2. Diagrammatic representation of neutrophil function.

Adherence

Migration and chemotaxis

Recognition of opsonized micro-organisms

Phagocytosis

Killing

Digestion

The neutrophil granules are discharged into the phagocytic vacuoles and the cell undergoes a respiratory burst with the production of superoxide and hydroxyl radicals. The oxidative burst causes the pH within the phagocytic vacuoles to rise to 7·8–8·0 and at this pH the cationic proteins from the azurophil granules are actively microbicidal. Dead micro-organisms are digested and degraded materials are excreted into the surrounding medium. Lactoferrin, vitamin B_{12} binding protein and lysozyme are also secreted.

FUNCTION OF EOSINOPHILS

Eosinophils phagocytose particles, degranulate and kill micro-organisms; they are particularly effective in killing parasites. They may also modulate hypersensitivity reactions by release of prostaglandins, histaminase, arylsulphatase, phospholipase, eosinophil basic protein and eosinophil plasminogen.

FUNCTION OF BASOPHILS AND MAST CELLS

The basophils and mast cells are secretory cells involved in the pathogenesis of immediate hypersensitivity reactions and allergic states. These cells release histamine when IgE becomes fixed to their surface leading to increased vascular permeability and smooth muscle contraction.

MONOCYTE/MACROPHAGE FUNCTION

Monocytes are phagocytic cells, and are also involved in the immune function of both T and B lymphocytes (*see* Chapter 16).

QUANTITATIVE ABNORMALITIES OF GRANULOCYTES

The causes of neutrophilia, neutropenia, eosinophilia, eosinopenia and basophilia are enumerated in Chapter 2.

Cyclical Neutropenia

Cyclical neutropenia is a congenital disorder of unknown mechanism that is often familial (autosomal dominant). There is cyclical neutropenia lasting 3 or 4 days every 3–7 weeks. If severe, the neutrophil count may fall to less than $0.2 \times 10^9/l$ and there is often oral and skin infection with fever which settles rapidly when the neutrophil count rises. Mild lymphadenopathy and splenomegaly may occur. Many cases are mild and do not produce significant clinical problems. The disorder is at the stem cell level and also affects erythroid and platelet precursors; the peripheral red cell and platelet counts do not fall significantly because of their longer life spans. Serial bone marrow examinations show a fall in granulocytic precursors before the onset of neutropenia. There is frequently a compensatory monocytosis and eosinophilia.

Periodontal disease may be severe but the disease is hardly ever fatal. The disease tends to improve after 10 years of age. Steroids may increase the neutrophil count but their role in treatment is unproven.

ABNORMALITIES OF NEUTROPHIL FUNCTION

Movement

1. Intrinsic Neutrophil Defects. Decreased motility and chemotaxis is seen in neonates, in chronic renal failure, diabetes, malnutrition and some adults prone to gingivitis, dermatitis and respiratory tract infections. A congenital disorder associated with defective chemotaxis and random migration has been described—the 'lazy leucocyte' syndrome.

2. Inhibitors of Neutrophil Motility and Deficiencies of Chemotactic Factors. These have been demonstrated in immune complex disease, graft versus host disease, Hodgkin's disease, other tumours and with steroid therapy.

Recognition

Abnormalities of recognition are usually due to deficiency of opsonins such as immunoglobulins, C_3b and C_2 rather than neutrophil receptor deficiency.

Phagocytosis

Decreased phagocytic capacity is seen in severe malnutrition and vitamin E deficiency.

Degranulation

Chédiak–Higashi Syndrome. This is an autosomal recessive disorder with oculocutaneous albinism, frequent pyogenic infections, a bleeding tendency and often progressive neurological impairment. In some cases an accelerated phase develops with lymphoid and histiocytic infiltration of the lymphoreticular organs and bone marrow causing pancytopenia and death. The primary defect is probably in the function of the microtubules such that phagocytic activity is poor. Giant secondary lysosomes are seen in the neutrophils, monocytes, fibroblasts and some other cells. Platelets fail to release storage ADP when stimulated. Some cases may be helped by ascorbic acid.

Killing

Chronic Granulomatous Disease. This disorder may be X-linked (most common) or autosomal recessive. It presents in infancy with chronic and recurrent infections of the skin, lungs, bone and other viscera; both abscesses and granuloma form. The infections are with gram-positive and gram-negative organisms which normally possess catalase activity. The primary abnormality is deficient or non-functioning neutrophil cytochrome b which is an integral part of the neutrophil oxidase system. The metabolic burst associated with phagocytosis does not occur, there is no superoxide/hydroxyl radical production, no reduction of nitroblue tetrazolium, no rise in phagocytic vacuole pH and no bacterial killing. There is no specific therapy.

Myeloperoxidase Deficiency. Myeloperoxidase is involved in the production of hydrogen peroxide and superoxide and deficiency can increase the risks of bacterial infection. Many cases are asymptomatic.

Others. Decreased killing has also been documented in G-6-PD deficiency, severe iron deficiency and after irradiation.

ASSESSMENT OF NEUTROPHIL FUNCTION

Batteries of tests are available to study most aspects of neutrophil function but only specialized laboratories can offer these tests. Recurrent severe or chronic infections, especially with unusual organisms, are an indication for detailed studies but the more common hypogammaglobulinaemia should first be excluded. Clearly defined neutrophil defects are rarely found. Abnormalities in systemic diseases such as renal failure or diabetes are common but the precise nature of the abnormality is difficult to define. The laboratory tests do not correlate with prognosis in individual patients.

QUANTITATIVE ABNORMALITIES OF MONOCYTES

The causes of peripheral blood monocytosis and monocytopenia are described in Chapter 2.

Increase of Tissue Monocytes (Macrophages or Histiocytes)

This may be classified as:
1. Reactive hyperplasia associated with:

    1.1 Conditions producing peripheral blood monocytosis (Chapter 2).

    1.2 Direct response to tissue infection by: (i) certain bacteria (tuberculosis, leprosy, brucellosis); (ii) fungi; (iii) parasites.

    1.3 Increased cell destruction, especially in the spleen, with some haemolytic anaemias and immune thrombocytopenias and, in the lungs, in pulmonary haemosiderosis.

    1.4 Response to certain chemicals in tissues, such as silica, carbon and beryllium.

    1.5 Granulomatous diseases, sarcoid and Wegener's granulomatosis.

    1.6 Lipid and other storage disorders (*see* Chapter 3).

    1.7 Sea-blue histiocytes.

    1.8 Iron overload—haemochromatosis.

2. Malignant proliferation of histiocytes occurs in:

    2.1 True histiocytic lymphoma (*see* Chapter 16).

    2.2 Possibly Hodgkin's disease.

    2.3 Histiocytic medullary reticulosis.

    2.4 'Histiocytosis X' spectrum.

An attempt to integrate a spectrum of disease, varying in severity and unknown aetiology, under the title 'histiocytosis X' may not be justified. The disorders are unifocal eosinophilic granuloma, multifocal eosinophilic granuloma or Hand–Schüller–Christian disease, and massive histiocytic infiltration of tissues and bone, the Letterer–Siwe syndrome.

Unifocal eosinophilic granuloma occurs most commonly in children and is more frequent in males. Bone lesions present with pain, occasionally as a pathological fracture. Treatment by curettage or radiotherapy is usually curative. Extra-osseous sites include lung and gastrointestinal tract; the symptoms may be severe and mimic other organic lesions.

Multifocal eosinophilic granuloma usually presents before 5 years, males being more frequently affected. About 25 per cent develop the triad of bone lesions, exophthalmos and diabetes insipidus; hepatosplenomegaly may also occur. Skin and mucous membrane lesions similar to those of Letterer–Siwe syndrome may occur. Focal lesions are treated by curettage or radiotherapy. Systemic therapy includes cytotoxic drugs and steroids, but induction of a permanent remission is very rare.

Letterer–Siwe syndrome occurs in infants and is characterized by marked hepatosplenomegaly, lymphadenopathy, localized bone lesions, a papular scaling rash, a normochromic, normocytic anaemia and sometimes thrombocytopenia. Weight loss is marked and fever common. Diagnosis may be made by splenic aspiration demonstrating non-lipid-containing histiocytes. Treatment with cytotoxic drugs, steroids and antibodies may result in partial remission. Similar responses have been reported after treatment with crude thymic extract. Severe cases before 2 years of age usually die within a few months, but children over 3 years with mild symptoms may survive for many years.

Reduction of Macrophages

This occurs following irradiation and in aplastic anaemia.

ABNORMALITIES OF MONOCYTE/MACROPHAGE FUNCTION

1. Chronic granulomatous disease.
2. With malignant histiocytosis.
3. With steroid therapy.
4. Sometimes in tuberculosis, leprosy and moniliasis. Whether this is a primary or secondary abnormality is uncertain.

Osteopetrosis (Albers–Schönberg's Disease)

This is a rare inherited disorder characterized by abnormally dense bone. The inheritance may be autosomal dominant or autosomal recessive; the latter form is more severe. The major complications are obliteration of the bone marrow cavity with leuco-erythroblastic anaemia, cranial nerve palsies, including blindness and deafness, and a propensity to develop fractures.

The precise aetiology is unknown but bone resorption is reduced and the disorder may be a defect of the osteoclast. In some patients monocyte function is abnormal and the osteoclast and macrophage may be closely related. Some cases have been successfully treated by bone marrow transplantation and the establishment of donor osteoclasts in the host has been demonstrated.

Selected Further Reading

Metcalf D. (1977) *In Vitro Cloning of Normal and Leukaemic Cells.* Berlin, Springer-Verlag.
Webster A. D. B. (ed.) (1982) Phagocytic and bacteriocidal defects in neutrophils. In: *Clinics in Immunology and Allergy,* Vol. 1. London, Saunders.

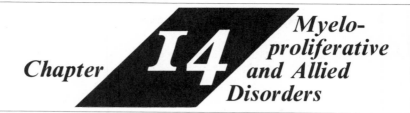

Chapter 14

Myelo-proliferative and Allied Disorders

The myeloproliferative diseases are a spectrum of neoplastic disorders in which there is proliferation of the myeloid stem cell or its derivatives (*see Fig. 3.1,* p. 17). This grouping of diseases recognizes that the proliferations of the myeloid series are not usually restricted to one cell line and that transitions and different combinations of cellular proliferations occur in individual patients. Precise diagnoses can be difficult. Furthermore, it is apparent that some myeloproliferative disorders occur at the level of the multipotent stem cell (e.g. chronic granulocytic leukaemia) and that lymphocytes are also involved in the neoplastic proliferation.

The myeloproliferative disorders are subdivided according to the predominant cell type present in the blood and/or marrow (*Table 14.1*).

Table 14.1. The myeloproliferative disorders

Predominant cell series involved	Predominant cell type	Disease entity
Granulocytic	Myeloblasts	Acute myeloid leukaemia
	Neutrophils	Chronic granulocytic leukaemia
Erythroid	Erythroblasts	Erythroleukaemia
	Red cells	Polycythaemia rubra vera
Megakaryocytes	Platelets	Primary thrombocythaemia
	Megakaryoblasts	Acute megakaryoblastic leukaemia / Acute myelofibrosis
Fibroblasts*	Fibroblasts in marrow	Myelofibrosis / Agnogenic myeloid metaplasia

*Fibrosis is reactive, not a primary neoplastic proliferation.

ACUTE MYELOID LEUKAEMIA

See Chapter 15.

ACUTE ERYTHROID LEUKAEMIA

See Chapter 7.

CHRONIC GRANULOCYTIC LEUKAEMIA (CGL OR CML)

Pathogenesis

At least 85 per cent of cases are associated with a consistent chromosome abnormality in the malignant clone. The Philadelphia chromosome is present in the granulocytic, erythroid and megakaryocytic lines and possibly some of the lymphoid cells. It is a defect of the long arm of chromosome 22 with a translocation of it, in most cases to chromosome 9 (9p + 22q—*see* Chapter 28). No normal myeloid cell clones can usually be demonstrated.

Incidence

Approximately 20 per cent of all leukaemias.

Clinical Features

Usually occurs in the over 30-year-olds; M : F equal. There is gradual onset of anorexia, weight loss and symptoms of anaemia. Splenomegaly is almost in-variable, usually 1–8 cm. Spleen pain often due to splenic infarction may be present. Usually the 'chronic phase' lasts 18 months—4 years before transition to an accelerated phase or 'blastic' crisis, which is usually either intractable anaemia with predominant myelofibrosis or an acute leukaemia.

Blood Picture

The haemoglobin is often normal at diagnosis, but tends to fall in relation to increasing leucocyte count. The leucocyte count is almost invariably elevated, usually with a significant left shift, i.e. many circulating promyelocytes, myelocytes and metamyelocytes. Up to 5–10 per cent of the leucocytes may be myeloblasts at diagnosis. Eosinophils and basophils are frequently increased. The neutrophil alkaline phosphatase (NAP) score is usually low during the chronic phase. Platelets are usually normal or may even be elevated at diagnosis.

The following have been described as poor prognostic indicators at diagnosis, though this has not been confirmed in all studies: thrombocytopenia, more than 5 per cent basophils, more than 10 per cent blast cells, second chromosome abnormality in addition to Ph[1], very large spleen.

Signs of transition to accelerated phase include:
1. Increasing unexplained anaemia.
2. Unexplained fever.
3. Sudden rise in basophils.
4. Significant increase in numbers of blasts.
5. Emergence of bone pain.
6. Extramedullary deposits of disease.
7. Lack of response of leucocyte count to chemotherapy.
8. Sudden increase in spleen size.
9. Emergence of further chromosome abnormality.

Bone Marrow

Very hypercellular with massive myeloid hyperplasia—often $M:E$ ratio $50:1$ (normal $2\cdot5:1$ to $10:1$).

Differential Diagnosis of CGL

Idiopathic Myelofibrosis. CGL has a greater left shift, low NAP (high in myelofibrosis) and the presence of Ph^1.

Chronic Myelomonocytic Leukaemia (CMML). Monocytoid cells are prominent in CMML and eosinophils and basophils are not usually a feature. There is often rapid progression to acute leukaemia. The Ph^1 chromosome is not present. Splenomegaly usually less.

Leukaemoid Reactions. These are not usually associated with splenomegaly. The leucocyte count is usually not as high as in CGL and an associated basophilia is rare. The high leucocyte count usually does not persist for a long period in leukaemoid reaction and the left shift is not as great as in CGL. The NAP score is usually high. There is no Ph^1 chromosome in leukaemoid reactions.

Treatment in Chronic Phase

1. Supportive therapy including allopurinol, blood transfusion, when necessary, and vigorous treatment of infections.

2. Busulphan 2–6 mg/day (or other alkylating agents), sometimes in combination with thioguanine (80 mg/day), is used to slowly bring down the white count over several months. The haemoglobin often rises and the spleen size decreases. Side effects of busulphan therapy include prolonged marrow suppression, skin pigmentation and pulmonary fibrosis. Such therapy improves the quality of life, but has not been shown to delay blast crisis.

3. Leukopheresis will rapidly, though transiently, reduce the white count and may be useful when thromboembolic phenomena occur secondary to massive leucocytosis.

4. Aggressive 'acute leukaemia type' induction regimes have been used to induce a Ph^1-negative state, but such 'remissions' are usually short-lived.

5. Recent reports of allogeneic bone marrow transplantation in chronic phase CGL from several centres are most encouraging.

Treatment of Acute Phase CGL

Myelofibrotic Type. Transfusion and haematinics for anaemia. Analgesia or splenic irradiation for splenic pain. Splenectomy may be indicated for massive splenomegaly or hypersplenism.

Acute Leukaemia Type. Most cases resemble acute myeloid leukaemia and are treated as such. In about 20 per cent of cases, however, the leukaemic blasts carry the cALL antigen and these cases respond best to ALL therapy. Occasionally both myeloid and lymphoid blasts are found simultaneously.

The response is poor in myeloid blast crisis; in lymphoid blast crisis the initial response is often good, but is invariably short-lived.

Ablative chemotherapy or irradiation followed by infusion of cryopreserved chronic phase peripheral blood leucocytes has been attempted in blast crisis and in the myelofibrotic crisis. This therapy is very costly and benefits only a few patients.

CHRONIC MYELOPROLIFERATIVE DISORDERS IN CHILDHOOD

These are rare, accounting for 2–5 per cent of childhood leukaemias. At least three distinct entities may be recognized.

1. Juvenile Chronic Granulocytic Leukaemia

This usually presents in infancy with anaemia, recurrent infections, lymphadeno-pathy, hepatosplenomegaly and distinct facial rashes. There is usually a leuco-cytosis ($15–100 \times 10^9$/l) with a prominent monocytosis. The HbF is usually raised to between 40 and 85 per cent. The red cells also bear fetal antigens. There is no Ph^1 chromosome but other karyotypic anomalies occur. The disease is rapidly progressive, death usually occurring due to bone marrow failure rather than blastic transformation. Specific therapy is ineffective.

2. Adult Type Chronic Granulocytic Leukaemia

This usually occurs in older children and is Ph^1 positive. The disease is identical to the adult form with frequent termination in blast crisis.

3. Monosomy 7

A chronic myeloproliferative disorder associated with monosomy 7 in the myeloid cells usually presents in infancy with recurrent respiratory infections, anaemia and hepatosplenomegaly. There may be a leucoerythroblastic anaemia, leucocytosis or thrombocytopenia. The marrow is hypercellular and left shifted. Marked dys-erythropoiesis may be prominent. HbF is normal or only slightly raised. The disease usually progresses to an acute leukaemic stage. Therapy is unsatisfactory.

PHILADELPHIA POSITIVE ACUTE LEUKAEMIA

The Ph^1 chromosome is found in approximately 2 per cent of childhood ALLs, 3 per cent of AMLs and up to 30 per cent of adult ALLs. Ph^1 is a poor prognostic feature in ALL with only about 50 per cent of cases achieving a complete remission. Those cases achieving remission mainly revert to a normal karyotype, but some cases develop a Ph^1-positive remission phase, suggesting that they have presented with a blast crisis of CGL. Other cases have partial remissions with mixed karyotypes.

POLYCYTHAEMIA RUBRA VERA (PRV)

Pathogenesis

There is excessive production of red cells in the presence of low levels of erythropoietin. In vitro culture studies suggest that the neoplastic clone is not erythropoietin independent, but is sensitive to extremely low levels of this hormone. At high erythropoietin levels in vitro, normally quiescent, non-neoplastic erythroid clones can still be demonstrated.

There is usually also granulocytic and megakaryocytic proliferation and the disease frequently terminates as myelofibrosis or acute leukaemia.

Clinical Features

Presentation usually over 40 years of age. Slightly more common in males. Higher incidence in European Jews; rare in Negroes. Symptoms are due to the increased blood volume and blood viscosity. There is insidious onset of headaches, dizziness, tinnitus, visual disturbances, pruritus, gout and thrombotic problems. Peptic ulceration occurs in 10–20 per cent of cases and gastrointestinal haemorrhage is common.

On examination one-third of patients are hypertensive. There is ruddy cyanosis of the mucous membranes, hepatomegaly in 35 per cent and splenomegaly in 75 per cent.

A chest radiograph often shows increased pulmonary vascular shadows.

Peripheral Blood Findings

Haemoglobin 18–24 g/dl, RBCs $8-12 \times 10^9/l$. RBCs normochromic and normocytic, but may become hypochromic and microcytic due to iron deficiency secondary to blood loss. The WBC is raised in 75 per cent, usually about $15 \times 10^9/l$, but may be up to $50 \times 10^9/l$. The NAP score is raised. Platelets are raised in about 50 per cent and may be up to $1000 \times 10^9/l$. The ESR is usually low. The serum vitamin B_{12} may be raised due to increased B_{12} binding protein; the red cell folate is usually normal; the serum iron is often low. The serum uric acid is raised in 75 per cent.

Bone Marrow Findings

A hypercellular aspirate with marrow extending into the fat spaces. Clumps of normoblasts are seen. The M : E ratio is often low but myelopoiesis is also active and megakaryocytes are readily seen.

Diagnosis

1. Demonstration of an increased red cell mass is essential for the diagnosis of polycythaemia. The plasma volume is usually normal or slightly increased (*see* Chapter 28).

A raised Hb or PCV due to a low plasma volume with a normal red cell mass can occur in relative or 'stress polycythaemia'. Stress polycythaemia is seen with dehydration, heart failure and prolonged bed rest. It is more common in heavy smokers, hypertensives and possibly in those with an anxious disposition. It is not a benign condition and thrombotic events are the major cause of morbidity and mortality. In stress polycythaemia the WBC and platelet count are not raised, the NAP score is normal and there is no splenomegaly.

2. To differentiate primary from secondary polycythaemia may be very difficult as nearly 20 per cent of PRV cases have a normal WBC and platelet count and the

WBC is often raised in secondary polycythaemia, e.g. chronic infective lung disease. The high NAP score suggests primary polycythaemia but this is also raised in infective conditions. Splenomegaly is usually indicative of PRV. Serum erythropoietin levels are high in secondary polycythaemia and low in PRV, but the 'exhypoxic polycythaemic mouse assay' for erythropoietin is technically very difficult and reliable immunoassays for erythropoietin are only available in a few centres.

Frequently the diagnosis of PRV must be by exclusion of secondary poly-cythaemia and the investigations should include: ESR, chest radiograph, arterial gases, intravenous pyeolgram, oxygen dissociation curve, Hb electrophoresis, and any other pertinent investigation suggested by the history and examination.

Treatment

1. Repeated venesection relieves symptoms and will increase survival. Iron deficiency may result, causing microcytosis and a very high red cell count with relatively higher viscosity in relation to the haemoglobin level. The platelet count often rises further after venesection and may become troublesome.

2. ^{32}P 100–300 MBq (3–8 mCi) i.v. can be given to suppress erythropoiesis. The effect on erythropoiesis may take 6–8 weeks to become apparent whereas the WBC and platelets may fall several weeks earlier. The injections can be repeated after 3–6 months if necessary. The platelet count usually influences the dosage and frequency of injections.

3. Busulphan (or another alkylating agent) 2–6 mg daily or higher doses in intermittent courses. Great care is required as prolonged hypoplasia may follow.

4. Supportive therapy

      4.1 Allopurinol to prevent gout.

      4.2 Pruritus treated with antihistamines or cimetidine.

      4.3 Management of bleeding and thrombotic complications.

      4.4 Iron to treat iron deficiency.

      4.5 Folic acid to treat secondary megaloblastosis.

Course and Prognosis

Untreated the median survival is only 2 years; with treatment it is 13 years. Thrombosis and haemorrhage are the major causes of death. About one-quarter of cases terminate with acute myeloid leukaemia or myelofibrosis with myeloid metaplasia. It is controversial whether the incidence of acute leukaemia is higher after ^{32}P therapy than cytotoxic therapy.

SECONDARY POLYCYTHAEMIA

Hypoxaemic Polycythaemia

1. Physiological. Newborn or at a high altitude (above 6000 feet).

2. Cyanotic heart disease, e.g. Fallot's tetralogy, Eisenmenger's syndrome.

The resultant polycythaemia increases the oxygen-carrying capacity until whole blood viscosity compromises blood flow and the oxygen-carrying capacity begins to fall.

3. Respiratory failure.
4. Abnormal haemoglobins.
> 4.1 Hereditary methaemoglobinaemia. These very rarely cause erythrocytosis (*see* Chapter 10).
> 4.2. Haemoglobins with increased oxygen affinity (*see* Chapter 10).

Variant substitutions interfere with the sub-unit and ligand interactions and shift the conformational stability in favour of oxy-forms, e.g. Hb Chesapeake. The shift of the oxygen dissociation curve to the left results in reduction of tissue oxygen tension, a hypoxic stimulus and erythrocytosis. Some cases of familial polycythaemia are due to this. Some of these high affinity haemoglobins are electrophoretically silent, so that an oxygen dissociation curve is an essential part of the study of a patient with polycythaemia of obscure origin.

Polycythaemia associated with Inappropriate Erythropoietin Production

1. Various renal lesions include hypernephroma, Wilms's tumour, polycystic kidneys, hydronephrosis, renal TB, renal adenoma.
2. Tumours including cerebellar haemangioblastoma, ovarian tumours, uterine fibroids, phaeochromocytoma, hepatoma and carcinoma of the bronchus. Erythropoietin-like substances can sometimes be extracted from these lesions.

Polycythaemia is said to occur in Cushing's syndrome, but the evidence for this is poor.

ESSENTIAL THROMBOCYTHAEMIA
(Idiopathic thrombocythaemia, essential haemorrhagic thrombocythaemia)

Pathogenesis

This occurs mainly in the middle-aged and elderly. It is a myeloproliferative disorder in which a very elevated platelet count predominates. It is closely related to myelofibrosis; some cases overlap with a polycythaemia rubra vera and Ph^1-positive essential thrombocythaemia may occur.

Clinical Features

These fall into two major groups:
1. Symptoms and signs of a myeloproliferative disorder: anaemia, splenomegaly and bone pain. The spleen may not be enlarged because repeated infarction with splenic atrophy is common.
2. Features associated with a massively high platelet count: recurrent arterial and venous thromboses and tendency to haemorrhage, especially from the gastrointestinal tract. Peptic ulcer is very common. Often these patients have significant iron deficiency.

Blood Picture

The haemoglobin is increased if there is a polycythaemic element, but is often normal or decreased, especially if there is iron deficiency. The WBC count is usually increased as in any myeloproliferative disorder, but may be normal. If increased, it may be associated with a leucoerythroblastic picture. The NAP score is usually increased. The blood picture may show the features of auto-splenectomy secondary to infarction, with Howell–Jolly bodies and target cells in addition to massive drifts of platelets. The platelet count is usually over $1000 \times 10^9/l$ and may be over $5000 \times 10^9/l$. Platelet function tests are frequently abnormal as in other myeloproliferative disorders. Poor aggregation with adrenaline is the most common aggregation defect.

Bone Marrow

Can be difficult to aspirate because of associated myelofibrosis, but is hypercellular with megakaryocytes and drifts of platelets being the dominant features. Biopsy often shows significant myelofibrosis.

Treatment

This is required for:

1. The very high platelet count and qualitative platelet defects. Cytotoxic drugs, particularly busulphan, are useful. Cyclophosphamide and chlorambucil are useful second-line drugs. ^{32}P may also be used. Antiplatelet aggregating agents may be indicated, especially if there is digital ischaemia.

2. Iron deficiency associated with gastrointestinal bleeding. Oral iron and cimetidine if there is an associated peptic ulcer.

3. Splenomegaly—this may disappear with recurrent infarction. If very large, cytotoxic drugs may be used or splenic irradiation considered. Splenectomy when the platelet count is very high should be avoided since it may result in a count which is higher still with a consequent thromboembolic catastrophe.

4. Bone marrow failure. This may occur later in the disease process and may require blood transfusion. Folate deficiency must be excluded.

Course and Prognosis

Patients may survive many years, but progression to marrow failure or acute leukaemia may occur.

MEGAKARYOCYTIC LEUKAEMIA

This entity is increasingly recognized with the aid of electron microscopy, platelet specific peroxidase and monoclonal anti-megakaryocyte antibodies (*see* Chapter 15).

The usual presentation is of pancytopenia with aggressive myelofibrosis. Many of the cases of so-called 'malignant myelofibrosis' are probably acute megakaryocytic leukaemia.

'PRIMARY MYELOFIBROSIS'

Pathogenesis

'Primary myelofibrosis' is a myeloproliferative disease in which fibrosis of the marrow and myeloid metaplasia predominate. After allogeneic bone marrow grafts, fibroblasts remain of recipient origin and analysis of fibroblasts for G-6-PD activity in heterozygous females with myeloproliferative disorders indicates that the fibroblastic proliferation is reactive and not a clonal expansion. The reason for this excessive 'fibrosis' in some myeloproliferative syndromes is not clear, but it is often associated with marked megakaryocytic proliferation. Myeloid metaplasia is probably due to the primary haemopoietic stem cell disorder rather than marrow replacement.

Treatment

Essentially for alleviation of symptoms, e.g. allopurinol for the prevention of gout, blood transfusions. Steroids are often given if the platelet count is low. Splenectomy may be valuable if there is marked hypersplenism, but the operation is often technically difficult in these elderly patients. Splenic irradiation is an alternative. Local irradiation may help severe bone pains.

Course and Prognosis

The course is extremely variable with a mean survival from diagnosis of about 5 years. Death is usually due to marrow failure and about 5 per cent of cases terminate in acute myeloid leukaemia.

A few patients have a very aggressive 'acute myelofibrosis' and this is often due to acute megakaryocytic leukaemia.

TRANSITIONS IN MYELOPROLIFERATIVE DISORDERS

Many of these disorders display overlapping features from the outset and obvious transitions from one kind to another often occur. For instance, a patient with a high haemoglobin, raised red cell mass, high WBC count and splenomegaly may show obvious fibrosis on biopsy of the marrow at diagnosis. As the disease 'burns out' the spleen may enlarge, the haemoglobin falls without treatment and a straightforward diagnosis of myelofibrosis can be made. Other patients may have obvious myelofibrosis except for a platelet count of $750–800 \times 10^9/l$ and lie somewhere between idiopathic myelofibrosis and thrombocythaemia. This can all be understood if these diseases are thought of as representing proliferation of a myeloid stem cell which is still pluripotent as far as red cells, platelets and granulocytes are concerned. The fibrosis is probably reactive. The terminal stage of many of the chronic myeloproliferative syndromes is an acute leukaemia, usually acute myeloid leukaemia but occasionally erythroleukaemia, or transformation to acute megakaryoblastic leukaemia or acute lymphoblastic leukaemia in CGL.

Selected Further Reading

Berlin N. I. (ed.) (1976) Polycythaemia. *Semin. Hematol.* **13**, 1.

Canellos G. P. (1976) Chronic granulocytic leukaemia. *Med. Clin. North Am.* **60**, 1001.

Fialkow P. G., Jacobson R. J. and Papayannopoulou T. (1977) Chronic myelocytic leukaemia: clonal origin in a stem cell common to the granulocyte erythrocyte platelet and monocyte/macrophage. *Am. J. Med.* **63**, 125–132.

Jacobson R. B. (1978) Agnogenic myeloid metaplasia. *Blood* **51**, 189.

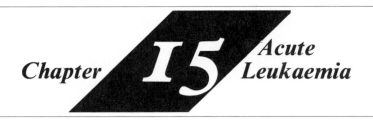

Chapter 15 Acute Leukaemia

Definition

Leukaemia is a malignant proliferation of the blood-forming tissues with quantitative and qualitative changes in the blood. The term 'acute leukaemia' implies that the leukaemic cells are morphologically immature and does not necessarily imply that the disease has a rapid onset with relentless progression.

Incidence

The yearly incidence of acute leukaemia is 3·5/100 000 and is apparently rising in the Western world. It is slightly more common in males.

Aetiology

The precise mechanism of leukaemogenesis is unknown, but is thought to be multifactorial. The following have been implicated.

1. Hereditary factors. (a) There is a greatly increased risk of acute leukaemia in a variety of hereditary disorders, e.g. trisomy 21, Bloom's syndrome, Fanconi's anaemia, ataxia telangiectasia and congenital agammaglobulinaemia. (b) There is a high frequency (25 per cent) of concordant leukaemia in monozygous twins, though this mainly applies to infantile leukaemia. The increased risk in non-identical twins is only fivefold. (c) Some high-risk families for leukaemia have been reported.

2. Ionizing radiation. There appears to be a near-linear relationship between risk and cumulative dose received between about 1–9 Gy (100–900 rad). Both acute lymphoblastic and acute myeloblastic leukaemia can occur. The mechansim may be direct chromosomal damage, but induction of oncogenic viral replication or generalized immunosuppression may be significant.

3. Chemicals. This is best documented for benzene, toluene and the alkylating agents but many other chemicals and drugs have been implicated. Alkylating drugs may be especially leukaemogenic when given in combination with radiotherapy.

4. Viruses. Certain animal leukaemias appear to be virally induced, but the evidence in man is more tenuous and includes (a) the finding of apparent viral particles in the cells of some cases of acute leukaemia; (b) the finding of reverse transcriptase in some acute leukaemic cells; (c) the occasional transference of acute leukaemia to donor cells after bone marrow transplantation.

5. Acquired haematological disorders predisposing to acute leukaemias include the myeloproliferative disorders and probably Hodgkin's disease and multiple myeloma.

Pathogenesis

It is thought that the leukaemic stem cell fails to differentiate so that there is an accumulation of primitive cells which do not die as rapidly as normally maturing cells. These leukaemic cells probably do not divide more rapidly than normal cells. The primitive cells replace the normal marrow elements and spill into the blood. In addition, there is probably a specific inhibition of normal haemopoiesis. Various factors known as 'leukaemia-associated inhibitors' have been isolated from leukaemic blast cells which are capable of suppressing normal haemopoietic progenitor cell growth (CFU-GM) in vitro.

Classification

Acute leukaemia is divided into acute lymphoblastic leukaemia (ALL) and acute myeloblastic leukaemia (AML) each of which can be further subdivided according to the morphology of the leukaemic cells. Rarely there may be a pronounced leukaemic element in other haematological malignancies such as myeloma and some lymphomas.

Clinical Features

The presentation of AML and ALL is frequently similar with a fairly sudden onset of the symptoms of marrow failure, namely lassitude, infection and bleeding. Bone and joint pain may occur, most often in ALL when a diagnosis of juvenile polyarthritis may be suspected. Lymphadenopathy and hepatosplenomegaly occur in all types of acute leukaemia though are usually more prominent in ALL. Infiltration of other tissues such as skin, gums and perineum occurs occasionally and often indicates a monocytic element. Central nervous system disease is rare at presentation (approximately 4 per cent in ALL and 1 per cent in AML). Metabolic disturbances including hypokalaemia (especially in monocytic leukaemias where a specific renal tubular lesion occurs), hyperkalaemia, hyponatremia, hypocalcaemia and hypomagnesaemia and uricaemia, are not infrequent and may be exacerbated by treatment.

ACUTE LYMPHOBLASTIC LEUKAEMIA

Incidence

ALL accounts for nearly 20 per cent of all leukaemias and is the commonest malignant disease of childhood. The incidence of ALL peaks in childhood between the ages of 2 and 9 years, is relatively low in adolescence and then rises steadily with age. The ratio of males to females is $1·3:1$, the excess of males being found mainly in young boys.

Clinical Features

The onset is nearly always acute with no preleukaemic phase. The clinical features have been described previously. Approximately 50 per cent of cases with T cell

ALL have also a mediastinal mass on chest radiography. This is not seen in other types of ALL.

Peripheral Blood

Marked anaemia is almost invariable at diagnosis. It is usually normocytic.

The total leucocyte count is most frequently raised, but is normal or low in 30 per cent of cases. The granulocyte count and platelet count are usually depressed. The neutrophils have normal or even high neutrophil alkaline phosphatase (NAP) activity. Lymphoblasts are usually seen in the blood, though this is not invariable (so-called aleukaemic leukaemia).

Marrow

The marrow is hypercellular and almost totally replaced by lymphoblasts. Fibrosis is seen in 10–15 per cent of cases and is especially common in those with bone pain.

Morphology and Differential Diagnosis

The diagnosis is usually straightforward with typical lymphoblasts being seen with Romanowsky stains (*see* Chapter 3). The distinguishing morphological and cytochemical features of lymphoblasts and myeloblasts are shown in *Table 15.1*.

Table 15.1. Morphological and cytochemical features of leukaemic blast cells

	Lymphoblast	*Myeloblast*
Nucleoli	1 or 2	Often more than 2
Nuclear chromatin condensation around nucleoli and nuclear membrane	Present in some cases	Absent
Cytoplasm	Scanty	Abundant
Auer rods	Absent	Present
Sudan black	Negative	Often positive
Peroxidase	Negative	Often positive
Non-specific esterase	Negative	Faint positivity—not inhibited by fluoride
PAS	Often positive, often in large blocks	Negative or faint tinge

ALL can be divided into three groups on morphological criteria—French American British (FAB) Classification. In L_1 type over 90 per cent of the blasts are small, with scanty cytoplasm and regular round or clefted nuclei with indistinct nucleoli and often some chromatin condensation. In L_2 type the cells are larger with more cytoplasm, oval-round and often clefted and folded nuclei with fine chromatin and prominent nucleoli. There is often considerable heterogeneity of cell size and morphology. In L_3 type the blasts are large and homogeneous with finely stippled nuclei, one or more nucleoli and deep basophilic abundant cytoplasm with prominent vacuolization (variably present to a lesser degree in type L_1 and L_2).

At electron microscopy, Rieder cells with conspicuous microtubules are frequently seen and there is an absence of myeloid differentiation granules.

Occasionally, infections (e.g. infectious mononucleosis, cytomegalovirus and toxoplasmosis) may resemble acute lymphoblastic leukaemias as may the lymphocytic lymphomas, neuroblastomas and occasionally other metastatic tumours. A full clinical examination, and bone marrow aspirate and biopsy, will usually resolve the issue, but in doubtful cases cell marker studies may be particularly helpful, e.g. mature suppressor T cell phenotype in infectious mononucleosis, light chain restricted surface immunoglobulins in lymphocytic lymphomas.

Cell Marker Studies in ALL

The study of leukaemic cell phenotypes has added greatly to the understanding of normal haemopoiesis and to malignant disease in general. The clonal concept of cancer has been upheld, and the antigen expression of leukaemic cells has been shown to reflect the phenotype of normal haemopoietic precursor cells. Cancer-specific markers have not been found. It should be noted that the phenotypic expression of leukaemic cells does not identify the target cell for the disease, but merely the level of 'differentiation block'. The concept of de-differentiation is not currently popular.

Using a panel of markers it is possible to divide ALL into four major groups, reflecting different stages of lymphocyte differentiation. Among the most useful markers are:

1. Nuclear terminal deoxynucleotidyltransferase (Tdt) which can be measured chemically or detected by immunofluorescence.

2. Anti-Ia serum. This detects part of the HLA-Dr complex and is found on normal myeloid progenitor cells, B-lymphocyte progenitors and mature B lymphocytes and monocytes.

3. Anti-common ALL antiserum which probably detects an antigen (cALL) on B and T lymphocyte precursors.

4. Surface immunoglobulin (SmIg) which is found on maturing B cells.

5. The sheep red blood cell rosette receptor (E) which is found on thymocytes and peripheral T lymphocytes.

6. A variety of monoclonal and heterologous polyclonal thymocyte and T cell antisera (T) (*see* Chapter 2).

Fig. 15.1 illustrates the phenotypes of the major subdivisions of ALL.

Most of the common ALLs are probably pre B cell neoplasms; one-third of them have intracytoplasmic chains and most others have putative B cell markers defined by monoclonal antisera.

The approximate incidence of the major subgroups in children and adults has been assessed by M. F. Greaves et al. and is shown in *Table 15.2*.

Phenotypic shifts between null cell ALL and common ALL occur frequently at relapse, but shifts between putative B cell and T cell ALL do not occur.

The rare B cell ALL has L_3 morphology and the other immunological subgroups are distributed among the FAB L_1 and L_2 groups.

Chromosomes in ALL

Cytogenetic abnormalities of all kinds are present in 45 per cent of cases. Hyperdiploidy is particularly common. One to two per cent of childhood ALLs

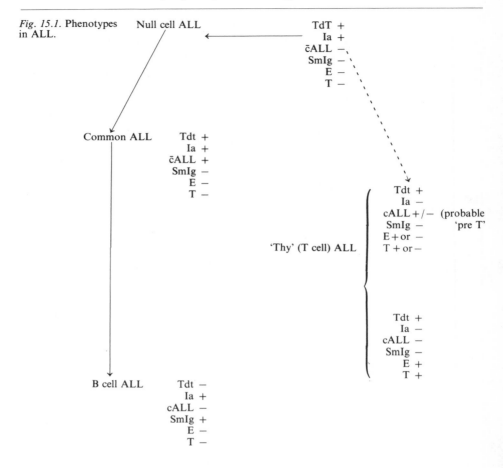

Fig. 15.1. Phenotypes in ALL.

Table 15.2. Incidence of different phenotypes in ALL

	Children	Adults
Null cell ALL	12%	38%
Common ALL	75%	50%
B cell ALL	< 1%	2%
T cell ALL	12%	10%

and up to one-quarter of adult ALLs have the Ph[1] chromosome. The significance of this is discussed in the previous chapter.

Treatment

1. Supportive therapy
Blood transfusion, control of infection and the arrest of bleeding are often necessary at presentation. The importance of adequate psychological support for both patients and close relatives must be emphasized.

2. Remission induction

Vincristine and prednisone (dosages variable according to specific regimes) are the mainstay of treatment and remission can be obtained in over 85 per cent of children. The addition of daunorubicin increases the remission rate to about 97 per cent; some centres use daunorubicin from the outset and others reserve it for vincristine- and prednisone-resistant cases, because of the considerable toxicity of the anthracyclines. L-Asparaginase, mercaptopurine and methotrexate have been included in remission induction regimes but are of lesser value. The remission rate in adult ALL is less than that for childhood ALL—approximately 75 per cent.

3. Maintenance therapy

Remission is defined as less than 5 per cent blasts in a cellular marrow with normal blood cell counts. The residual leukaemic cell mass may still be as high as 10^8 cells, however, and maintenance therapy is intended to reduce this residual disease. Many regimes are used, but most include cyclical courses of mercaptopurine, methotrexate and cytosine arabinoside and often further courses of vincristine and prednisone. Maintenance therapy is discontinued after 2–3 years of sustained remission.

4. Craniospinal prophylaxis

Disease of the central nervous system develops in over 50 per cent of those surviving more than 2 years if no prophylaxis is given. A combination of irradiation and intrathecal chemotherapy is usually employed. Irradiation is given to the cranium including the optic nerves and cervical spine. 24 Gy (2400 rad) are commonly given in 2 Gy (200 rad) daily fractions. Repeated injections of intrathecal methotrexate or cytosine arabinoside are given, rather than including the spine in the irradiation field because this can cause troublesome myelosuppression and will affect growth of the axial skeleton in children. Cranial irradiation causes cerebral calcification in some cases.

When central nervous system disease occurs, intrathecal methotrexate is probably the optimum treatment. If there is raised intracranial pressure it may be necessary to implant a shunt and a subcutaneous reservoir (Ommaya reservoir) into which the drugs may be given.

5. Testicular prophylaxis

Testicular biopsies in remission have shown that in approximately 10 per cent of boys there is occult leukaemic infiltration and further cases have testicular relapses. Prophylactic irradiation of the testes is therefore recommended in some centres though this does cause hypogonadism as well as sterility. The incidence of testicular relapse is markedly reduced but not the incidence of bone marrow relapses.

Prognosis

Approximately 40 per cent of childhood cases have remissions exceeding 5 years and many of these children are probably cured. The following factors at presentation are independently associated with a good prognosis: (*a*) low peripheral blood white cell count; (*b*) age between 2 and 10 years; (*c*) female sex; (*d*) more than 75 per cent of blasts type L_1 (FAB classification); (*e*) normal chromosomal karyotype.

The duration of remission is related to the immunological phenotype of the leukaemic blasts in that patients with common ALL have a better prognosis than those with null cell ALL which is better than those with T or B cell leukaemia.

However, this effect on prognosis disappears if one takes into account the fact that T cell leukaemia tends to present with a higher white cell count than null cell ALL which tends to present with a higher white cell count than common ALL. The one exception may be that those with a 'pre-T' phenotype tend to present with lower white cell counts and yet have the very poor prognosis of T cell ALL. The prognosis in adult ALL is less good than in children and this may be in part due to the fact that common ALL is less common. Some centres claim that the prognosis for adult-common ALL approaches that of childhood-common ALL, but other centres have claimed that the prognosis for adult ALL is as poor as that for adult AML.

Bone Marrow Transplantation in ALL

Although second remissions are frequently obtained in ALL, the ultimate prognosis following relapse is very poor and allogeneic bone marrow transplantation from a matched sibling during second remission is probably the treatment of choice (*see* Chapter 6). Fifty per cent of transplanted cases relapse, and the long-term survival is only about 30 per cent. It may be appropriate to graft poor-prognosis patients in first remission, but few centres do this at present. Allogeneic grafting in relapse does produce some long-term survivors, but the mortality is extremely high.

ACUTE MYELOID LEUKAEMIA

Incidence

Acute myeloblastic leukaemia or acute non-lymphoblastic leukaemia accounts for approximately 25 per cent of all leukaemias and is commonest in the middle-aged and elderly.

Clinical Features

These have been discussed previously. Although the onset is usually acute, 10–20 per cent of cases are preceded by a smouldering or preleukaemic phase. Infiltration of the gums and perineum occurs in monocytic leukaemias and severe bleeding due to disseminated intravascular coagulation may be the presenting feature of acute promyelocytic leukaemia and occasionally of acute monocytic leukaemia.

Peripheral Blood

There is anaemia, either normocytic or macrocytic, often with anisocytosis and poikilocytosis. The reticulocyte count is not usually raised, but the occasional normoblast may be seen.

The white cell count is usually, though not invariably, raised and blast cells predominate. Neutrophils are usually reduced in numbers with relatively few intermediate forms between the myeloblast and the neutrophil (cf. chronic granulocytic leukaemia). The neutrophil alkaline phosphatase score is nearly always low.

The platelet count is usually low especially if there is consumption as well as marrow failure.

Bone Marrow

The marrow is hypercellular and may produce a 'dry tap'. The majority of cells are usually blasts of the myeloid series and the red cell precursors often show dyserythropoiesis and megaloblastic change. Ringed sideroblasts may be seen on the iron stain. Megakaryocytes are markedly reduced.

Morphology

The morphological and cytochemical features of the myeloblast are shown in *Table 15.1*. The coalescent primary granules known as Auer rods are pathognomonic of AML (*Fig. 15.2*). They are more conspicuous with a peroxidase and Sudan black

Fig. 15.2. Myeloblast.

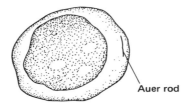

Auer rod

stain. Varying degrees of myeloid differentiation (granulocytic, monocytic or erythroid) may be apparent, and this is used as a basis for further categorization:

1. Acute undifferentiated myeloid leukaemia (M1—FAB nomenclature). Myeloblasts with no signs of maturation.

2. Acute myeloid leukaemia with evidence of maturation (M2). Of the granulocytic cells 10–20 per cent are beyond the promyelocyte stage.

3. Acute promyelocytic leukaemia (M3). The predominant leukaemic cell is the promyelocyte often with prominent bundles of Auer rods known as 'faggots'. Occasionally hypogranular varieties of acute promyelocytic leukaemia occur. There is typically a dumb-bell shaped nucleus and a mistaken diagnosis of monocytic leukaemia may be made. It is an important distinction because disseminated intravascular coagulation is likely in acute promyelocytic leukaemia either at presentation or at initiation of treatment. Cytochemistry shows very strong peroxidase or Sudan black activity in these cells with little non-specific esterase activity.

4. Acute myelomonocytic leukaemia—Naegeli type (M4). Monoblasts as well as myeloblasts are found. The monoblasts have voluminous cytoplasm with folded nuclei and 3–5 nucleoli. The cytoplasm contains fine PAS and Sudan black granules and very strong non-specific esterase activity that is inhibited by fluoride. The serum and urinary muramidase (lysozyme) are raised.

5. Acute monoblastic leukaemia—Schilling type (M5). There is a pure monoblastic proliferation. Whether this represents one end of a spectrum or is a distinct entity from acute myelomonocytic leukaemia is uncertain and whether Auer rods are found in this condition is controversial.

6. Acute erythroid leukaemia (M6). Over 30 per cent of the blast cells are erythroblasts. Anaemia is usually severe with marked anisocytosis and poikilocytosis. Large numbers of normoblasts are usually seen in the peripheral blood, often

showing megaloblastoid change with atypical and bizarre forms and ringed sideroblasts. The erythroblasts frequently show strong block PAS positivity. *Table 15.3* summarizes the incidence of the different AML variants as reported in the literature. This, we believe, exaggerates the proportion of M2 cases as strictly defined by the FAB classification criteria.

Table 15.3. FAB classification of AML

M1	20%
M2	37%
M3	7%
M4	23%
M5	9%
M6	4%

It should be noted that acute megakaryoblastic leukaemia also occurs. The blast cells have very basophilic cytoplasm and may be mistaken for myeloblasts or lymphoblasts. The clinical picture is often that of 'acute myelofibrosis'. The megakaryoblasts can be recognized by their staining with platelet myeloperoxidase, their characteristic electron microscopy appearance and their staining with monoclonal 'anti-platelet' antibodies.

Electron microscopy may also help in the differentiation of lymphoblastic and myeloblastic leukaemias, but is not routinely required.

Cell Marker Studies in AML

Leukaemic myeloblasts are usually Ia positive whereas acute promyelocytic leukaemia is Ia negative. Various antisera to granulocytic differentiation antigens are available, but they are usually only positive in cases that show obvious maturation on light microscopy.

AML cells do not have surface immunoglobulin, E receptors, T cell antigens or the common ALL antigen. Nuclear Tdt is usually absent. In those cases where it is found, it either indicates a mixed lymphoid/myeloid leukaemia or that the leukaemic phenotype is very immature and that by inference Tdt is a stem cell marker. Regardless of the biological significance of Tdt positivity in AML it appears that these patients fare badly.

The erythroblasts of acute erythroid leukaemia have red cell antigens on their surface (glycophorins and Band 3) which can be detected with a variety of antisera. A small group of undifferentiated leukaemias and some chronic granulocytic blast crises have also been found to carry these erythroid markers.

Some cases of presumed megakaryoblastic leukaemias react with monoclonal anti platelet antisera (*see above*).

Chromosomes in AML

Chromosomal abnormalities are seen in about 50 per cent of cases by Giemsa banding analysis. Hypodiploidy is particularly common. Methotrexate banding after culture is said to reveal abnormalities in nearly all cases.

Bone Marrow Culture Studies in AML

Varying patterns of abnormal colony growth are seen in AML. There are usually few or no colonies (aggregates with more than 40 cells) and often many clusters (aggregates less than 40 cells). The number of clusters obtained from the blood is frequently high. These colonies and clusters do not grow autonomously but require, in general, higher levels of colony-stimulating activity than normal progenitor cells. Karyotype analyses have shown that all the colonies and clusters are derived from leukaemia progenitor cells and not residual normal cells. The leukaemic cells, in fact, produce inhibitory factors that suppress normal colony growth (LAI = leukaemia-associated inhibitors).

Various studies have correlated the pattern of colony growth at presentation with the prognosis but this has not proved to be clinically useful. Abnormal growth patterns in remission may antedate a clinical and haematological relapse by a few weeks but this knowledge is not presently of value.

Treatment

1. Supportive therapy (*see* Chapter 6)
The level of support required to treat AML is greater than that for ALL as far greater periods of hypoplasia are encountered. Disseminated intravascular coagulation, if present, is treated with low dose heparin 10 000–20 000 units/24 hours by continuous infusion) and clotting factor replacement.

2. Remission induction
Whereas vincristine and prednisone show selectivity in their cytotoxic action towards the leukaemic lymphoblasts, the drugs used to treat AML have a similar cytotoxic effect on normal and leukaemic myeloid cells. It is unusual therefore to obtain remission without first producing a hypoplastic marrow. The normal cells regenerate more rapidly than the leukaemic cells and this is probably the main principle behind AML therapy. The most effective drugs are the anthracyclines (daunorubicin and adriamycin), cytosine arabinoside and thioguanine and these are often all given in combination. A typical regime is illustrated in *Table 15.4*.

Table 15.4. A course of induction therapy for AML

Day:	1	2	3	4	5
Daunorubicin 50 mg/m^2 i.v.	↓				
Cytosine arabinoside 100 mg/m^2 i.v.	↓↓	↓↓	↓↓	↓↓	↓↓
Thioguanine 100 mg/m^2 p.o.	↓↓	↓↓	↓↓	↓↓	↓↓

Following the above cytotoxic course the maximum cytopenia (nadir) occurs after about 5 days. The patient is reassessed 7–10 days after such a regime. If there are still blasts in the blood a further course of chemotherapy is given. If there are no blasts in the blood a bone marrow is performed. If blasts are present a further course is given immediately, but if the marrow shows normal cellular elements (i.e. remission) further treatment is not given until the peripheral blood count has recovered. Frequently the marrow is aplastic and under these circumstances one should wait a week and then repeat the marrow examination. With this type of regime, 70–80 per cent of patients will achieve remission. Most patients who achieve remission do so in less than five courses of chemotherapy and if there has been no response after four cases the pros and cons of more intensive chemotherapy versus palliative therapy must be weighed carefully.

   3. Consolidation

It is conventional to give further courses of intensive therapy to reduce residual disease. This is repeated in some centres after one year to 18 months.

   4. Maintenance therapy

Cycles of less intensive therapy are given every 3 or 4 weeks for about 2 years if the patient remains in remission. Anthracyclines are usually reduced or excluded from maintenance cycles because of cumulative cardiac toxicity. The accepted maximum cumulative dose is 550 mg/m². Myocardial assessment by ECG prior to anthracycline administration is routinely performed though incipient damage is better detected by echocardiography. As well as cytosine arabinoside and thioguanine, mercaptopurine and methotrexate are often used. Immunotherapy has been used, but has generally not been found helpful. The value of maintenance therapy is largely unproven and the comfort and convenience for the patient should be given high priority.

   5. Craniospinal prophylaxis

Improved remission rates have led to an increase in cerebrospinal disease and some centres recommend craniospinal prophylaxis in younger patients.

Prognosis

Although remission rates have improved considerably in recent years, the median duration of remission is only about 1 year. There are generally few long-term survivors though exceptions have been reported from some centres, with up to one-quarter of those entering remission becoming long-term survivors. Most centres claiming such good results have used very intensive induction or maintenance regimes, and it is as yet uncertain whether regimes similar to that illustrated in this chapter will result in a significant tail of long survivors (5 years plus).

   Various factors have been said to affect the prognosis in terms of remission rates and length of remission. Young patients do better than the elderly because they are able to tolerate more intensive therapy and those patients presenting without severe thrombocytopenia may also have a better prognosis. There is no agreement in the literature on the significance of the morphological type but an overall impression is that monocytic and erythroid differentiation are poor prognostic features. Acute promyelocytic leukaemia is associated with early deaths due to disseminated intravascular coagulation, but if this crisis can be averted or overcome then the prognosis is at least as good as for other forms of AML. The presence of Tdt or chromosomal abnormalities is said to be a poor prognostic feature.

   After relapse second remission can be induced in 25–50 per cent of cases but this is almost invariably brief.

Bone Marrow Transplantation in AML

Allogeneic grafting in first relapse produces long-term survival in about 10 per cent of cases and is no longer considered to be a reasonable approach. Allogeneic grafting in first remission, however, produces long-term survival in over 50 per cent of cases and it is hoped that many of these patients will be cured. Most deaths are due to 'graft problems' rather than recurrent leukaemia (10–20 per cent) though the relapse rate may be higher when cyclosporin A is used for GVHD prophylaxis. The results are less satisfactory for grafts in second remission. Interestingly, the recurrence of leukaemia after syngeneic marrow transplants was reported to be higher in Seattle, suggesting that either post-transplantation methotrexate or graft versus host disease has significant antileukaemic activity.

It must be pointed out that at present allogeneic transplantation is only appropriate for the under 40 years with an HLA identical sibling or a sibling or parent with only a single locus mismatch which excludes the vast majority of patients with AML.

The infusion of autologous cryopreserved marrow harvested in remission, after lethal ablative therapy in relapse has been tried in some centres. Second remissions are obtained though these are usually brief.

PRELEUKAEMIA

This refers to the syndrome of haemopoietic dysfunction that precedes the classic manifestations of acute myeloid leukaemia in about 10 per cent of cases. The diagnosis can, of course, only be made retrospectively. A preleukaemic syndrome prior to ALL has only rarely been reported. By definition, congenital disorders with an increased risk of developing leukaemia, such as Down's syndrome and Fanconi's anaemia, are excluded from the preleukaemic syndrome. Other acquired marrow dyscrasias such as paroxysmal nocturnal haemoglobinura and primary sideroblastic anaemia may be considered 'preleukaemic'.

Patients usually present with symptoms of cytopenia (one or more cell lines) and rarely fever and bone pain. A spleen may be palpable in some cases. Anaemia is usual and anisocytosis, poikilocytosis and macrocytosis are frequent. Occasionally, there is a striking reticulocytosis. The HbF level may be normal or slightly raised. The neutrophil count is often low and Pelger–Huët forms may be seen. The NAP score is low or normal. Monocytosis may be a feature of preleukaemia. The platelet count is often reduced and giant and bizarre forms may be seen. The marrow is usually hypercellular except in those patients who have had previous exposure to leukaemogenic drugs or ionizing radiation. Erythropoiesis often appears megaloblastic and granulopoiesis is frequently left shifted with a modest increase in myeloblasts (refractory anaemia/cytopenia with an excess of blasts = RAEB). Auer rods are not usually seen and their presence is often said to be indicative of leukaemia rather than preleukaemia. Chromosomal abnormalities are detected in 50–60 per cent of cases.

The features of preleukaemia are thus protean and non-specific and it is very difficult to be sure which cases of dyshaemopoiesis will evolve into leukaemia. Even in RAEB only one-third of patients develop overt leukaemia although this is largely because of the elderly age of many patients. Culture studies in dyshaemo-poietic states may be normal or have a leukaemic growth pattern and in the latter group the risk of death from progressive marrow failure or overt leukaemia is much higher. The presence of a chromosomal abnormality in dyshaemopoietic states is also a poor prognostic factor.

It is generally accepted that patients with preleukaemia should not receive specific leukaemia therapy until overt leukaemia arises even though the prognosis of the overt leukaemia is then particularly poor.

SMOULDERING ACUTE LEUKAEMIA

This is a term sometimes used to describe a cytopenia in which the marrow is found to have a marked increase in blast cells (usually about 50 per cent). There is usually anaemia and a few blast cells may be present in the blood but the clinical and haematological state remains stable for variable periods of time, occasionally for several years. Specific treatment is withheld until an increase in blasts or a progressive impairment of normal haemopoiesis occurs.

CHRONIC MYELOMONOCYTIC LEUKAEMIA

There is an increase of monocytes and often also neutrophils in the blood. The marrow is left shifted and the number of monocyte precursors is often less than would be expected from the peripheral blood. Megaloblastosis is frequently present. The serum and urinary lysozyme levels are raised. This disorder presents insidiously with symptoms of anaemia, fever, anorexia and weight loss and is therefore often classified with the preleukaemic syndromes.

DI GUGLIELMO'S SYNDROME

There is a spectrum of diseases characterized by primary refractory anaemia, macrocytosis, megaloblastoid erythroid hyperplasia and ineffective erythropoiesis and Damashek has suggested that Di Guglielmo's syndrome should refer to this spectrum rather than any one disease entity:

Refractory   Chronic   Acute   Acute
sideroblastic — erythraemic — erythraemic — erythroid
anaemia   myelosis   myelosis   leukaemia

'Preleukaemia'   — — — — — — — — — — — →   Overt leukaemia

Selected Further Reading

Catovsky D. (ed.) (1981) *The Leukaemic Cell*. Edinburgh, Churchill Livingstone.
Thomas E. D., Buckner C. D., Clift R. A. et al. (1979) Marrow transplantation for acute nonlymphoblastic leukaemia in first remission. *N. Engl. J. Med.* **301**, 597–599.

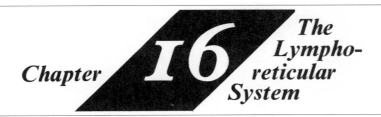

Chapter *16* *The Lymphoreticular System*

The lymphoreticular system refers to those organs involved in the surveillance and elimination of foreign antigens from the body. The major primary lymphoreticular organs in which stem cells become committed to forming immunocompetent cells are the bone marrow and thymus. The lymphoid aggregates throughout the body, particularly the lymph nodes, spleen and Peyer's patches, are known as secondary lymphoid organs.

STRUCTURE OF THE LYMPHATIC SYSTEM

A small proportion of tissue fluids, plus any cellular debris or pathogens, transudes into the lymphatic capillaries where it is drained by the lymphatic vessels, through lymph nodes and on to the great veins at the root of the neck whence it joins the bloodstream. The lymph nodes also have a rich blood supply allowing delivery of blood-borne foreign antigens to the nodes and a rapid exchange of small lymphocytes between the lymph node and the bloodstream. *Fig. 16.1* is an

Fig. 16.1 Structure of a normal lymph node

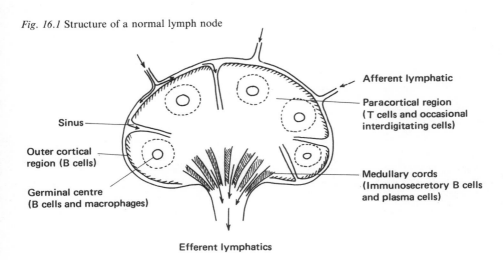

Afferent lymphatic

Paracortical region
(T cells and occasional interdigitating cells)

Sinus

Outer cortical region (B cells)

Germinal centre
(B cells and macrophages)

Medullary cords
(Immunosecretory B cells and plasma cells)

Efferent lymphatics

illustration of the normal lymph node architecture. Unstimulated lymph nodes vary in size between that of a pin head and a small cherry.

FUNCTIONS OF LYMPH NODES

1. Phagocytosis

Damaged cells and organisms in the lymph pass into the lymph node sinuses where they are removed by histiocytic 'reticulum' cells.

2. Lymphocyte Reservoir

The lymph nodes form a large lymphocyte reservoir which is in continual flux with the blood lymphocyte pool. Small lymphocytes pass through the endothelial cells lining the blood venules and into the paracortex. They then enter the medulla and filter into the efferent lymphatics from where they are returned to the blood. A similar migration occurs in Peyer's patches, spleen and other lymphoid aggregates. Most of the long-lived circulating lymphocytes are T cells.

3. Immune Response

The structure of the lymph nodes enables foreign antigens to be readily presented to immunocompetent cells in an appropriate environment for a proliferative response. The cells of the lymph nodes can be divided into at least three major groups:

> 3.1 The B cells which produce antibody.
>
> 3.2 The cells which by definition are thymus dependent. They serve many functions including: (i) cell-mediated immunity; (ii) delayed hypersensitivity reactions and graft rejection; (iii) regulation of antibody production by B cells.

Mature T cells can be subdivided into at least two groups by their staining pattern with monoclonal antisera and functional properties; a helper/inducer subset and a suppressor/cytotoxic subset.

> 3.3 The monocytic/histiocytic cells. These cells are: (i) phagocytic (micro-organisms and senescent or damaged host cells); (ii) involved in antigen presentation to lymphocytes (afferent limb of immune response); (iii) have 'killer' activity which is often antibody dependent (efferent limb of immune response); (iv) involved in the regulation of many T cell functions.

STRUCTURE OF THE SPLEEN

The spleen may be considered as a large lymph gland interposed within the circulation. Dimensions in health are $2.5 \times 7.5 \times 12.5$ cm; weight 100–200 g; with a blood flow of 150–200 ml/minute. It is situated inferior to the diaphragm beneath ribs 9, 10 and 11 and is surrounded by peritoneum. It is innervated by the phrenic nerve (C2, C3 and C4) and hence the pain of splenic infarcts is often referred to the shoulder.

The splenic artery, arising from the coeliac axis, enters the hilum and branches into five or more trabecular arteries which supply segments of the spleen; absence of anastomosis between these branches predisposes to infarction. When subdivisions of the trabecular arteries attain 200 μm diameter they enter the splenic tissue. At about 50 μm diameter the arteries pass into the red pulp to become the straight penicilliary arteries which terminate as capillaries just proximal to the splenic sinuses. In health, half of the splenic mass is composed of lymphocytes. The splenic arterioles are surrounded by a cuff of predominantly T lymphocytes which intersperse the germinal follicles consisting of a central zone with a high proportion of T cells, and an outer zone comprised predominantly of B lymphocytes with plasma cells at the periphery (marginal zone) (*Fig. 16.2*).

The splenic sinuses are composed of endothelial-lined channels and are surrounded by pulp cords which are a meshwork of fibrillary reticulum cells (*Fig. 16.3*). In health most red cells pass directly from the arterial capillaries through the

Fig. 16.2 The relationship of lymphoid tissue to the arterial circulation in the spleen.

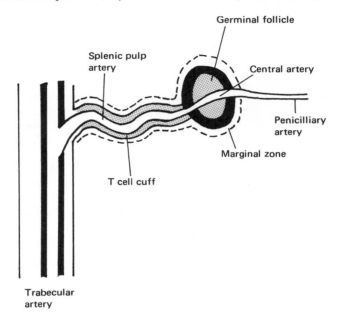

Fig. 16.3. Sinusoidal circulation of the spleen. (Reproduced by courtesy of the publishers of *Hospital Medicine*.)

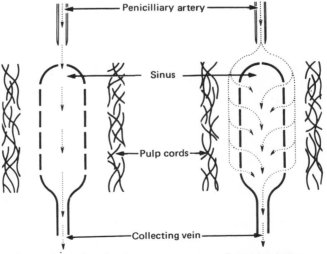

Sinusoidal (closed) pathway
Red cells enter directly into
sinuses from penicilliary artery

Open circulation
Red cells enter sinuses via
slits in walls from pulp cords

sinuses; less than 10 per cent of the red cells enter the pulp cords. To re-enter the circulation the red cells must pass through slits in the sinus walls. In hypersplenism considerable numbers of red cells become 'pooled' in the pulp cords. The sinuses empty into collecting veins, thence via trabecular veins to form the splenic vein at the hilum.

FUNCTIONS OF THE SPLEEN

1. Blood Formation

1.1 Red cells are produced in utero from $3\frac{1}{2}$ to 5 months. In childhood, marrow hyperplasia cannot always meet increased demand, thus splenic extramedullary erythropoiesis may occur readily with chronic haemorrhage, severe haemolysis, polycythaemia associated with cyanotic heart disease and also osteopetrosis and myelofibrosis. In adults, splenic erythropoiesis occurs only in severe anaemias, such as thalassaemia major, acquired haemolytic anaemias and pernicious anaemia; splenic haemopoiesis also occurs in the myeloproliferative disorders (myeloid metaplasia) and with severe marrow infiltration or replacement.

1.2 White cells: neutrophils are produced in utero from $1\frac{1}{2}$ to $6\frac{1}{2}$ months in small numbers. Lymphocytes proliferate in the spleen throughout life.

1.3 Platelets: megakaryocytes are found in utero from $1\frac{1}{2}$ to $6\frac{1}{2}$ months; after that date they are only found in association with myeloid metaplasia and allied disorders, e.g. megakaryocytic myelosis.

2. Reservoir Function

2.1 Red cells: in man the healthy spleen only contains some 20–60 ml of red cells, but in disease 10–20 per cent, and occasionally 40 per cent of the total red cell mass may be present. Reticulocytes are selectively segregated in the spleen possibly because they are covered with transferrin.

2.2 White cells: the spleen does not act as a reservoir for neutrophils, but hypersplenism may be associated with neutropenia as trapped neutrophils are not released from the spleen. The spleen is a large lymphocyte reservoir.

2.3 Platelets: one-third of total platelet mass is present in an exchangeable pool in the spleen. The platelets may be discharged into the circulation when the autonomic sympathetic system is stimulated. Considerable sequestration may occur in immune thrombocytopenic purpura and other causes of hypersplenism.

3. Phagocytosis, Culling and Pitting

Phagocytosis by macrophages in pulp cords with cytoplasmic projections through fenestrations between sinus endothelial cells has been demonstrated by electron microscope (EM) studies. Sinus endothelial cells are not very active in phagocytosis. Bacteria, especially pneumococci and encapsulated gram-negative bacilli, are removed from the circulation. Effete red cells are removed by the reticulo-endothelial cells of the pulp cords as may be neutrophils and platelets. Removal of whole cells has been termed 'culling'. Removal of particles from the cytoplasm of intact red cells has been termed 'pitting', e.g. iron granules of siderocytes and Heinz bodies, Howell–Jolly bodies and malarial parasites.

4. Immune Response

The microcirculation of the spleen enables blood-borne antigens to come into close proximity with lymphoid follicles, where T cells, B cells and antigen-presenting cells can cooperate to initiate an immune response. Infections are prone to occur following splenectomy, more so in childhood and especially before the age of 2 years. Polyvalent pneumococcal vaccine and prophylactic penicillin should be given to all patients following splenectomy. The risk of infection is greater if the underlying disorder necessitating splenectomy is serious, such as thalassaemia major, portal hypertension due to cirrhosis and the Wiskott–Aldrich syndrome, compared with disorders such as hereditary spherocytosis and immune thrombocytopenia.

5. Factor VIII Production

A significant amount of Factor VIII-related antigen may be synthesized by the reticulo-endothelial cells of the spleen.

LYMPHOCYTOSIS

See Chapter 2.

MONOCYTOSIS

See Chapter 2.

INFECTIOUS MONONUCLEOSIS

Infectious mononucleosis may have pronounced haematological effects giving rise to diagnostic difficulties.

Aetiology

Infectious mononucleosis is due to infection with a herpesvirus known as the Ebstein–Barr virus (EBV), usually in late childhood or early adulthood. Infections in young children are usually subclinical. The disease is not highly contagious and the incubation period is often as long as 30–50 days.

Clinical Features

In typical cases there is a prodromal period of non-specific malaise, anorexia and headaches followed after several days by fever, sore throat (often exudative) and lymphadenopathy affecting particularly the posterior cervical nodes and not the occipital nodes (cf. rubella). The spleen is just palpable in 40 per cent of cases, usually in the second and third weeks of the disease. Hepatomegaly is present in about 10 per cent of cases and jaundice in about 5 per cent, but raised transaminases are found in nearly all cases and may be a useful diagnostic pointer. A maculopapular rash is seen in about 10 per cent of cases and may be precipitated by ampicillin administration. Rare complications of infectious mononucleosis include pneumonitis, a variety of neurological manifestations, immune haemolytic anaemia and immune thrombocytopenia.

The EBV genome is found in the tumour cells of Burkitt's lymphoma and nasopharyngeal cancer together with very high anti-EBV antibody titres.

Peripheral Blood Findings

A moderate leucocytosis ($10–20 \times 10^9$/l) usually develops in the second week and may occasionally be as high as 50×10^9/l.

The increased cells are lymphocytes and many have an atypical appearance; the cells are larger than normal lymphocytes, have a lobulated or indented nucleus with a mature condensed chromatin pattern, though nucleoli may be present, and the cytoplasm is basophilic and often foamy or vacuolated. These cells have the phenotype of suppressor T lymphocytes and are Ia positive which probably represents T cell activation. These atypical lymphocytes are also seen in other infections, including toxoplasmosis and cytomegalovirus infections. During the acute phase of infectious mononucleosis there is severe depression of cell-mediated immunity. Occasionally Coombs' positive haemolytic anaemia or immune thrombocytopenia occurs.

Diagnosis

The diagnosis depends on the clinical and haematological findings and the transient appearance of sheep and horse red cell agglutinins and ox cell haemolysins. Antibodies to EBV persist, but are rarely measured. Various commercial screening tests for sheep or horse cell agglutinins are available, e.g. Monospot. A full 'Paul–Bunnell' requires the testing of serial serum dilutions for sheep (or horse) cell agglutinins before and after absorption with guinea pig kidney cells and ox cells. The heterophil antibody is absorbed by ox cells, but not the guinea pig kidney cells. A titre greater than 1 in 16 is diagnostic, but it is usually higher. Heterophil antibodies are present in some normal sera, but these are absorbed by guinea pig cells.

Treatment

Treatment is largely symptomatic. Bed rest is recommended if there is marked hepatitis or splenomegaly. Steroids are given for life-threatening respiratory obstruction, neurological lesions, haemolytic anaemia and immune thrombocytopenia.

LYMPHOPENIA

See Chapter 2.

MONOCYTOPENIA (*see* Chapter 2)

See Chapter 2.

IMMUNODEFICIENCY DISEASES

The major primary immunodeficiency diseases may be classified as follows:
1. Primary B-cell deficiencies
    1.1 X-linked agammaglobulinaemia (Bruton's disease).
    1.2 Selective immunoglobulin deficiencies.
    1.3 Transient hypogammaglobulinaemia of infancy.
2. Primary T-cell deficiencies
    2.1 Wiskott–Aldrich syndrome.
    2.2 Congenital thymic aplasia (Di George's syndrome).
3. Mixed T- and B-cell deficiencies
    3.1 Severe combined immunodeficiency.
    3.2 Hereditary ataxia telangiectasia (defect in cellular immunity and lack of IgA).
    3.3 Common variable unclassifiable immunodeficiency.
4. Complement deficiency diseases
This classification is somewhat arbitrary in that primary T-cell disorders may affect B-cell proliferation and function; the primary defect in many of the above disorders has not been characterized.

LYMPHADENOPATHY

Lymphadenopathy may be classified as shown:
1. Localized lymphadenopathy
    1.1 Infective.
    1.1.1 Acute infections, such as tonsillitis, giving rise to cervical lymphadenopathy.
    1.1.2 Chronic infections, such as cervical TB, cat-scratch disease, lymphogranuloma venereum.
    1.2 Carcinomatous.
    1.3 Lymphomatous. Hodgkin's disease usually presents with localized lymphadenopathy especially in the neck; non-Hodgkin's lymphoma presents less commonly with localized lymphadenopathy.
2. Generalized lymphadenopathy
    2.1 Infections; both acute and chronic.
    Infections may be bacterial (e.g. brucellosis, syphilis) viral (e.g. infectious mononucleosis), rickettsial, fungal (e.g. histoplasmosis) or parasitic (toxoplasmosis).
    2.2 Malignant lymphoreticular disorders (*see* Chapter 17).
    2.3 Autoimmune disorders including immune haemolytic

anaemia (particularly in children), rheumatoid arthritis, systemic lupus erythematosus. A pseudolymphomatous condition is described in association with Sjögren's syndrome.
2.4 Hypersensitivity reactions.
2.5 Sarcoidosis.
2.6 Some storage disease, e.g. Niemann–Pick disease, sea-blue histiocyte syndrome, rarely Gaucher's disease (*see* Chapter 3).
2.7 Dermatopathic lymphadenitis—seen with chronic skin lesions.
2.8 Hyperthyroidism.
2.9 Sinus histiocytosis. A rare disorder presenting mainly in children and young adults with often massive generalized lymphadenopathy especially affecting the neck. Fever and leucocytosis may occur. The condition is usually benign though node enlargement may persist for years.

Clinical Approach to Lymphadenopathy

A thorough history and examination are essential. Particular attention must be paid to the drainage area of localized lymph nodes. Inguinal lymphadenopathy, for example, should prompt a thorough search of leg, buttock, lower abdominal wall, external genitalia and the anal canal. Other lymph node areas and the liver and spleen must be carefully palpated.

All patients should have a full blood count with examination of the blood film (leukaemic cells, atypical mononuclear cells, etc.), liver function tests, a chest radiograph (primary tumour, TB, sarcoid) and syphilis serology. Other investigations are dictated by the site or sites of involvement and the history and examination. For example, hard supraclavicular nodes will prompt barium studies of the upper gastrointestinal tract. Lymph node biopsies should be performed early rather than late. A whole affected gland should be removed and this should be as central as possible. Inguinal node biopsies particularly give equivocal results.

SPLENOMEGALY

This may be classified as follows:
1. Due to abnormalities of the peripheral blood.
    1.1 Red cells, e.g. hereditary spherocytosis, thalassaemia, haemoglobinopathies and autoimmune haemolytic anaemia.
    1.2 White cells, e.g. immune neutropenia (as in SLE) and drug-induced neutropenias.
    1.3 Platelets, e.g. immune thrombocytopenic purpura. The splenomegaly is only slight to moderate.
2. Due to primary splenic disorders.
    2.1 Chronic congestive splenomegaly, e.g. portal cirrhosis, hepatic vein thrombosis (Budd–Chiari syndrome) and portal vein thrombosis.

2.2 Lymphoproliferative disorders, e.g. malignant lymphomas, chronic lymphocytic leukaemia and hairy cell leukaemia.
2.3 Myeloproliferative disorders, e.g. chronic myeloid leukaemia, myelofibrosis and acute myeloid leukaemia.
2.4 Storage disorders
2.5 Infections, e.g. tuberculosis, brucellosis, typhoid, septicaemia and tropical infections.
2.6 Collagen vascular diseases.
2.7 Sarcoidosis.

HYPERSPLENISM

Defined as a reduction of one or more of the cellular components of the peripheral blood which returns to normal following splenectomy. Mechanisms possibly responsible for hypersplenism include:
1. Pooling within the spleen.
2. Reduction of cell life-span.
3. Increase in plasma volume.
4. Decreased cell production in the bone marrow.

Pooling or sequestration within the spleen may be caused by a primary haematological disorder in which the spleen removes abnormal cellular components from the blood, or by a primary splenic disorder responsible for architectural changes altering the splenic circulation; the haematological effects being secondary.

A reduction of cell life span may occur in both types of hypersplenism. Expansion of the plasma volume has been demonstrated in association with many causes of splenomegaly. There is no proven evidence that a hormone produced in the spleen affects marrow activity; however, many systemic disorders producing hypersplenism also may be associated with marrow depression; usually the bone marrow shows compensatory increased cellularity.

BLOOD CHANGES FOLLOWING SPLENECTOMY

Red Cells

Howell–Jolly bodies, siderocytes, leptocytes, including target cells, and the occasional normoblast may be present. After haemorrhage, numerous normoblasts may be seen.

White Cells

Leucocytosis usually reaches a maximum in 3–7 days; commonly $10–15 \times 10^9$/l, but sometimes up to 30×10^9/l. It gradually falls over weeks or months, but occasionally remains high for years. The initial leucocytosis is chiefly due to neutrophils, later to lymphocytes and monocytes. In splenectomized patients infections are often associated with a marked left shift of the neutrophils; myelocytes and also normoblasts may be present in the peripheral blood.

Platelets

Thrombocytosis may occur within a few hours, but may not develop for several days. It may reach a maximum of $2000–3000 \times 10^9/l$ before falling within the normal range over the next few weeks or months. Occasionally a thrombocytosis persists indefinitely.

HYPOSPLENISM

The peripheral blood findings are identical with those occurring after splenectomy.

Aetiology

1. Congenital absence.
2. Sickle-cell disease (resulting from multiple infarcts).
3. Associated with enteropathies—coeliac disease and dermatitis herpetiformis and occasionally with longstanding ulcerative colitis.
4. Idiopathic thrombocythaemia.
5. Spleen may become atrophied in old age.
6. Systemic lupus erythematosus.

ASSESSMENT OF SPLENIC FUNCTION

1. Indirect investigations.
> 1.1 Peripheral blood count: in the presence of splenomegaly, a reduced count of red cells, neutrophils or platelets may suggest hypersplenism.
> 1.2 Determination of the red cell mass by ^{51}Cr technique and plasma volume by ^{125}I-or ^{131}I-labelled albumin.
2. Direct surface counting over the spleen may
> 2.1 Demonstrate 'pooling' uptake curve of hypersplenism
> 2.2 Demonstrate red cell sequestration; the spleen : heart ratio rising to $2:1$ or more if there is significant 'pooling'. There is a poor correlation between the degree of increased splenic counts and the benefit of splenectomy because smaller spleens are counted more efficiently, there is variation of organ depth and absorption of radiation by overlying tissue and because red cell ^{51}Cr loss with subsequent take-up by splenic reticulo-endothelial cells varies widely.
3. Scanning spleen with isotope-labelled spherocytic cells; cells may be heat damaged or chemically damaged. The scanning is carried out by a rectilinear scanner or gamma camera.

4. Clearance of labelled spherocytes (damaged cells) is reduced in hyposplenism; the $T\frac{1}{2}$ is normally 5–15 min.

5. Measurement of splenic red cell volume. Injection of undamaged red cells labelled with $^{99}Tc^m$ or ^{14}C-carbon monoxide using a calibrated dual-headed rectilinear scanner. Splenomegaly due to myelosclerosis, polycythaemia rubra vera or hairy cell leukaemia contain proportionately more red cells than with lymphomas.

6. Transferrin labelled with ^{59}Fe or ^{52}Fe will demonstrate extramedullary erythropoiesis. Normal splenic tissue (like rest of reticulo-endothelial systems) will not take iron from transferrin. In myeloproliferative disorders there is poor correlation between splenic uptake and organ size. In the myeloproliferative disorders, erythropoiesis is ineffective and transferrin-labelled ^{59}Fe uptake by the spleen does not reflect useful haemopoiesis.

Selected Further Reading

Fudenberg H. H., Stites D. P., Caldwell J. L. et al. (1978). *Basic and Clinical Immunology,* 2nd ed. California, Lange.

Reinherz E. L. and Schlossman S. F. (1981) The characterization and function of human immunoregulatory T lymphocyte subsets. *Immunology Today* **2**, 69–75.

Richards J. D. M. (1976) Hypersplenism. *Br. J. Hosp. Med.* **15**, 505.

GENERAL CONSIDERATIONS

The normal response of the lymphoreticular system to antigenic or inflammatory challenge is a proliferative one, but providing the primary cause is apparent and the response is self limiting it does not cause confusion with a malignant disorder (*see* Chapter 16). Occasionally, however, such benign proliferations may be chronic and the distinction of a reactive from a neoplastic state may be very difficult. The demonstration of monoclonality has proved to be a useful criterion of malignancy in B-cell proliferations, but it is not always possible to show this and there are no clonal markers for T cells or

Fig. 17.1. Normal B cell maturation and corresponding malignancies.

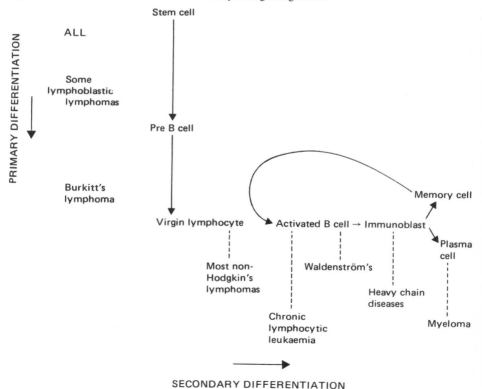

monocytes. Furthermore, there is often a reactive and polyclonal response to a monoclonal malignant proliferation. Frequently, therefore, a diagnosis must be made on the appearance of a lymph node biopsy without pathognomonic features of malignancy. Effacement of normal node architecture, extension beyond the original confines of the node and replacement by uniform or abnormal cells all suggest malignancy, but considerable experience with both normal and diseased tissues is essential.

Malignant change within a cell line results in the accumulation of cells with a common phenotype and this phenotype, which corresponds to a normal developmental stage in that cell line, correlates closely with the disease entity produced. The cell phenotype does not represent the target cell for malignant change, but merely the level of arrested differentiation.

The assignment of some of these malignancies to these positions on the differentiation pathway is controversial. This is particularly true of Burkitt's lymphoma and chronic lymphocytic leukaemia.

Fig. 17.2. Normal T cell maturation and corresponding malignancies.

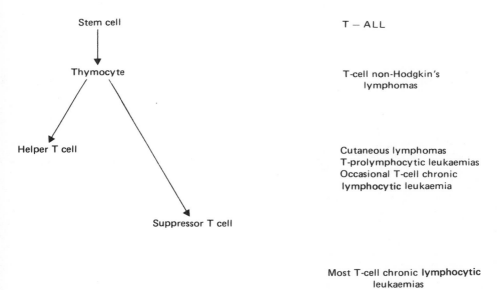

Histiocytes are probably tissue-based monocytes and originate from the bone marrow. The proliferative potential of tissue histiocytes is uncertain as is the developmental sequence.

Most so-called histiocytic lymphomas are really B-cell lymphomas, though occasional true histiocytic lymphomas occur. Histiocytic medullary reticulosis, and Hodgkin's disease may also have a histiocytic derivation.

Those malignant lymphoreticular malignancies that predominantly affect the peripheral blood are referred to as leukaemias and those that affect the tissues as lymphomas though in some cases the distinction is arbitrary. Those B-cell

Fig. 17.3. Normal monocyte maturation and corresponding malignancies.

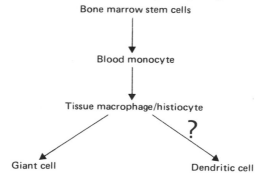

neoplasms that synthesize significant quantities of immunoglobulin are referred to as immunoproliferative disorders and are discussed in Chapter 18. Acute lymphoblastic leukaemia is discussed in Chapter 15.

HODGKIN'S DISEASE

Pathogenesis

Hodgkin's disease is a malignant neoplasm that usually arises in a group of lymph nodes and spreads to other adjacent nodes before metastasizing to non-lymphoid organs. The spread is probably contiguous by the lymphatic channels. The malignant cell in Hodgkin's disease is the Reed–Sternberg giant cell and its mononuclear counterparts, as has been demonstrated by the frequent finding of aneuploidy and clonal marker chromosome abnormalities in these cells. The origin of Reed–Sternberg cells is uncertain, but they are possibly derived from the histiocytic or dendritic cell series; the cells morphologically resemble histiocytes. They have microfibrils and small lysosomes which are seen at electron microscopy; they bear Ia antigen; the cells phagocytose immunoglobulin and they have no monoclonal surface immunoglobulin or other lymphocyte specific markers. They do not, however, exhibit non-specific esterase activity which is usually taken to be a hallmark of monocytic/histiocytic cells. The tumour cells are usually associated with reactive lymphocytes (mainly T lymphocytes), plasma cells, eosinophils, neutrophils, histiocytes and fibroblasts such that the malignant cells are often quite sparse. The cause of Hodgkin's disease is unknown. A viral aetiology has been proposed, but not substantiated.

Incidence

Hodgkin's disease accounts for 45 per cent of all malignant lymphomas in the UK. It is uncommon prior to puberty, but then quickly reaches a plateau between the ages of 20 and 40 years, with a further peak in the elderly. It is more common in males.

Clinical Features

Patients usually present with lymphadenopathy most frequently affecting the cervical nodes. The nodes may be tender or non-tender and grow rapidly, slowly or even fluctuate in size. Alcohol-related pain is very occasionally described. The spleen may be palpable. Constitutional symptoms may be present at diagnosis and include anorexia, weight loss, fever, malaise, sweats and pruritus. Almost any organ can be ultimately affected by Hodgkin's disease so the possible presentations are protean. In general, younger patients tend to present with localized nodes and feel well, and older patients with systemic symptoms and disseminated disease.

Histology

The diagnosis must always be confirmed by biopsy of an affected node. A large central node should be removed in toto and whenever possible nodes from the inguinal area or in the drainage area of a local infection should be avoided. The presence of the Reed–Sternberg cell in a background of reactive cells is central to the diagnosis, but the finding of Reed–Sternberg cells is itself not sufficient to make the diagnosis of Hodgkin's disease.

The Reed–Sternberg cell is characteristically large and binucleate with vesicular nuclei and prominent eosinophilic nucleoli (owl's eyes appearance). The cells may appear to lie in 'laminae' probably due to fixation artefact. The whole node is generally replaced by a mixture of malignant and reactive cells and it is principally the differences in composition of the reactive component on which the histological classification is based (Lukes–Butler):

1. Nodular Sclerosis. This category has two principal characteristics:

      1.1 Frequent occurrence of 'laminar cells'.

      1.2 Subdivision of the node by bands of granulation tissue. This type of Hodgkin's disease is especially common in young women and particularly affects the mediastinal nodes; it has a good prognosis.

2. Lymphocyte Predominant. The large numbers of reactive lymphocytes may obscure the presence of Reed–Sternberg cells and as the nodal architecture may be partially preserved, the correct diagnosis may be overlooked. The prognosis of this variant is favourable.

3. Lymphocyte Depleted. The effaced nodes contain large numbers of Reed–Sternberg type cells and few reactive lymphocytes. Extensive fibrosis and necrosis may be present. The prognosis is poor.

4. Mixed Cellularity. This variant is somewhere between the lymphocyte-predominant and lymphocyte-depleted variants. The abnormal mononuclear and giant Reed–Sternberg cells are readily seen and there are reactive lymphocytes, neutrophils, eosinophils and plasma cells. The prognosis is intermediate.

Within individual patients there is a tendency to progress to a more malignant histological variety:

Lymphocyte predominance $\longrightarrow$ Mixed cellularity $\longrightarrow$ Lymphocyte depleted

Other Investigations

Anaemia is present in one-third and does not invariably indicate marrow involvement. In advanced disease haemolysis may be present, usually but not always associated with a positive direct antiglobulin test (DAT). The neutrophil and sometimes the eosinophil count may be raised in active disease, though the neutrophil count may be low if there is extensive marrow infiltration or hypersplenism.

There may be thrombocytopenia related to marrow replacement, hypersplenism or occasionally an immune thrombocytopenia.

The serum albumin is often low and the serum globulin raised. Rarely a nephrotic syndrome occurs.

The serum calcium and alkaline phosphatase are occasionally raised.

There is often a deficit of cell-mediated immunity even in early stages of the disease. Low total T-cell numbers defined by sheep red blood cell rosetting have been reported, but is probably due to a serum factor rather than a primary lymphocyte abnormality. The response of T cells to mitogens such as PHA is reduced, however, as are delayed hypersensitivity reactions. The mixed lymphocyte reaction is reported to be low by some groups and may be due to inhibitory monocytes. Whatever the significance of these in vitro results there is in vivo an increased susceptibility to certain bacterial, viral (particularly herpes zoster) and fungal infections.

Staging

Accurate staging gives a good guide to prognosis and indicates the appropriate therapy. The Ann Arbor staging system is usually used.

Stage I. Single lymph node region or a single extra-lymphatic organ or site (I_E).

Stage II. Two or more node regions on one side of the diaphragm or one node region plus one extra-lymphatic site on the same side of the diaphragm (II_E).

Stage III. Nodes on both sides of the diaphragm which may be accompanied by extralymphatic involvement (III_E), splenic involvement (III_S) or both (III_{SE}).

Stage IV. Diffuse or disseminated involvement of one or more extralymphatic organs.

Each stage is divided into A or B according to the absence or presence of systemic symptoms. These include a sustained fever (over 38 °C), night sweats and weight loss of more than 10 per cent in 6 months. Pruritus does not merit a B classification.

Staging includes a thorough history and examination, including inspection of Waldeyer's ring. A chest radiograph and lymphangiogram are usually performed if there are no contraindications to the latter (chronic obstructive airways disease, previous radiotherapy to the lungs, right-to-left shunts, pregnancy, iodide sensitivity). A bone marrow aspirate and biopsy should be performed. Liver and spleen scans, abdominal ultrasound and computerized axial tomography may be performed according to local preference and availability; even so the accuracy of such staging is poor. Only half of the palpable spleens are histologically involved and histological involvement of the spleen is present in 25 per cent of cases without splenomegaly; lymphangiography gives false positive results and does not visualize the high para-aortic glands; all non-invasive techniques are poor at detecting diffuse hepatic involvement without hepatomegaly. A surgical laparotomy including splenectomy, wedge and needle biopsy of the liver and multiple nodal biopsy (para-aortic, iliac, coeliac, mesenteric) should therefore be performed, *providing* the information obtained will dictate the therapy given; the aim being to give the minimum treatment that offers the maximum chance of cure. Staging laparotomy results in a change of stage in approximately one-third of patients. When to perform a staging laparotomy is thus dictated by the treatment policy in a given centre, but in general it is performed on patients with Stage I→IIIA in whom radiation therapy can be considered as the optimal initial treatment. A further advantage of splenectomy is that it reduces the radiation field required and prevents the possible development of hypersplenism.

Treatment

1. Radiotherapy. Megavoltage therapy is the treatment of choice for most cases staged as I–IIIA; 35–40 Gy (3500–4000 rad) are given in divided doses over a period of 4–5 weeks. An extended field is used to irradiate those nodes contiguous with the involved nodes, such that a 'mantle field' is used to treat supradiaphragmatic disease Stages I and II and an 'inverted Y field' to treat infradiaphragmatic disease Stages I and II. An additional field area is frequently added to the inverted Y to include the splenic bed (*Fig. 17.4*). The relapse rate for Stages

Fig. 17.4. Radiotherapy fields in Hodgkin's disease.

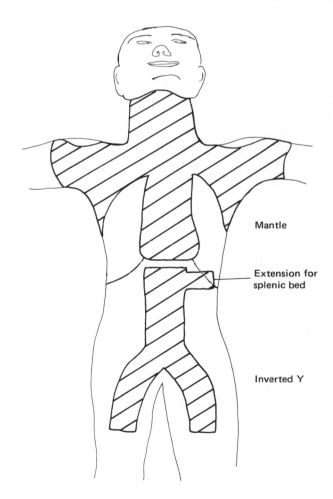

Mantle

Extension for splenic bed

Inverted Y

IB and IIB is higher than for Stages IA and IIA which are usually cured by such treatment and most centres therefore irradiate the para-aortic nodes for 'B' subjects as well as the mantle field in supradiaphragmatic disease. For Stage IIIA total nodal irradiation (mantle and inverted Y) is used. Mantle treatment is very well tolerated though dryness of the throat, epilation in the posterior cervical region and oesophagitis frequently occur to the end of therapy. Some pneumonitis is inevitable, but does not usually cause clinical problems. Infradiaphragmatic irradiation is generally less well tolerated and irradiation of the cord may cause transient paraesthesiae. With total nodal irradiation, thrombocytopenia and neutropenia may occur and rarely necessitate the interruption of treatment.

2. Chemotherapy

2.1 Initial Definitive Therapy. Combination chemotherapy is routinely used as initial therapy for Stages IIIB and IV disease and for those relapsing after radiotherapy. Some centres have also used chemotherapy as first line treatment for Stages IIB and IIIA disease.

Mustine hydrochloride	$6\,\text{mg/m}^2$	(Days 1 and 8)
Vincristine	$1\cdot4\,\text{mg/m}^2$	(Days 1 and 8)
Procarbazine	$100\,\text{mg/m}^2$	(Days 1–14)
Prednisone	$50\,\text{mg/m}^2$	(Days 1–14; often only first and fourth cycles)

This course of therapy (MOPP) is given monthly, usually for a total of 6 courses. There is no evidence that further 'maintenance' reduces the relapse rate. Chemotherapy is much less well tolerated than radiotherapy; mustine-induced nausea and vomiting may be severe, hair loss occurs in 30 per cent (always reversible) and paraesthesiae frequently occur due to vincristine toxicity. Procarbazine has a monoamine oxidase inhibitory effect and patients must be warned not to take alcohol, narcotics, antihistamines, tranquillizers, sympathomimetics, etc. during therapy. Most men are rendered azoospermic and semen should be cryopreserved in those who have not yet completed their families.

A complete remission is obtained in approximately 80 per cent of cases (nearly 100 per cent of those with only A symptoms). Even after a radiation treatment relapse, 50 per cent of cases will have a prolonged remission with MOPP or an equivalent regime.

2.2 Tumour Reduction prior to Radiotherapy. Chemotherapy is also used to reduce large mediastinal nodes that cannot be encompassed within a mantle field prior to radiotherapy.

2.3 Relief of Vital Structures. Where there is pressure on a vital organ a large single dose of mustine hydrochloride will often relieve symptoms very rapidly.

3. Combined Modality Treatment. Low-dose radiotherapy followed by MOPP may be useful in the treatment of children as it will not retard axial bone growth, but in general a cautionary approach should be adopted to the use of adjuvant chemotherapy to radiotherapy. Longer survival has not yet been demonstrated, the response of radiation-treated relapses to chemotherapy is still good, the morbidity of chemotherapy is greater than radiotherapy and there appears to be an increased incidence of leukaemia and non-Hodgkin's lymphoma in those who have received combined modality treatment.

4. Salvage Chemotherapy after MOPP Failure. If relapse occurs after a remission of more than 1 year a further complete remission may be obtained with MOPP in 40 per cent of cases. If the remission was less than 1 year a potentially non cross-resistant regime should be tried, the most common one used being ABVD (adriamycin, bleomycin, vinblastine, imidazole carboxamide). The majority respond and a few have a sustained complete remission.

Prognosis

Overall, the 10-year survival is about 60 per cent. Stages I and II, nodular sclerosis and lymphocyte-predominant histology and a normal haemoglobin are good prognostic features. Stages III and IV, the presence of B symptoms and lymphocyte-depleted histology are inter-related poor prognostic features, but even in Stages IIIB and IV over half of those who enter a complete remission will be alive at 10 years. Of all relapses 80–90 per cent occur in the first 2 years and 95 per cent of those alive and well at 5 years will be cured.

NON-HODGKIN'S LYMPHOMAS (NHL)

Pathogenesis

No aetiological agent can be implicated in most cases of NHL though certain factors are known to predispose to its development.

1. Immunodeficiency disorders including:

   1.1 Primary immunodeficiency states.

   1.2 Immunosuppressed patients, particularly after renal transplantation.

   1.3 Collagen vascular diseases, such as systemic lupus erythematosus and rheumatoid arthritis. The increased risk is small.

Chronic antigenic stimulation may be the common factor and it is interesting that α heavy chain disease may initially be 'benign' in that it will occasionally respond to antibiotic therapy (*see* Chapter 18). 'Immunoblastic lymphadenopathy' is often associated with drug allergies or auto-immune diseases and in about 20 per cent of cases progresses to a frank malignancy.

2. Irradiation. An increased incidence of NHL was seen after the atom bomb at Hiroshima and after irradiation for ankylosing spondylitis. The increased risk only appears after relatively heavy exposure.

3. Chemical carcinogens have been implicated by some, but firm data is generally lacking.

4. Viruses.

   4.1 The Ebstein–Barr virus (EBV) has been implicated in the case of African type Burkitt's lymphoma. African Burkitt's lymphoma and EBV infection have been linked by sero-epidemiological studies, and EB viral DNA and an EBV-associated nuclear antigen are found in the cells of these lymphomas. Although the data is compelling the case is not fully proven.

   4.2 In the X-linked immunoproliferative syndrome there is an apparent inability to cope with EBV infection leading to a progressive (? malignant) lymphoreticular proliferation.

5. Chromosomal alterations. The NHLs usually have a diploid chromosome number (cf. hyperploidy in Hodgkin's disease) and over half of the B-cell lymphomas have translocations involving chromosome 14. In Burkitt's lymphoma, the donor chromosome is No. 8, but no consistent pattern is observed in the other types of NHL.

Incidence

There are approximately 5 cases per 100 000/year. It is slightly more common in males. There is a pre-adolescent peak followed by a late teenage nadir and then a logarithmic increase with age.

Clinical Features

The majority of patients have obvious lymphadenopathy at presentation. Spread is not contiguous via the lymphatic channels as in Hodgkin's disease so that patterns of nodal involvement are not predictable. Widespread disease with hepatomegaly and splenomegaly are common at diagnosis. Patients with 'low-grade histological disease' tend to present with few symptoms whereas patients with 'high-grade histological disease', tend to be symptomatic with fever, anorexia, malaise, abdominal pains, etc.

Laboratory Investigations

Anaemia is not uncommon and may result from haemorrhage (thrombocytopenia), hypersplenism, auto-immune haemolysis which is more common than in Hodgkin's disease, but less common than in chronic lymphatic leukaemia, and from marrow replacement. Neutropenia and thrombocytopenia occur for similar reasons and may be exacerbated by therapy.

Hypoalbuminaemia and hypergammaglobulinaemia are common, especially in the small lymphocytic and small cleaved cell lymphomas. M bands are seen in approximately 15 per cent of these cases compared to 7 per cent in CLL and 3 per cent in the large-cell lymphomas.

In the early stages of NHL there is little increased susceptibility to infection or evidence of an impaired immune response, but this becomes apparent as the disease progresses.

Histological and Immunological Classification

The classification of NHL is far from simple and the large number of histopathological classifications available is a reflection of this.

The Rappaport classification has been most widely used and an early version of it is tabulated below. This classification recognizes that follicular or nodular lymphomas have a better prognosis than diffuse lymphomas, and that the same applies for tumours composed of well-differentiated cells with the appearance of lymphocytes rather than histiocytes.

Rappaport Classification of Lymphomas

Favourable prognosis
  Nodular well-differentiated lymphocytic (NWDL)
  Diffuse well-differentiated lymphocytic (DWDL)
  Nodular poorly-differentiated lymphocytic (NPDL)
  Nodular mixed lymphocytic-histiocytic (NM)

Unfavourable prognosis
  Nodular histiocytic (NH)
  Diffuse poorly-differentiated lymphocytic (DPDL)
  Diffuse mixed (DM)
  Diffuse histiocytic (DH)
  Diffuse undifferentiated
    (Burkitt's and non-Burkitt's type) (DU)

This classification has been criticized on several grounds. First, it does not relate in a rational way to the morphological or immunological phenotypes of the normal cell counterparts. The well-differentiated lymphocytic lymphomas consist of small–medium-sized lymphocytes with few atypical forms and very few mitoses. The cell is identical to that of chronic lymphocytic leukaemia and probably represents an early immunosecretory B cell. It is virtually never truly nodular and apparent nodularity should raise the suspicion of lymphocytic predominant Hodgkin's disease. Nodular lymphomas arise from cells like those seen in normal lymph node follicles: small B cells (larger than in DWDL) with variation of nuclear size and shape with frequent notches or clefts and usually a single distinct nucleolus; and larger B cells with vesicular nuclei, prominent nucleoli and amorphic cytoplasm which may appear syncytial. Thus, all the nodular histiocytic lymphomas are 'activated B cells' and not monocyte/histiocyte derived. Of the diffuse histiocytic lymphomas about 60 per cent are of B cell origin, 10–15 per cent of T-cell origin and the remainder are nearly all unclassifiable. True histiocytic lymphomas with appropriate enzymes within the cells account for only a small percentage. They are particularly common in the gut lymphomas complicating coeliac disease.

Secondly, the DPDL group and the DH group account for approximately 20 per cent and 30 per cent of all cases respectively and both of these groups are heterogeneous. The DPDL group contains tumours composed of small cleaved cells as seen in the follicular lymphomas and also tumours composed of lymphoblasts like those seen in lymphoblastic leukaemia. Most of these tumours have convoluted cells which are of early T-cell phenotype and often present with mediastinal masses. The non-convoluted lymphoblastic tumours consist of both T- and B-cell tumours. Lymphoblastic lymphomas in adults have a very poor prognosis. The DH category contains tumours with large cells and also tumours with large cells showing immunoblastic differentiation, the latter having a poor prognosis.

To overcome some of these problems with the Rappaport and other classifications an expert international panel has proposed a working formulation for the NHL.

New Formulation of NHL

	Rappaport equivalent	
Low grade		
Small lymphocytic	WDL	Favourable prognosis
Follicular predominantly small cleaved	NPDL	
Follicular mixed small cleaved and large cells	NM	

Intermediate grade
Follicular predominantly large cell   NH ⎫
Diffuse small cleaved cell   DPDL ⎪
Diffuse mixed small and large cell   DM ⎪
Diffuse large cell   DH ⎪   Unfavourable
High grade   ⎬   prognosis
Large cell—immunoblastic   DH ⎪
Lymphoblastic—convoluted   DPDL ⎪
         —non-convoluted   ⎪
Small non-cleaved cell   DU ⎭

Miscellaneous, including mycosis fungoides,
composite lymphomas

The small (larger than small lymphocyte lymphomas) non-cleaved lymphomas include both Burkitt's and non-Burkitt's varieties. The cells are monomorphic, 15–25 μm in size with round or oval nuclei with a prominent nuclear membrane and 2–5 prominent basophilic nucleoli. The cells may appear cohesive, but each cell has a distinct rim of amorphic/basophilic and intensely pyrininophilic cytoplasm with vacuole-like spaces within it. Interspersing with benign macrophages gives the characteristic but not pathognomonic (also seen in lymphoblastic lymphomas) 'starry sky' appearance. The non-Burkitt's small non-cleaved cell lymphomas tend to have a degree of nuclear variation and pleomorphism, but there is no uniformity as to the diagnosis of Burkitt's lymphomas. In Europe, the term Burkitt's lymphoma usually implies the 'African variety' with Ebstein–Barr virus nuclear antigen within the cells and surface immunoglobulin and C_3 receptors on the surface. In America the term is applied to similarly appearing tumours which have no EBV antigen and often no surface immunoglobulin or C_3 receptors.

Reactive elements are less pronounced than in Hodgkin's disease, but do occur particularly in some of the immunoblastic lymphomas. In a rare subgroup of the mixed small- and large-cell lymphomas which have immunoblastic differentiation there are plentiful eosinophils and plasma cells and there is often an associated monoclonal or polyclonal gammopathy with severe systemic symptoms. Even in a B-cell follicular lymphoma up to 40 per cent of the cells in a diseased node suspension may be T cells.

Staging

The Ann Arbor staging system is used as for Hodgkin's disease, though it is clinically less useful in the NHL. The majority of patients are Stage III or IV at diagnosis, and localized disease is most common in the large-cell lymphomas despite the fact that these tumours generally have a worse prognosis than the small-cell lymphomas. Staging includes thorough examination with inspection of Waldeyer's ring (involved in 25 per cent), full blood count, liver function tests, chest radiograph and usually liver and bone scans. Abdominal ultrasound and CAT scans are used where available. A lymphangiogram will be positive in about half of patients with follicular lymphomas previously thought to be localized (Stage I or II), in most cases of diffuse small-cell lymphomas, but in less than 10 per cent of apparently localized diffuse large-cell lymphomas. A liver biopsy is positive in about 20 per cent of cases and a bone marrow biopsy is positive in about 10 per cent of large-cell lymphomas and 30–50 per cent of the remainder.

Unless local radiotherapy is being considered or the patient is being entered into a trial in which knowledge of patient comparability is essential, the more invasive investigations such as liver biopsy and lymphangiography may be omitted as they will not affect therapy.

Laparotomy should only be performed to make the diagnosis in local abdominal disease, if there are local gut problems that merit surgical attention in disseminated disease, or in the rare localized supradiaphragmatic disease in which radiotherapy alone is deemed to be appropriate definitive therapy.

Treatment

Patients with low-grade disease should not be treated unless they are symptomatic or have functional impairments (e.g. anaemia, deranged liver function tests) as there may be long periods of relatively static disease and there is no evidence that early treatment prolongs survival. Patients with intermediate or high-grade disease are usually symptomatic, the disease progresses rapidly and treatment should be started as soon as possible. The optimal therapy for the NHL is not defined and many different regimes are in use.

1. Radiotherapy

1.1 Follicular Lymphomas. In patients with follicular lymphomas Stages I–III, good results can be obtained with radiotherapy, providing an adequate dose and field is employed.

1.2 Localized Diffuse NHL. In adults this is mainly large-cell lymphomas. Pathological Stages I and IE are as highly curable with either radiotherapy or chemotherapy alone whereas the results of treating Stages II and IIE with radiotherapy are considerably less good than with chemotherapy. Many centres argue that chemotherapy is the optimum treatment for all cases as the number of patients with Stages I and IE are small and many extensive staging procedures can be avoided. In childhood lymphomas Stages I and IE affecting the head and neck chemotherapy (with or without radiotherapy) should be given whereas resectable abdominal lymphomas can be adequately treated with whole abdominal irradiation (24 Gy; 2400 rad).

1.3 Local Control. Radiotherapy will produce excellent local control of troublesome tumours in patients with advanced disease, but its precise role in patients also receiving chemotherapy is yet to be defined.

2. Chemotherapy

2.1 Low-grade Histology. Single agent therapy with chlorambucil (2–4 mg/day) or cyclophosphamide, or combination chemotherapy regimes such as COP (*see below*) produce a satisfactory response in most patients.

Cyclophosphamide	400 mg/m^2 p.o.	(Days 1–5)
Vincristine	1·4 mg/m^2 i.v.	(Day 1)
Prednisone	100 mg/m^2 p.o.	(Days 1–5)

The above regime given every 21 days produces a response in 90 per cent and a complete remission in about 50 per cent. The majority of patients ultimately relapse and this is often associated with transition to more unfavourable histology.

2.2 Diffuse Small Cleaved Cell Lymphomas. COP produces few complete remissions (about 15 per cent) but the addition of adriamycin (CHOP) or adriamycin and bleomycin (BACOP) gives better complete response rates—50–80 per cent.

2.3 Large-cell Lymphomas. Pathological stages I and IE may be curable with radiotherapy, but more advanced stages require combination chemotherapy. Combinations should include an anthracycline, but the value of cyclophosphamide is less clear cut than in the diffuse small cleaved cell lymphomas. CHOP is the most commonly used regime and a typical intensive regime is shown below.

Cyclophosphamide	$750\,mg/m^2$ i.v.	(Days 1 and 8)
Adriamycin	$25\,mg/m^2$ i.v.	(Days 1 and 8)
Vincristine	$1{\cdot}4\,mg/m^2$ i.v.	(Days 1 and 8)
Prednisone	$100\,mg/m^2$ p.o.	(Days 1–5)

Complete remission rates between 40 and 70 per cent have been obtained. Bleomycin, high-dose methotrexate and cytosine arabinoside have been added to this basic regime in varying doses and combinations and excellent results have been obtained in small series.

2.4 Lymphoblastic Lymphomas. Anti-leukaemia type therapy is used, employing combinations of drugs such as vincristine, prednisone and adriamycin, with intrathecal methotrexate and cytosine arabinoside as cranial prophylaxis.

2.5 Small Non-cleaved Cell Lymphomas. Some of the best results in Burkitt's lymphoma have been achieved with regimes not employing an anthracycline. The following regime was described by Ziegler et al. (COMP).

Cyclophosphamide	$1\,g/m^2$ i.v.	(Day 1)
Vincristine	$1{\cdot}4\,mg/m^2$ i.v.	(Day 1)
Prednisolone	$1\,g/m^2$ i.v.	(Days 1–5)
Methotrexate	$12{\cdot}5\,mg/m^2$ i.v.	(Days 1, 3, 4)
Methotrexate	$12{\cdot}5\,mg/m^2$ i.t.	(Days 2 and 5)

The best treatment for non-Burkitt's small-cell lymphoma has not been clearly defined, but either COMP or CHOP may be used.

Maintenance Chemotherapy. Continuation of chemotherapy when in complete remission has not yet been shown to be of value and most centres stop treatment several courses after complete remission is obtained. The continued relapses in patients with low-grade histological disease suggest that some form of maintenance would be of value, though no evidence of this has been obtained.

2.7 First-line Therapy Failures. Patients who do not respond to one of the primary induction regimes are unlikely to survive 2 years. None the less, regimes such as M-BACOD (as BACOP with methotrexate and dexamethasone instead of prednisone) are usually tried in CHOP failure. Failure of nodes to respond should always raise the suspicion of concomitant tuberculosis or fungal infection.

3. Combined Modality Therapy. Combined radiotherapy and chemotherapy is used in many clinical settings in the NHL. The reason is mainly historical in that chemotherapy was added on to radiotherapy which was already known to be partially successful. There have been few studies to determine whether adjuvant radiotherapy is of any value when combination chemotherapy is given.

Prognosis

Patients with low-grade histological disease have a favourable prognosis with a median survival of approximately 7 years, yet the disease is nearly always disseminated at presentation, is at present incurable and most patients eventually die of their disease. In the higher grade histological diseases most patients used to die within 2 years, but intensive therapy has produced more encouraging results. Many studies suggest that complete remission rates in excess of 50 per cent can be obtained and that a high proportion of these patients will still be disease-free at 2 years. Survival curves appear to plateau, suggesting that many of these patients are cured. In the British National Lymphoma Investigation study of poor prognosis histology lymphomas treated with CHOP the complete remission rate was approximately 50 per cent and the projected 5-year survival approximately 25 per cent. These results are less satisfactory than some smaller studies and probably reflect the means of patient selection and differences in histologically grading some tumours.

Childhood Lymphomas

The phenotype of childhood lymphomas differs from that of adults with childhood tumours generally having a more immature cell type. Lymphoblastic lymphomas with an early thymic phenotype account for one-third of cases and 30–40 per cent of cases are composed of small non-cleaved lymphocytes. These small non-cleaved (undifferentiated) lymphoma cells are B cells with variable surface immunoglobulin and C_3 receptor expression. It has been suggested that the normal counterpart is a primary undifferentiated B cell whereas in the adult most B cell lymphoma counterparts are found on the secondary differentiation pathway. Childhood lymphomas do not secrete paraproteins. Diffuse large-cell lymphomas occur in childhood, but follicular lymphomas are virtually never encountered (always suspect nodular Hodgkin's disease).

The different histological types typically present in different ways. Lymphoblastic lymphomas present with supradiaphragmatic disease, often with mediastinal involvement; African Burkitt's lymphomas have a predilection for the jaw, but other types of small non-cleaved lymphoma tend to present with abdominal disease; the diffuse large-cell lymphomas present with disease of the gut, Waldeyer's ring and other extranodal sites. Extranodal disease is thus common and the tumours of all types usually proliferate rapidly.

The childhood lymphomas are potentially curable with appropriate radiotherapy or combination chemotherapy regimes (*see* previous section) and overall actuarial survivals of 60–80 per cent at 5 years have been reported. Burkitt's lymphoma remains a poor prognosis disease. Cranial prophylaxis is usually given in childhood NHL as this is a common site of relapse.

CUTANEOUS T-CELL LYMPHOMAS

Pathogenesis

This category of lymphomas includes mycosis fungoides and the Sezary syndrome which is essentially a leukaemic variant of mycosis fungoides. T cell CLL which may be associated with cutaneous infiltration is considered as a separate disorder. The malignant cell in both mycosis fungoides and the Sezary syndrome is a T cell which bears the Fc receptor for IgM and stains positively with monoclonal antisera for helper/inducer T cells. The disease is relatively marrow sparing and it should be noted that the majority of normal bone marrow T cells stain with monoclonal antisera against suppressor/cytotoxic T cells. The malignant cells have been shown at least in some cases to be capable of promoting the differentiation of B cells into plasma cells. Mycosis fungoides often begins as a non-specific eczematous eruption and there is considerable controversy as to whether this is a premalignant phase or the first manifestation of malignancy.

Clinical Features

The cutaneous T-cell lymphomas occur most commonly in middle-aged males. Mycosis fungoides typically starts as non-specific scaly eruptions and progresses to plaques, tumours and fungating ulcers. In the early stages the lesions may fluctuate and tend to regress when exposed to sunlight: In the later stages there may be generalized erythroderma. Lymphadenopathy is common, but hepatosplenomegaly is rare unless there is a leukaemic element (Sezary syndrome). Fever occurs in the advanced stages of the disease. In the Sezary syndrome, there is leukaemia, lymphadenopathy and hepatosplenomegaly with infiltration of the skin. There is typically an exfoliative erythroderma often affecting the face, palms and soles; it is highly pruritic.

Peripheral Blood

In the Sezary syndrome there is a leucocytosis varying between 10 and $250 \times 10^9/l$, and the leukaemic cells have a distinctive morphological appearance; they are typically large mononuclear cells with large hyperchromatic grooved and folded nuclei with a small rim of cytoplasm; the nucleus appears cerebriform on electron microscopy. A small cell variant may also be seen. Similar cells can also be seen in the blood in mycosis fungoides if a thorough search is made. There is often a moderate eosinophilia.

Skin Biopsy

Biopsies of affected skin in both mycosis fungoides and the Sezary syndrome are indistinguishable with infiltration of tumour cells in the dermis and the presence of 'Pautrier's microabscesses'.

Treatment

Mycosis fungoides apparently localized to the skin can be treated with topical nitrogen mustard, topical steroids, psoralens and long-wave ultraviolet light or electron beam therapy. If visceral involvement is apparent or skin lesions fail to respond to local therapy then systemic chemotherapy is given. Single agents such as cyclophosphamide, methotrexate and vincristine have been used as has combination chemotherapy (COP). There is little comparative data on these treatment regimes. In the Sezary syndrome traditional treatment is with chlorambucil (2–6 mg/day) and prednisone. Leucopheresis will reduce a high white count and ameliorate the skin lesions though the effect is temporary.

Prognosis

The cutaneous T-cell lymphomas are eventually fatal and once a histological diagnosis of mycosis fungoides has been made the median survival is approximately 5 years. The prognosis is much worse if there is obvious visceral involvement. Septicaemia is the commonest cause of death despite a usually normal neutrophil count.

CHRONIC LYMPHOCYTIC LEUKAEMIA (CLL)

Pathogenesis

The incidence of CLL is increased in some families and in those with either congenital or acquired immune deficiencies. The incidence of CLL is not increased by ionizing radiation. The vast majority of CLLs are B-cell neoplasms; the cells bear monoclonal surface immunoglobulin (light chain restricted) which is usually IgM with or without IgD. The density of surface immunoglobulin is usually low and the cells also have receptors for C_3 and the Fc portion of IgG. This phenotype probably corresponds to an early immunosecretory B cell though this is not certain.

Incidence

CLL accounts for 25 per cent of all leukaemias in the UK. It is nearly twice as common in men and occurs mainly in the elderly.

Clinical Features

CLL typically presents with insidious onset of anaemia and lymphadenopathy. Many cases are discovered on an incidental blood test. Splenomegaly occurs but is less prominent than in chronic granulocytic leukaemia and hepatomegaly is generally a late feature. There is an increased incidence of bacterial infections. Haemorrhagic complications usually indicate advanced disease.

Staging

The Rai staging system has gained general acceptance though it is of limited value.
Stage 0. No physical signs; peripheral blood lymphocyte count $10 \times 10^9/l$ or higher (immunology important in doubtful cases). Marrow aspirate must be > 30–40 per cent lymphocytes. Biopsy to confirm diffuse infiltration.
Stage I. Lymphocytes $> 10 \times 10^9/l$ plus palpable nodes—multiple small nodes at several sites or two or more larger nodes at one or more sites.
Stage II. Blood and marrow as above plus palpable spleen $\pm$ liver. Nodes palpable or not.
Stage III. Blood and marrow as above plus Hb $< 10\,g/dl$ (excluding iron deficiency, haemolysis or megaloblastic change). Physical signs as I or II or absent.
Stage IV. Blood and marrow as above, but platelets $< 100 \times 10^9/l$ (excluding autoimmune thrombocytopenia). Physical signs as I or II or absent.

Laboratory Features

There is frequently a normocytic anaemia though this is usually mild unless there is advanced disease or autoimmune haemolytic anaemia. Autoimmune haemolytic anaemia occurs in 5–10 per cent of cases and a positive Coombs' test can be detected at some stage in up to 25 per cent of cases. The lymphocyte count is usually markedly raised (30–$300 \times 10^9/l$). Most of the lymphocytes are unremarkable except that there are usually a few larger cells and prolymphocytes and a large number of smudge cells. The platelet count only drops with advanced disease unless there is an immune thrombocytopenia.

The bone marrow is heavily infiltrated and in advanced stages there may be an increase of mast cells and some megaloblastoid erythropoiesis. Biopsy of an involved lymph node is identical to a small lymphocytic cell lymphoma (*see* NHL secretion).

About 35 per cent of cases have hypogammaglobulinaemia and this may be present at diagnosis. M bands are found in 3–5 per cent of cases and these are usually IgM in type. Problems with hyperviscosity or cryoprecipitation are rare. Cell-mediated immunity is also reduced, but the absolute number of T cells is often increased. These cells mainly have a suppressor cell phenotype as defined by monoclonal antisera and have Fc receptors for IgG.

Treatment

Asymptomatic static disease, Stages 0–II, does not require therapy. Symptoms, or progression of the disease, should be treated early. Chlorambucil 2–6 mg/day is often effective therapy. Prednisone 20–40 mg/day is sometimes also given and is very useful for the control of immune haemolysis. In good responders it is often possible to stop treatment, and aggressive therapy to obtain a complete remission should not be attempted. In non-responders, combination chemotherapy with cyclophosphamide, vincristine and prednisone is usually tried. Ultimately all patients suffer haematological and immunological deterioration that is unresponsive to chemotherapy and fractionated total body irradiation may have a role in this situation.

Prognosis

The mean survival is about 5 years. Patients with Stages 0 and I disease may survive 10 years or more whereas most Stages III and IV disease are dead within 2 years.

CHRONIC LYMPHOCYTIC LEUKAEMIA VARIANTS

1. T Cell CLL

Probably 1–3 per cent of CLLs are T-cell neoplasms. The cells are morphologically mature, but sometimes have nuclear indentations or numerous cytoplasmic azurophilic granules; they usually stain with suppressor/cytotoxic T-cell subset antisera. If T-cell prolymphocytic leukaemias are excluded the white count is usually only moderately raised and in the absence of marked organomegaly a diagnosis of malignancy may be difficult as there are no clonal markers for T cells. Many cases of supposed T-CLL are probably benign proliferations. Massive splenomegaly and cutaneous infiltration are sometimes seen. The bone marrow tends to be only moderately infiltrated compared to B-CLL yet profound anaemias or neutropenias are common; this may represent immune suppression. The prognosis overall is good, with many patients having a remarkably static course. Occasionally a Richter-like syndrome or 'blast crisis' may develop.

2. Prolymphocytic Leukaemia

This is an unusual variant of CLL in which the characteristic cell in the blood is a relatively large lymphoid cell with a large prominent nucleolus, relatively well-condensed nuclear chromatin and a moderate amount of cytoplasm. Both T and B cell cases occur. The B cell cases have denser surface immunoglobulin than in the usual B-CLL and they do not form rosettes with mouse red blood cells. Some T cell cases have both helper and suppressor markers on the cell surface; other cases have a more mature phenotype The disease tends to present with a very high lymphocyte count, massive splenomegaly and very little, if any, lymphadenopathy. The response to usual CLL therapy is poor and splenectomy may be of value in some cases. Survival after diagnosis is in most cases quite short. In the terminal stages of B-CLL, cells with similar appearances (prolymphocytoid) accumulate in the blood. These cells, however, maintain the same phenotype as the original B-CLL lymphocyte.

HAIRY-CELL LEUKAEMIA

Pathogenesis

The nature of the pathognomonic hairy cell remains obscure. The cells have features common to monocytes, B lymphocytes, T lymphocytes and null cells though they are probably of B-cell origin. The cells are adherent, weakly phagocytic, and have strong Fc receptors for IgG; they are strongly Ia positive and they synthesize and secrete immunoglobulin; in occasional cases the cells bear the sheep red blood cell receptor (E^+) and this can be expressed in vitro in other cases after stimulation with phytohaemagglutinin. No aetiological factors have been clearly identified.

Clinical Features

This uncommon disease typically occurs in middle age. It is four times more common in males. Most patients present with the non-specific symptoms of weakness, shortness of breath and weight loss; others present with infections or haemorrhage. Splenomegaly is almost invariable, but hepatomegaly occurs in less than half and lymphadenopathy is unusual.

Laboratory Features

Pancytopenia is characteristic. The anaemia is often macrocytic. The neutrophil and monocyte counts are nearly always reduced, but eosinophil numbers are normal. Hairy cells can usually be found in the peripheral blood and sometimes there are sufficient numbers to cause a leucocytosis. Typical hairy cells are mononuclear cells with an irregular nucleus, a moderate amount of cytoplasm with fine surface projections seen best under phase contrast. The cells have tartrate-resistant acid phosphatase activity. On electron microscopy pathognomonic 'ribosome-lamellar complexes' are seen in some cases. In some cases a partial remission (spontaneous or response to splenectomy) is associated with a rise in circulating T cells. In all stages there is a relative increase in T cells bearing the Fc receptor for IgG.

A bone marrow aspirate is often 'dry' and biopsy reveals fibrosis and a diffuse infiltrate of well separated mononuclear cells with a 'halo' appearance. Myelopoiesis is depressed. Immunoglobulin alterations are not usually seen.

Differential Diagnosis

This includes CLL, NHL, aplastic anaemia and myelofibrosis.

Treatment

Patients with marked splenomegaly usually benefit from its removal as splenic red cell pooling is particularly prominent in the 'pseudosinuses' found in the red pulp.

Other forms of therapy are usually unhelpful and aggressive chemotherapy is hazardous.

Prognosis

This is a chronic disease with marked fluctuations in the course of the disease. The mean survival is approximately 5 years, but occasional patients survive for over 20 years.

HISTIOCYTIC MEDULLARY RETICULOSIS

This is a rare malignant proliferation of monocytic/histiocytic cells seen in children and adults. A familial form has been described. The disorder typically presents with fever and pancytopenia. There is severe anaemia with a modest reticulocytosis and a negative Coombs' test. Lymphadenopathy and hepatosplenomegaly frequently occur. Clinical and laboratory features of disseminated intravascular coagulation are often seen. Bone marrow examination reveals abnormal histiocytic cells which exhibit phagocytosis of erythrocytes and leucocytes. Even with aggressive combination chemotherapy the prognosis remains very poor.

Selected Further Reading

Berard C. W., Greene M. H., Jaffe E. S. et al. (1981) A multidisciplinary approach to non-Hodgkin's lymphomas. *Ann. Intern. Med.* **94**, 218.
Canellos G. P. (ed.) (1979) The lymphomas. *Clin. Haematol.* **8**, 3.
Catovsky D., Linch D. C. and Beverley P. C. L. (1982) T cell disorders in haematological diseases. *Clin. Haematol.* **11**, 3.
Kaplan H. S. (1981) Hodgkin's disease—biology, treatment, prognosis. *Blood* **57**, 813.
Lennert K. (1978) *Malignant Lymphomas.* Berlin. Springer-Verlag.
Lutzner M., Edelson R., Schein P. et al. (1975) Cutaneous T cell lymphomas. *Ann. Intern. Med.* **83**, 534–552.
Sweet D. L. and Golomb H. M. (1980) The treatment of histiocytic lymphoma. *Semin. Oncol.* **7**, 302–309.

MYELOMA

Definition

A neoplastic B-cell proliferation of the bone marrow in which the predominant cell types are immature and mature plasma cells. The plasma cells usually secrete monoclonal immunoglobulins or light chains and there is an associated immune-paresis.

Incidence

Approximately 3/100 000; slightly more common in males; mean age at diagnosis is 62 years and rare under 40 years.

Clinical Features

The clinical manifestations of myeloma relate to the multiple pathology.
1. Skeletal destruction frequently gives rise to:
        1.1 Bone pain.
        1.2 Hypercalcaemia with its symptoms of thirst, polyuria, constipation, abdominal pains, lethargy, confusion and even coma. Skeletal radiography show purely osteolytic lesions or diffuse osteoporosis in most cases. The alkaline phosphatase is not raised and a $^{99}Tc^m$ bone scan is usually normal. The pathogenesis of bone destruction is uncertain, but may be due to release by myeloma cells of an 'osteoclast-activating factor' (OAF).
2. Haemopoietic dysfunction leading to symptoms of anaemia, leucopenia and thrombocytopenia. Anaemia can only partly be accounted for by marrow replacement and some inhibition of haemopoiesis seems likely. The plasma volume is often raised if there is a high paraprotein level giving disproportionately severe anaemia.
3. Plasma protein abnormalities include immuneparesis as well as a paraprotein. Infections are very common. A hyperviscosity syndrome occasionally occurs especially with IgA, IgD and IgM myelomas (these immunoglobulins are capable of aggregation). Patients complain of lethargy, confusion and may become comatose. Gangrene of the extremities, blurring of vision and blindness due to venous occlusion may occur. Fundal examination shows venous congestion. There may be a haemorrhagic tendency with purpura, epistaxes and ecchymoses.

Hyperviscosity symptoms usually indicate a plasma viscosity greater than 4·0 Pa.s. Some paraproteins are cryoglobulins and Raynaud's phenomena may be present.

4. Renal dysfunction arises from multiple causes including:

    4.1 Light chain precipitation in the renal tubules.

    4.2 Amyloid deposition in the glomeruli.

    4.3 Hypercalcaemia.

    4.4 Hyperuricaemia.

    4.5 Renal tract infections.

    4.6 Rarely, myelomatous infiltration of the kidney.

Patients may present with acute or chronic renal failure.

5. Neurological dysfunction:

    5.1 Cord compression may result from extraosseous myeloma deposits or vertebral collapse.

    5.2 Cranial nerve palsies are usually due to myeloma deposits.

    5.3 Peripheral neuropathies may be due to amyloid infiltration, but are often a 'non-metastatic manifestation of malignancy'. Motor symptoms often predominate.

6. Soft-tissue myeloma deposits are particularly common in the skin, pleura, lung, retroperitoneal and retro-orbital tissues.

Laboratory Investigations

1. Rouleaux formation and a very high ESR are the rule. Anaemia, leucopenia and thrombocytopenia are variable. The anaemia is occasionally leuco-erythroblastic. A careful search shows plasma cells in the peripheral blood in about 5 per cent of cases.

2. The bone marrow typically shows a plasmacytosis greater than 10 per cent and often greater than 30 per cent. Some plasma cells may appear normal, but they are often multinucleate and contain vacuoles and a variety of cytoplasmic inclusion bodies (*Fig. 18.1*). Some myeloma cells have a reddish tinge and are known as 'flaming plasma cells'.

Fig. 18.1. Myeloma cells.

 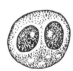

3. Skeletal radiographs show osteoporosis, crush fractures or lytic lesions in 80 per cent of cases. The skull is frequently involved.

4. The total serum protein is usually raised and may be greater than 100 g/l. The gammaglobulin level is usually raised and the albumin level is often reduced. Plasma protein electrophoresis usually shows a narrow monoclonal band (*see* Chapter 28). IgG paraproteins are usually in the gammaglobulin region but IgA paraproteins are often broader and found in the betaglobulin region. Measurement of immunoglobulin levels shows a raised IgG in about 50 per cent of cases and IgA in about 25 per cent. IgD myelomas account for only 2 per cent of

myelomas and IgE and true IgM myelomas and are very rare. In 20 per cent of cases the plasma cells secrete only light chains, and as these are rapidly metabolized and excreted, an M band is usually not apparent on an electrophoretic strip. Occasionally no monoclonal protein can be demonstrated ('non-secretory myeloma') and rarely two monoclonal proteins are produced. These usually have the same light chain and are thought to arise from the same cell clone. IgG paraprotein levels are usually greater than other immunoglobulin types reflecting the longer half-life of IgG rather than a higher myeloma cell mass. The other immunoglobulin levels are frequently reduced.

5. Detection and quantitation of urinary light chains (Bence Jones protein) should be performed by immunoelectrophoresis (*see* Chapter 28). Positive results are obtained in 70 per cent of cases compared to about 40 per cent by heat coagulation testing.

6. Serum calcium, phosphate, urea, creatinine, uric acid and a creatinine clearance are required for assessement of hypercalcaemia and renal function.

7. Plasma β-microglobulin is nearly always raised.

Diagnostic Criteria

Diagnosis is not usually a problem. Lytic lesions, bone marrow plasmacytosis and an M band occur individually in other conditions, but the combination of all three are pathognomonic of myeloma. Various diagnostic criteria are defined for marginal cases which vary considerably from centre to centre. Bone marrow plasmacytosis (10–30 per cent) may be seen in chronic infections and inflammation, hepatitis and cirrhosis, Hodgkin's disease and hypernephroma. M bands are also seen in macroglobulinaemia, heavy chain disease, cryoglobulinaemia occasionally in lymphomas, chronic lymphocytic leukaemia, myelofibrosis, and in essential or benign monoclonal gammopathy. This latter diagnosis is initially one of exclusion and should not readily be made unless the haemoglobin and serum albumin are normal, there are less than 10 per cent plasma cells in the marrow, little or no Bence Jones protein in the urine and no osteolytic lesions. The paraprotein level should remain constant and below 35 g/l for IgG and 20 g/l for IgA; it is usually < 10 g/l. Other immunoglobulins are not usually depressed. Benign monoclonal gammopathy is found in 3 per cent of those over 70 years and less than 10 per cent of these will develop a myeloma.

Staging

Various criteria can be used, but the most discriminating in terms of prognosis are the blood urea after rehydration, the haemoglobin and the performance status.

I	Good prognosis	Urea < 8 mmol/l
		Hb > 10 g/dl
		Few or no symptoms
II	Intermediate	Not I or III
III	Poor prognosis	Urea > 10 mmol/l
		+ restricted activity
		or Hb ⩽ 7·5 g/dl
		+ restricted activity

Estimates of myeloma cell mass can be made by computation of the serum and urine M component, the haemoglobin, plasma and urinary calcium and a 'skeletal survey score'. Such estimates are more useful for monitoring treatment than initial staging.

The level of the plasma β-microglobin (corrected for the level of plasma creatinine) correlates well with the myeloma cell mass.

Treatment

Relief of pain is paramount. Local radiotherapy is often strikingly effective (12–15 Gy; 1200–1500 rad) and intravenous mithramycin may be of value, in addition to analgesic therapy. Attention must be paid to level of hydration, as azotaemia is often partially pre-renal in origin and even severe established renal impairment can be reversed with prolonged high fluid administration. Hypercalcaemia is treated in the normal way with fluids, loop diuretics and steroids, in addition to cytotoxic chemotherapy. Mithramycin is often used. Infections are common and must be treated vigorously. Transfusions may be necessary. Hyperviscosity syndrome can be alleviated with plasmapheresis.

Alkylating agents are used initially; usually intermittent oral melphalan and prednisone, e.g. melphalan 0·15 mg/kg and prednisone 0·6 mg/kg per day for 7 days every 3 weeks providing there is an adequate leucocyte and platelet count. Cyclophosphamide is equally effective though generally less well tolerated. A 1–2 log cell-kill is frequently observed and many of these patients enter a fairly stable or plateau phase after some months of therapy. This is best assessed by estimation of the myeloma cell mass. At this stage the myeloma is kinetically quiescent and continued treatment is probably unhelpful. Therapy is restarted at the first sign of progression. If the myeloma does not respond to first-line therapy other drugs can be tried, including vincristine, adriamycin and BCNU. Split whole-body irradiation is being assessed in some centres.

Prognosis

The prognosis remains very poor with a median survival of less than 2 years though long-term survivors do occur. The 2-year survival of Stage I patients is about 75 per cent, 50 per cent in Stage II and 10 per cent in Stage III. The type of myeloma protein does not correlate well with the course and prognosis of the disease, though patients with light chain disease have an increased risk of developing renal failure. Acute myeloid leukaemia occurs in a significant number of patients. Alkylating agents may contribute, but some patients present with both disorders suggesting that they are related in the natural history of the disease.

SOLITARY PLASMACYTOMAS

These are treated by local surgery or irradiation. A careful search must be made for multiple myeloma and if an M band persists or reappears after eradication of the plasmacytoma then systemic chemotherapy should be given. In many cases of solitary plasmacytoma, the apparently normal plasma cells have been shown to be light chain restricted indicating their clonal and hence neoplastic origin. None the less, the prognosis is good and long remissions and even cures occur. Regular follow-up is essential.

WALDENSTRÖM'S MACROGLOBULINAEMIA

Definition

A low grade B-cell malignancy in which the predominant cell type is a small lymphocyte with variable plasmacytoid differentiation. The tumour cells secrete monoclonal IgM, usually in high titres with associated hyperviscosity. Differentiation from chronic lymphocytic leukaemia or lymphocytic lymphoma with an IgM paraprotein can be subtle and is usually based on the cell morphology, tissue distribution of the cells, the level of paraprotein and the clinical picture.

Incidence

A rare disease occurring mainly in the elderly. Twice as many males as females are afflicted.

Clinical Features

Lethargy and haemorrhage are the commonest presenting symptoms. The haemostatic defect is related to the hyperviscosity and involves platelet dysfunction (possibly due to IgM coating), inhibition of fibrin monomer aggregation and depression and inhibition of coagulation factors. Hyperviscosity may also cause a variety of neurological symptoms including headaches, vertigo, transient pareses, coma, visual failure, Raynaud's phenomena and thromboses. Weight loss is common. Lymphadenopathy is found in 30 per cent of patients and hepatosplenomegaly in 40 per cent. Cardiac failure secondary to an increased plasma volume frequently occurs. Bone pain and lytic lesions on radiography are rarely encountered.

Laboratory Investigations

Anaemia and a high ESR are usually present. The leucocyte count and platelet count are frequently normal. The bone marrow reveals a diffuse increase in small lymphocytes with some plasmacytoid forms. Mast cells may be seen. Lymph node biopsy shows a lymphocytic infiltration without destruction of the reticulin pattern. The IgM paraprotein is usually high and the other immunoglobulins may be depressed. The plasma viscosity is almost invariably raised. Cryoglobulin is detected in 30 per cent of cases and Bence Jones protein in 25 per cent. Renal failure is much less common than in myeloma.

Treatment

An expectant policy can be taken in asymptomatic patients with non-progressive disease. Repeated plasmapheresis usually combined with chlorambucil therapy

(2–6 mg/day) is used to treat hyperviscosity symptoms. Cyclophosphamide and steroids may also be useful.

Prognosis

The median survival is about 5 years from diagnosis.

HEAVY CHAIN DISEASES

These are rare lymphocytic/plasma cell neoplasms in which the cells secrete defective heavy chains and no light chains. These disorders are classified according to the class of heavy chain produced.

α-Heavy Chain Disease

This is the commonest variety. It occurs mainly in people under 50 years, mainly in Asia, S. America and the Mediterranean areas. It is slightly more common in men. It presents with chronic diarrhoea and malabsorption without lymphadenopathy or hepatosplenomegaly. The gut mucosa is heavily infiltrated with lymphocytes and the peritoneal nodes are enlarged. Diagnosis requires demonstration of a serum component that will react with anti-IgA, but not anti-κ or anti-λ antibodies. Remissions have been reported in the early stages of the disease with tetracycline and this should be tried. Standard lymphocytic lymphoma therapy is tried, but is usually ineffective, the disease ultimately proving fatal in most cases.

γ-Heavy Chain Disease

Occurs mainly in the elderly. It presents with symptoms of anaemia and general malaise. There is lymphadenopathy (may initially wax and wane) and often hepatosplenomegaly. There is usually anaemia and often pancytopenia. Atypical lymphocytes may be seen in the blood and the marrow is infiltrated with these cells. The course is variable with death occurring from months to many years from the diagnosis. Standard lymphoma therapy is rarely effective.

μ-Heavy Chain Disease

This disorder is probably a rare variant of chronic lymphatic leukaemia. Abnormal μ chains are found in blood and urine, usually in addition to κ chains.

CRYOGLOBULINAEMIA

Definition

Cryoglobulins are antibodies which precipitate when cooled.

Classification

Three types are recognized, depending on the immunoglobulin composition.

Type I is due to a monoclonal immunoglobulin, most commonly IgM or IgG in type; rarely of IgA type or due to a Bence Jones protein.

Type II is associated with mixed monoclonal and polyclonal immunoglobulins. The polyclonal immunoglobulins are IgG; the monoclonal component is usually IgM, only rarely IgG or IgA.

Type III is due to mixed polyclonal immunoglobulins; this group accounts for 50 per cent of the patients. IgM/IgG combinations are the most common. The cryoglobulins in this group are usually present as immune complexes 'immunoglobulin–anti-immunoglobulin'; sometimes incorporating complement fractions or lipoproteins.

Aetiology

Type I is usually associated with lymphoproliferative disorders (except heavy chain disease); very occasionally associated with autoimmune disorders; a few are idiopathic.

Type II is usually associated with autoimmune disorders and occasionally with a lymphoproliferative disorder.

Type III is often transient and is most frequently associated with infections (bacterial, viral or parasitic) or is idiopathic. Only occasional cases are associated with lymphoproliferative or autoimmune disorders.

Clinical Features

(i) Vascular purpura, which is palpable, most common in lower limbs; (ii) Raynaud's phenomenon; (iii) cold urticaria; (iv) acrocyanosis; (v) bleeding from mucous membranes; (vi) arthralgia; (vii) renal failure due to glomerulo nephritis; (viii) hepatic impairment; (ix) isolated neurological lesions may cause deafness, blindness etc.

Laboratory Findings

Agglutination and marked rouleaux on blood films. False indices (often very high MCV) with electronic counters due to red cell aggregates. Falsely low ESR values occur at room temperature with the true raised level determined at 37 °C. Characteristic biochemical finding identified by immunological studies.

Treatment

1. General—the patient should be kept warm and avoid unnecessary standing.
2. Acute severe symptoms respond to plasmapheresis.
3. An underlying cause should be treated. Hydroxychloroquine may be of benefit if there is an associated collagen disorder.
4. Azathioprine, cyclophosphamide and chlorambucil have been used to reduce synthesis of cryoglobulins.
5. Steroid therapy is occasionally beneficial.

AMYLOIDOSIS

Definition

Amyloidosis is a generic term for a group of disorders characterized by a homogeneous waxy infiltration of the tissues. The deposits are eosinophilic and exhibit emerald green birefringence after staining with alkaline Congo red. Electron microscopy reveals that these deposits have a fibrillar nature and X-ray crystallography has shown that these fibrils form a crossed pleated sheet. It is this tertiary structure that imparts the tinctoral and optical properties to amyloid when stained with Congo red. The infiltration of tissues causes pressure atrophy and disruption of normal function. The amyloidoses can be classified as follows:
1. Immunocyte dyscrasias with amyloidosis.
2. Reactive systemic amyloidosis.
3. Heredofamilial amyloidosis.
4. Amyloid associated with endocrine tumours.
5. Amyloid of ageing.

1. Immunocyte Dyscrasias with Amyloidosis

This includes 'primary amyloidosis' and myeloma associated with amyloidosis, the difference between the two being the absence or presence of osteolytic bone lesions. **Pathogenesis of the Amyloid Deposits.** This type of amyloid has been shown to consist of homogeneous intact light chains or the N terminal V_L domain of the light chain, or both, and is designated AL. Various studies indicate that the amyloid light chains are monoclonal and a monoclonal protein can be demonstrated in the blood or plasma of nearly all patients either at diagnosis or on follow-up. It is not clear why some and not all light chains are amyloidogenic, but the presence of free light chain (Bence Jones protein) appears to favour amyloidosis. Between 6 and 15 per cent of all myelomas are associated with amyloidosis, and amyloid is also seen occasionally in association with Waldenström's macroglobinaemia, the heavy chain diseases and immunoblastic lymphadenopathy. **Clinical Features.** The mean age of presentation is approximately 60 years. The possible symptom complex is high, mirroring the possible widespread infiltration of the amyloid. The following features, however, should always raise the possibility of amyloidosis and prompt further studies.
1. Peripheral neuropathy often with prominent sensory and autonomic components.
2. Median nerve entrapment and carpal tunnel syndrome.
3. Macroglossia.
4. Malabsorption and protein-losing enteropathy. Bowel obstruction and haemorrhage can also occur.
5. Cardiomyopathy, often of restrictive type.
6. Polyarthropathy affecting particularly the large joints.
7. 'Pinch purpura', skin nodules and infiltrations.
8. Haemorrhage due to acquired Factor X deficiency. Acquired Factor X deficiency is only rarely seen in other circumstances.

The amyloid is usually widely distributed, but may occasionally be localized, e.g. skin or pulmonary nodules.

Diagnosis. The diagnosis of amyloidosis rests on the microscopic examination of a tissue specimen stained with alkaline Congo red, aided by electron microscopy. A clinically affected organ should be biopsied if possible but failing this a rectal biopsy or renal biopsy gives a high yield of positive results (75–90 per cent).

The clinical pattern of the disease is often highly suggestive of an immunocyte dyscrasia and there should be no preceding or concurrent disease likely to give rise to reactive systemic amyloidosis.

Attempts to demonstrate a monoclonal protein should be made and a bone marrow aspirate and skeletal survey performed.

Treatment

1. The primary treatment is supportive. Heart failure must be treated with great care as digoxin may precipitate a fatal dysrhythmia and diuretics can cause catastrophic hypotension. Elastic stockings may lessen any postural hypotension. Intestinal motility problems may give rise to bacterial overgrowth and a course of antibiotics may improve any malabsorption. Renal failure may in occasional cases merit dialysis and even transplantation. Macroglossia may necessitate gastrotomy and tracheostomy.

2. Cytotoxic therapy is worth a trial especially if there is obvious myeloma, but the results are disappointing.

3. Dimethylsulphoxide is an amyloid-fibril denaturing agent and in massive doses may have occasional clinical value.

Prognosis. The mean survival is between 14 and 28 months in different series and is probably less in the presence of overt myeloma.

2. Reactive Systemic Amyloidosis

Pathogenesis. This is associated with acute or chronic infections, inflammatory conditions and neoplastic disorders, especially hypernephroma and Hodgkin's disease. Rheumatoid arthritis is probably the commonest cause. The amyloid deposits consist of a protein designated AA. It is probably derived from an acute phase serum component, though small amounts of light chain are also found in the deposit.

Clinical. The amyloidosis appears some years after the primary disease and tends to affect the kidney causing nephrotic syndrome, the liver and the spleen (hepatosplenomegaly). The diagnosis of reactive systemic amyloidosis is made in an appropriate clinical setting after biopsy proof and failure to demonstrate an immunocyte dyscrasia.

Treatment. Primarily of the underlying disease, though in the collagen vascular disease cytotoxic therapy should be considered.

Prognosis. Better than amyloid in immunocyte dyscrasias with a 10-year survival of 50 per cent.

3. Heredofamilial Amyloidoses

This includes the type associated with familial Mediterranean fever (FMF) in which the amyloid is of the AA type and familial Portuguese nephropathy in which the amyloid is possibly derived from 'pre-albumin', as well as many other less common disorders. Colchicine is said to lessen the amyloid deposition in FMF.

4. Amyloid associated with Endocrine Tumours

Amyloid is found in some endocrine glands, particularly if they contain certain tumours, e.g. medullary carcinoma of the thyroid and in multiple endocrine adenomatoses Type II. The amyloid protein in medullary carcinoma of the thyroid is probably derived from precalcitonin.

5. Amyloid of Ageing

Amyloid deposits are frequently found at post-mortem in the elderly, particularly in the brain and heart.

Selected Further Reading

Brouet J. C., Clauvel J. P., Danon F. et al. (1974) Biological and clinical significance of cryoglobulins. *Am. J. Med.* **57**, 775.
Durie B. G. H., Russell D. H. and Salmon S. E. (1980) Reappraisal of plateau phase in myeloma. *Lancet* **2**, 65.
Glenner G. G. (1980) Amyloid deposits and amyloidosis. *New Engl. J. Med.* **302**, 1283.
Salmon S. E. (ed.) (1982) Myeloma and related disorders. *Clin. Haematol.* **11**, 1.

Chapter 19

Normal Haemostasis and its Laboratory Evaluation

Introduction

A complex sequence of events takes place when vascular endothelium is damaged and subendothelial structures are exposed to the blood. Platelets and thrombin interact in this damaged area to produce a platelet–fibrin mesh (a blood clot) which prevents undue bleeding and acts as a scaffold for the repair process. Other homeostatic limiting mechanisms come into play which limit the clot to the site of injury. Five major interacting systems contribute to this process:

1. The intrinsic coagulation cascade, activated when collagen is exposed to the blood.

2. The extrinsic coagulation cascade, activated when the blood meets the membrane-bound glycoprotein, traditionally called tissue factor.

3. The platelets which form primary haemostatic plugs and contribute to the coagulation cascade by the provision of platelet phospholipid (platelet Factor 3) during shape change, release of Factor V from platelet granules, and activation of Factors XII and XI following exposure to ADP and collagen.

4. The fibrinolytic system, which ultimately dissolves fibrin deposited on the vascular endothelium.

5. A system of coagulation and fibrinolysis inhibitors, including antithrombin, antiplasmin and α_2-macroglobulin. These modify and modulate the serine proteases which are central to the clotting sequences and the kinin and complement activating mechanisms which often accompany activation of the coagulation system.

THE COAGULATION SYSTEM

Coagulation takes place following a complex amplifying system in which an enzyme precursor is transformed into a serine protease which acts upon its substrate and converts it to a potent biologically active molecule, this process itself being modulated by inhibitory plasma components which complex the stable protease. Activation of Factor X to its active serine protease Xa, with the generation of thrombin, is the common end product of both the intrinsic and extrinsic pathways.

The Intrinsic Coagulation Cascade

This system is activated by exposure of damaged vessel wall to the blood (*Fig. 19.1*). The first factor activated is Factor XII (Hageman factor). This hydrolyses Factor XI and also converts prekallikrein to kallikrein and plasminogen to plasmin. The kallikrein in turn converts Factor XII to XIIa in a cyclic pathway. Factor XIIa converts XI to XIa which, in turn, converts Factor IX to IXa.

Fig. 19.1. The mechanisms of coagulation.

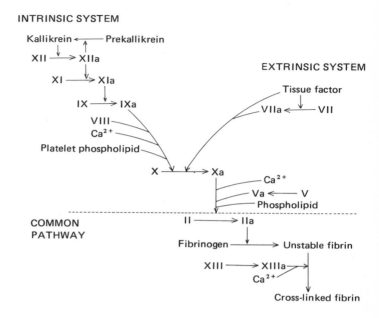

Factor IXa is responsible for the rapid activation of Factor X and its localization to the site of tissue injury. Factor X is a 2 chain structure of mol. wt 50 000 which becomes activated by the formation of multimolecular complexes at the sites of tissue injury. These complexes contain Factor IXa, Factor VIII, Factor X and Ca^{2+} ions and a platelet or phospholipid surface is required for their formation.

The Factor VIII complex consists of three parts (*Fig. 19.2*). The major structural component, as detected by immunoassay is known as Factor VIII RAG. The component concerned with clotting activity, which is defective in haemophilia, is Factor VIII C. Factor VIII C can be purified and used to raise antisera; the component detected by such antisera is referred to as Factor VIII CAG. Factor VIII C is only functional when combined with Factor VIII RAG. The third component facilitates the binding of platelets (binds to glycoprotein I) to the subendothelial structures and also is required for platelet aggregation by ristocetin; this factor is the von Willebrand factor (Factor VIII vWF or VIII RiCoF).

The Extrinsic Coagulation Cascade

The exposure of the blood to a foreign surface activates a tissue factor present on the surface of these cells which is a membrane-bound glycoprotein which complexes with Factor VII to produce active VIIa. Factor X binds to this complex with phospholipid and calcium ions similar to the process which occurs in the intrinsic system. Factor X is rapidly converted to Factor Xa by proteolytic cleavage.

The Common Pathway

In the common coagulation pathway the Factor Xa generated via the extrinsic and intrinsic cascades converts prothrombin (Factor II) to the disulphide-linked two-chain serine protease thrombin (Factor IIa). Prothrombin contains unique carboxyglutamic residues formed by a vitamin K-dependent post-ribosomal process. Oral anticoagulants interfere with this process in the synthesis of prothrombin and Factors VII, IX and X. If coumarins are ingested prothrombins are synthesized without adequate γ carboxyglutamic acid residues and cannot bind tightly to appropriate surfaces and be rapidly activated to thrombin. Thrombin generation from prothrombin is dramatically accelerated by Factor V, a glyco-protein co-factor which binds to Xa, prothrombin and Ca^{2+}, accelerating prothrombin conversion to thrombin 10 000–15 000 fold.

Fig. 19.2. Diagrammatic representation of the Factor VIII molecule.

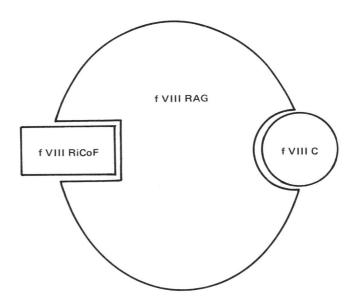

The Thrombin-fibrinogen Reaction and the Formation of the Fibrin Clot

When thrombin is formed via the common pathway it digests fibrinogen which is a 6 chain structure: 3 paired α, β and γ chains of total mol. wt around 340 000.

The fibrinogen molecule is transformed to fibrin by the action of thrombin, releasing fibrinopeptides A and B which may initiate fibrin polymerization. Fibrin, once formed, may combine with fibrinogen to form soluble fibrin–fibrinogen complexes or may interact with other fibrin molecules to form fibrin polymers.

The fibrin clot is ultimately stabilized by covalent cross-linking of polymers via a transpeptidase reaction catalysed by Factor XIIIa, the precursor of which is found in both plasma and platelets. This crosslinking involves binding of lysyl donor sites to glutamyl acceptor regions and if crosslinking is defective bleeding may occur.

PLATELETS

An arterial thrombus appears to develop in three phases which include platelet adhesion, platelet aggregation and activation of clotting factors.

Platelet Structure

The platelets are 6–10 fl in volume. They have a trilaminar covering membrane with a series of surface-connecting channels which greatly expand the surface of the platelet and are used for extrusion of secretory products. These membranes are the structural basis of platelet Factor III. The platelets have at least three different types of granules (*Fig. 19.3*).

1. Electron-dense bodies containing ATP, ADP, calcium and serotonin.
2. α granules containing platelet Factor IV, fibrinogen, β-thromboglobulin and acid hydrolases.
3. Small glycogen granules.

A few mitochondria are present in the cytoplasm. There is no nucleus.

Fig. 19.3. Platelet ultrastructure.

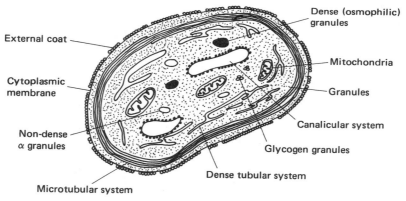

External coat

Cytoplasmic membrane

Non-dense α granules

Microtubular system

Dense (osmophilic) granules

Mitochondria

Granules

Canalicular system

Glycogen granules

Dense tubular system

Platelet Function

The platelets have a critical role in haemostasis and thrombus formation, sealing endothelial defects and forming plugs which initially arrest bleeding. This plug is formed via platelet adhesion and aggregation. The primary haemostatic plug becomes stabilized by fibrin formation. The platelets take part in the coagulation cascade by the provision of phospholipid.

Adhesion. Following endothelial damage, platelets adhere to subendothelial connective tissue structures, such as collagen, and degranulate. The adhesion is mediated via the von Willebrand factor which binds to a specific platelet receptor on glycoprotein I.

Aggregation and Release. Adherent platelets attract other platelets which build up to form the haemostatic plug. Collagen and ADP released from damaged tissues cause platelet aggregation by a direct effect on the platelet membranes. Following activation a calcium-dependent phospholipase releases arachidonic acid from the membrane which is converted by cycloxygenase to the unstable cyclic endoperoxidases (PG G_2 and PG H_2) (*Fig. 19.4*). Some of the endoperoxides are converted

Fig. 19.4. Diagrammatic representation of platelet–vessel wall interactions.

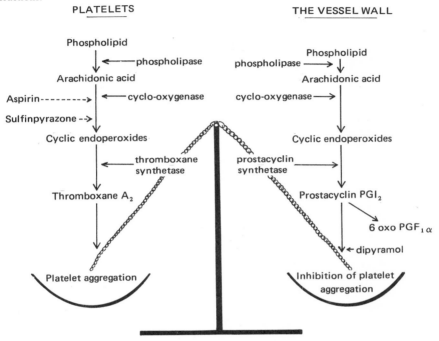

to thromboxane A_2 which causes release of dense granule contents and a rise in platelet intracellular calcium ions. ADP released from the dense granules perpetuates further platelet aggregation. Thromboxane A_2 is a potent vasoconstrictor and is rapidly degraded to thromboxane B_2, an inactive stable compound, which can be measured by radioimmunoassay. PG $F_{2\alpha}$ and PG D_2 are other conversion products of the endoperoxides the latter possibly acting as an inhibitor of aggregation. Malondialdehyde (MDA), a stable non-active compound, is also formed from the cyclic endoperoxides and reflects platelet prostaglandin synthesis.

The released free calcium ions are thought to bind to the protein calmodulin, and this complex is responsible for the phosphorylation and subsequent concentration of the platelet myosin fibres.

Antiplatelet drugs (*see* Chapter 24) may inhibit arachidonic acid production, thromboxane A_2 synthesis or increase cyclic AMP. Some common antiplatelet drugs are shown below.

1. Drugs affecting arachidonic acid production:

    1.1 Drugs blocking phospholipase enzymes—mepacrine, hydrocortisone, methylprednisolone.

    1.2 Inhibition of cyclo-oxygenase—aspirin, indomethacin, phenylbutazone, ibuprofen, naproxen.

    1.3 Inhibition of thromboxane synthetase—imidazole.

2. Drugs increasing cyclic AMP—dipyridamole.

During release of the contents of platelets and granules there is a parallel release of platelet factor IV (PF4) and β-thromboglobulin (βTG). PF4 is a small protein with heparin-neutralizing activity. βTG may be a stable proteolytic fragment of low affinity PF4 (LA-P F4).

Prostacyclin PGI₂

The vascular endothelial cells produce a unique prostaglandin, prostacyclin, PGI_2, which is a potent vasodilator and inhibitor of platelet aggregation and release. Thus, there is a delicate balance between platelet and endothelial cell production of prostaglandin compounds that regulate platelet aggregation and vessel constriction. The platelet inhibitory action of prostacyclin seems to be related to adenylate cyclase and increased platelet cyclic AMP with decreased platelet calcium. Many predisposing factors to atherosclerosis and thrombosis may be mediated by alteration of the thromboxane A_2–prostacyclin production equilibrium. PGI_2 is unstable, but its stable metabolite 6-oxo $PGF_{1\alpha}$ can be measured in the serum as an indicator of prostacyclin synthesis.

FIBRINOLYSIS

The dissolution of fibrin deposited on the vascular endothelium is mediated via the β-globulin pro-enzyme plasminogen, the central event being the transformation of the single chain plasminogen to the two-chain active serine protease, plasmin. Plasminogen can be activated through the intrinsic system via XIIa (thus triggering clot formation also triggers clot resolution) or via serine proteases in the extrinsic system. Fibrinolysis is usually carefully regulated with plasminogen activated only within the clot. Circulating antiplasmins restrict fibrinolytic activity to the clot itself except in some disease states when large amounts of plasmin are generated, which overwhelm antiplasmin, producing systemic fibrinolysis and proteolysis with accompanying degradation of Factors V, VIII, XIII and fibrinogen. Plasmin digestion of fibrin is a multistage process producing fragments X, Y, D and E. The split degradation products of fibrin and fibrinogen produced by plasmin are inhibitors of fibrin polymerization. They also potentiate the hypotensive effect of bradykinins, promote chemotaxis of monocytes and neutrophils, and impair lymphocyte activation.

BRADYKININ PRODUCTION

Fletcher factor (prekallikrein) circulates in the blood as a complex with a co-factor (Fitzgerald factor) and is cleaved by XIIa to form kallikrein which releases bradykinin from bradykininogen.

Bradykinin lowers the blood pressure, increases vascular permeability and is a vasodilator. Kallikrein exhibits chemotactic activity for neutrophils and monocytes and recruits them to sites of tissue injury.

THE INHIBITOR SYSTEM OF COAGULATION AND FIBRINOLYSIS

A family of discrete plasma proteins inhibit activated components of coagulation, fibrinolysis and kinin generation. These include:

1. Antithrombin III: deficiency causes severe thrombotic disease.
2. Antiplasmin: deficiency causes a bleeding disease.
3. C_1 inactivator: deficiency causes hereditary angioneurotic oedema.
4. α_1-antitrypsin: deficiency causes emphysema and liver disease.
5. α_2-macroglobulin.

Antithrombin III (AT III)

This is a major inhibitor of the coagulation cascade with a mol. wt of 56 000 and is an essential co-factor for the action of heparin. It neutralizes the activity of thrombin via an arginine serine interaction. Heparin binds to the lysyl residues on antithrombin III causing a conformational change of the AT III resulting in acceleration of thrombin inactivation.

In adults the level of AT III decreases with age, is low in women during the child-bearing period and the levels fall during the last trimester of pregnancy. Oestrogen therapy and liver disease also depresses the AT III level.

Antiplasmin

This is a protease inhibitor rapidly neutralizing any circulating plasmin. In certain pathological states more than half the circulating plasminogen may be converted to plasmin; this saturates the antiplasmin and any excess plasmin binds to α_2-macroglobulin.

α_2-Macroglobulin

This is a non-specific proteolytic inhibitor which can neutralize plasmin, trypsin, thrombin and kallikrein. These endopeptidases may be inactivated by a 1 : 1 or 2 : 1 stoichiometric complex of enzyme and inhibitor.

THE LABORATORY EVALUATION OF HAEMOSTASIS

The importance of a detailed history in the evaluation of a bleeding disorder cannot be overemphasized and in many cases a diagnosis can be reached before any laboratory tests are carried out. The signs and symptoms of disordered haemostasis can be divided into two main groups: cutaneous and mucosal bleeding usually suggests a vessel and/or platelet disorder whilst confluent skin ecchymoses and haemarthrosis are more often seen in disorders of coagulation factors. Disorders of coagulation factors and platelets may occur together (*Table 19.1*). In the laboratory the coagulation system, fibrinolytic system and the platelet number and function are evaluated by a series of tests which assess various components and functions individually.

Table 19.1. Clinical features of coagulation and vessel wall disorders

Findings	Coagulation disorders	Platelet or vessel disorders
Purpura	Rare	Typical
Haematomas	Typical	Rare
Haemarthrosis	Typical	Rare
Delayed bleeding	Common	Rare
Bleeding from minor superficial injury	Uncommon	Typical
Sex	In hereditary forms usually males	More common in females
Family history	Typical	Rare

COAGULATION TESTS

The prothrombin time (PT) which tests the extrinsic system and the partial thromboplastin time (PTT) or partial thromboplastin time with kaolin (PTT(K)) which tests the intrinsic system have replaced the whole blood clotting time which was a poor screening test of coagulation.

The Prothrombin Time (PT)

Method. Plasma is recalcified and the time to clot formation measured in the presence of excess tissue thromboplastin. The test bypasses the intrinsic coagulation cascade above Factor X. Normal range 10–14 sec. As in other coagulation assays a concurrent normal control is essential and the result is frequently expressed as a ratio of test sample : control.
Significance. A prolonged prothrombin time may indicate an abnormality of Factor II, V, VII or X. Factors II, VII and X are vitamin K-dependent and the test is abnormal in liver disease and widely used for the control of oral anticoagulants. Factor VII deficiency is demonstrated by an abnormal PT in the presence of a normal PTT. Heparin and other clotting inhibitors also prolong the PT. Both haemophilia (Factor VIII deficiency) and Christmas disease (Factor IX deficiency) have a normal PT.

The Partial Thromboplastin Time (Kaolin) (PTT (K))

This screens the intrinsic coagulation system.
Method. Platelet-poor plasma is incubated with kaolin (which standardizes contact activation) and cephalin (platelet lipid substitute) and the clotting time after recalcification is noted. Normal range 38–45 sec.
Significance. The test is prolonged in patients with deficiencies of clotting Factors XII, XI, IX, VIII, X, V, prothrombin or fibrinogen, but *not* VII. It is also prolonged by heparin and inhibitors of clotting factors.

The Thrombin Time (TT)

Method. Thrombin is added to plasma, bypassing the extrinsic and intrinsic cascades and the time to clot formation is a reflection of the thrombin–fibrinogen reaction.

Significance. The thrombin time is prolonged in patients with fibrinogen defects, quantitative or qualitative, and also by heparin and FDPs. These may be differentiated by clinical history, fibrinogen assays and the use of the snake venom 'Reptilase' which will cause conversion of fibrinogen to fibrin, even in the presence of heparin.

Table 19.2. The screening coagulation tests in common bleeding disorders

	PT	PTT	TT	Platelet count
Liver disease	↑	↑	usually N	initially N
Warfarin	↑	↑	N	N
Factor VII deficiency	↑	N	N	N
Haemophilia	N	↑	N	N
Christmas disease	N	↑	N	N
Heparin	↑	↑	↑	N
DIC	↑	↑	↑	↓

Assays for Specific Coagulation Factors

These are usually required to make an exact diagnosis following the detection of an abnormality in one or more screening tests, e.g. haemophilia A and Christmas disease have identical history, clinical features and screening coagulation abnormality, i.e. an isolated prolongation of the PTT in the presence of a normal PT and TT. (Here, assay of Factor VIII and/or IX level is diagnostically useful.) In assays for Factor VIII three different aspects are important:

1. The coagulation or 'procoagulant' activity VIII C (the antigenic activity of which is known as VIII CAG) is measured in the laboratory using one-stage assays which are a modification of the PTT, or two-stage assays which are modifications of the thromboplastin generation test. In the one-stage assays dilutions of pooled normal plasma are added to plasma devoid of Factor VIII and PTTs performed at different dilutions. A straight line calibration graph is plotted on double log graph paper and compared with a parallel straight line devised from the test plasma mixed with haemophilic plasma. Although one-stage assays have many disadvantages they are rapid and easy to perform. Two-stage assays, based on the thromboplastin generation test are more complex, but more reliable.

2. That part of the Factor VIII molecule which precipitates with a xenogeneic (heterologous) antibody usually raised against human Factor VIII in a rabbit. This is known as the Factor VIII-related antigen (VIII RAG) and is measured immunologically by the Laurell 'rocket' technique. VIII RAG is normal in haemophilia, but reduced to the same degree as VIII CAG in von Willebrand's disease.

3. The co-factor activity of Factor VIII necessary for platelet aggregation by ristocetin (VIII RiCoF or the von Willebrand factor). A calibration graph is plotted on double log paper from serial dilutions of normal pooled plasma (1 u/ml) against the change in optical density of a platelet suspension produced by ristocetin (measured in an aggregometer).

The coagulant activity of most other factors is generally performed by the addition of various dilutions of the patient's plasma (or serum if applicable) to a plasma devoid of the factor to be assayed, and testing the mixtures in a modified PTT or PT depending on whether the factor to be assayed is in the intrinsic or extrinsic pathway (*see above* for Factor VIII estimation).

Fibrinogen levels must often be determined to elucidate the cause of a prolonged TT and the most reliable method is to measure the thrombin–clottable protein.

PLATELET COUNT AND TESTS OF PLATELET FUNCTION

The Platelet Count

Platelets are now enumerated by fully automated electronic methods. Normal range $150–400 \times 10^9/l$.

The Bleeding Time

Method. Several methods are available, but in the 'template' method the skin of the forearm is punctured by a standard lance and the time taken to clot formation noted. Normal range 2–9·5 min.

Significance. Tests for competence of vessel wall and qualitative and quantitative platelet function. It is prolonged in moderate and severe thrombocytopenia, von Willebrand's disease and qualitative platelet disorders but it must be noted that the bleeding time is prolonged by aspirin ingestion, and the bleeding time is often normal in disorders attributed to abnormalities of the vessels.

Platelet Adhesion

Platelet adhesion is measured by a variety of methods, the most widely used being those in which fresh or anticoagulated blood is drawn through a plastic tube, the fall in platelet count across the tube being measured. The results are influenced by flow rate, haematocrit and von Willebrand factor; adhesion is classically reduced in von Willebrand's disease.

Platelet Aggregation

The most important in vitro platelet function tests relate to the aggregation of platelets with ADP, collagen, adrenaline, arachidonic acid and ristocetin. Aggregation is detected by decreased turbidity measured photometrically (*Fig. 19.5*). The patterns of aggregation tests in certain disorders are shown in *Table 19.3*.

TESTS OF FIBRINOLYSIS

The Euglobulin Lysis Time (ELT)—Screening Test for Fibrinolysis

The plasma euglobulin fraction (obtained by acetic acid precipitation) contains plasminogen activators, plasminogen, plasmin and fibrinogen, whilst antiplasmins

Fig. 19.5. Platelet aggregation.

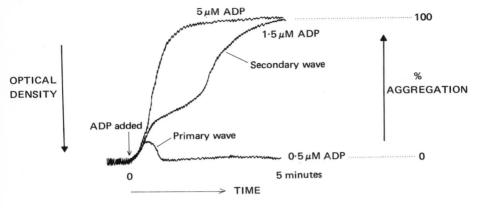

Table 19.3. Platelet aggregation patterns in qualitative platelet disorders

	ADP	Collagen	Arachidonic acid	Ristocetin
Glanzmann's disease	Nil	Nil	Severely reduced	Normal
Bernard–Soulier syndrome	Normal	Normal	Normal	Reduced
Storage-pool disease	1st phase only	Reduced	Normal or reduced	Normal or slight reduction in secondary wave

remain in the supernatant. The euglobulin lysis time, which is the rate of lysis of a fibrin clot prepared from the euglobulin fraction provides a means of measuring fibrinolysis in the absence of its inhibitors. The test measures mainly the activity of plasminogen activators.

Significance. Short ELT indicates fibrinolysis. Short ELT in presence of EACA indicates fibrinogenolysis since EACA inhibits plasminogen activators, but not free plasmin.

Fibrin Fibrinogen Degradation Products (FDPs)

These are protein fragments resulting from proteolytic action of plasmin on fibrin and fibrinogen.

Method. A variety of assays are available, based on red cell haemagglutination inhibition, staphylococcal agglutination or immunodiffusion.

Significance. Their presence reflects fibrinolysis and fibrinogenolysis; high levels are found in DIC. They prolong the TT in the presence of a normal fibrinogen. Serum FDPs are raised after major surgery, trauma and in renal failure.

MEASUREMENT OF INHIBITORS

Antithrombin III

Two methods for the assay of AT III are available: either determination of AT III antigen level or measurement of inhibitory activity towards thrombin and Factor Xa. In the latter the test sample is incubated with a standard amount of serine protease (thrombin or Xa) and after incubation residual enzyme activity is measured in a second stage.

Acquired Inhibitors

The most important inhibitor is the acquired Factor VIII antibody which occurs in 6–10 per cent of haemophiliacs, though inhibitors to other factors occur. Screening tests for inhibition are performed by incubating test plasma with a known concentration of Factor VIII. Loss of coagulant activity following incubation suggests the presence of an inhibitor. A variety of assay methods for Factor VIII inhibitors exist and in them either varying dilutions of Factor VIII are incubated with the test plasma, the inhibitor concentration being related in each case to residual Factor VIII activity after incubation.

Selected Further Reading

Biggs R. (ed.) (1976) *Human Blood Coagulation Haemostasis and Thrombosis*, 2nd ed. Oxford, Blackwell Scientific Publications.
Poller L. (ed.) (1981) *Recent Advances in Blood Coagulation*, 3rd ed. Edinburgh. Churchill, Livingstone.
Thomas J. M. (1980) *Blood Coagulation and Haemostasis*, 2nd ed. Edinburgh, Churchill Livingstone.

Platelet disorders are related to qualitative or quantitative abnormalities of platelets often associated with spontaneous bruising or bleeding and abnormalities of the bleeding time and platelet count.

QUANTITATIVE PLATELET DISORDERS

Thrombocytopenia is the commonest platelet disorder; there are two main groups:
1. Production thrombocytopenias.
2. Thrombocytopenias with increased platelet destruction.

PRODUCTION THROMBOCYTOPENIAS

Classification

Congenital or Hereditary
1. Fanconi's syndrome
2. Amegakaryocytic thrombocytopenia
   2.1 With absent radii
   2.2 'Fanconi-like'
   2.3 Other X-linked or autosomal conditions
   2.4 Associated with trisomies
3. Thrombopoietin deficiency
4. Wiskott–Aldrich syndrome
5. May–Hegglin anomaly
6. Bernard–Soulier syndrome

Acquired
1. Marrow hypoplasia
2. Marrow infiltration
3. PNH
4. Drug-induced generalized marrow suppression
5. Drug-induced platelet specific suppression
6. Viral infection
7. Nutritional deficiency

191

Fanconi's Syndrome
(Discussed in detail in Chapter 6)

Amegakaryocytic Thrombocytopenia

A group of congenital disorders with a cellular marrow and absent or decreased megakaryocytes.

The disorder may be due to an intra-uterine disturbance during the first 8 weeks and rubella has been implicated in some cases; these cases may be associated with circulating immune complexes active against megakaryocytes. Many cases are associated with other congenital anomalies.

Clinical Features. There are 3 groups.

1. Those with absent radii who may also have multiple congenital skeletal defects. Many of these die of cerebral haemorrhage in the first year of life. If they survive longer than this, prognosis is much better.

2. Those who have other features of Fanconi's anaemia and, unlike the first group, do not present with haematological problems until several years of age.

3. Those with trisomy 13, 15, or 18 and other X-linked or autosomal conditions usually associated with multiple abnormalities.

Diagnosis. Clinical picture and presence of amegakaryocytic thrombocytopenia with a marrow showing otherwise normal erythropoiesis and myelopoiesis.

Treatment. There is no specific treatment. Support with blood and platelet transfusions is given where necessary.

Wiskott–Aldrich Syndrome

An X-linked recessive disorder characterized by eczema, thrombocytopenia and recurrent infections. Thrombocytopenia is due both to ineffective thrombopoiesis and reduced platelet survival. Recurrent infections due to defective cellular and humoral immunity, with impaired delayed hypersensitivity, and reticular hyperplasia of lymph nodes with absent germinal centres and reduced T cells in paracortical areas.

Clinical Features. Bleeding in the first 6 months of life. Death usually occurs before 10 years from infection, bleeding or a lymphoproliferative disorder.

Laboratory Feature. Low platelet count with small-sized platelets. Platelet function is impaired; characteristically there is a 'storage pool' defect (*see later*).

Treatment. Steroids are not usually useful. Homologous platelet transfusions are indicated in emergencies. Allogeneic bone marrow transplantation may be curative.

May–Hegglin Anomaly

Rare autosomal dominant condition with giant platelets, basophilic inclusions in leucocytes (Döhle bodies) and thrombocytopenia in one-third. The aetiology is unknown. Most patients do not bleed and the condition is found incidentally.

Bernard–Soulier Syndrome
Discussed in section on qualitative platelet disorders (p. 198).

Acquired Thrombocytopenia

Marrow hypoplasia; Marrow infiltration; PNH and Drug-induced thrombocyto-penia with generalized marrow suppression are discussed elsewhere.

Drug-induced Thrombocytopenia with Platelet Specific Suppression

1. Thiazide diuretics: occasional patients on long-term therapy develop throm-bocytopenia with reduced numbers of megakaryocytes in the marrow.
2. Alcohol: probable direct toxicity to marrow megakaryocytes and also a reduction of platelet life span.
3. Prednisone and oestrogens: occasional reports of thrombocytopenia with decreased megakaryocytes.

Viral Infection

Thrombocytopenia may be associated with direct viral infection of mega-karyocytes. The following viruses have been incriminated: varicella, cytomegalo-virus, measles, rubella. All of these can also cause immune thrombocytopenia.

Nutritional Deficiency

B_{12}, folate and, very rarely, iron deficiency can all be associated with impaired platelet production.

THROMBOCYTOPENIAS WITH INCREASED PLATELET DESTRUCTION

In these syndromes, megakaryocytes are plentiful and platelets are destroyed or consumed either alone or with fibrinogen. They may be classified as:
1. *Immune thrombocytopenia*
   a. Immune thrombocytopenic purpura.
   b. Associated with other autoimmune syndromes
   c. Isoimmune neonatal thrombocytopenia
   d. Post-transfusion purpura.
   e. Drug-induced immune thrombocytopenia
2. *Microangiopathic platelet destruction*
   a. Haemolytic uraemic syndrome
   b. Thrombotic thrombocytopenic purpura
   c. Others
3. *Combined platelet and fibrinogen consumption*
   a. Disseminated intravascular coagulation
   b. Giant cavernous haemangioma
4. *Miscellaneous*
   Infections and following massive or exchange transfusions

IMMUNE THROMBOCYTOPENIA

Idiopathic Thrombocytopenic Purpura (ITP)

Aetiology. Many cases of ITP, at least in childhood, follow 2–3 weeks after a viral infection such as rubella, varicella, mumps, infectious mononucleosis, etc. It is possible in many cases to detect the presence of platelet-associated IgG (PA IgG) which may directly or by the involvement of immune complexes be responsible for the immune destruction of platelets. The platelet-associated antigen remains unknown and may be a normal membrane component. The antibody-coated platelets are destroyed predominantly by the RE cells of the spleen.

Clinical Features. The peak age in childhood is 2–5 years—males to females 1 : 1, though more females become chronic. The majority of childhood cases are of the acute type. Most adult cases are chronic—males to females 1 : 3.

Bleeding into the skin in the form of purpura and ecchymosis is the most common manifestation of ITP followed by epistaxis, haematuria and GI bleeding. Intracranial haemorrhage is an uncommon, but serious manifestation of the disease. The spleen is not palpable in over 90 per cent of cases and if it is felt, an alternative diagnosis should be considered.

Infants born to mothers with ITP may have thrombocytopenia due to transplacental passage of antibody. If the mother has been splenectomized her platelet count may be normal at this time.

Laboratory Features. Platelets are reduced, usually $< 40 \times 10^9/l$ whilst WBC and Hb levels are maintained, providing there has been no blood loss. The atypical lymphocytes of an associated viral infection are not uncommon. The marrow is cellular with normal or increased numbers of megakaryocytes which are poorly granulated and show little platelet budding, both these being features of very active thrombopoiesis.

Platelet-associated antibodies can be demonstrated by a variety of methods including serotonin release, binding assays and antiglobulin consumption. Some of these assays may be of value in the prediction of response to steroid therapy or splenectomy.

Treatment. Acute ITP in childhood is most often self-limiting and a conservative approach should be adopted. Treatment is more often required in chronic ITP and is directed towards depression of reticulo-endothelial activity and removal of antibody-producing cells.

When active treatment is needed, steroids are the treatment of choice, e.g. prednisolone or the equivalent at a dose of 0·5–2 mg/kg/day initially. If the response is good the dose can be tailed off but a modest maintenance dose may be necessary.

Splenectomy is beneficial in 65–80 per cent of patients refractory to steroid therapy; it removes a large lymphoid organ which is the site of much of the platelet destruction, and also removes a large number of antibody-producing cells. If possible, splenectomy is not carried out in very young children. Splenectomy may be required as an emergency if there is life-threatening haemorrhage despite steroid therapy. ITP in the first few months of pregnancy should be treated by splenectomy if steriods have not produced a full remission.

In the group of patients failing to respond to either steroids and/or splenectomy immunosuppressive agents are occasionally of value. They are not used in young children. Useful agents may include chlorambucil, azathioprine, cyclophosphamide and vinca alkaloids (occasionally injected after incubation with platelet concentrates).

The use of intravenous immunoglobulin has recently been reported in ITP. Most patients have an initial response, possibly due to reticulo-endothelial blockade, and some patients have a sustained remission. The precise role of immunoglobulin therapy is yet to be established.

Other Autoimmune Thrombocytopenias

Immune thrombocytopenia can occur in haemolytic anaemia (Evans' syndrome), Hodgkin's disease, non-Hodgkin's lymphoma, chronic lymphocytic leukaemia, rheumatoid arthritis and SLE. The latter is an important differential diagnosis, as thrombocytopenia alone may be the inital presentation of SLE.

Isoimmune Neonatal Thrombocytopenia

Aetiology. There is thrombocytopenia in the newborn due to passive placental transfer of alloantibodies made by the mother against specific antigens on the infant's platelets. These antigens are inherited from the father, and are absent from the mother's cells.

Clinical and Laboratory Features. Usually presents as a full-term, otherwise well, infant with isolated thrombocytopenia and a mother with a negative history for ITP or drug ingestion. Platelets are reduced but Hb, WBC and marrow are normal. The mother may lack the platelet A1 antigen, present in 98 per cent of population, but often the diagnosis must be made on clinical grounds by exclusion.

Treatment. In mild cases no treatment is necessary and the problem usually disappears in 8 weeks or so. Splenectomy is contraindicated and steroids are seldom of value.

If treatment must be given because of threatening haemorrhage then an infusion of maternal platelets is usually of benefit; these platelets lacking the target antigen.

Post-transfusion Purpura

There is rapid severe thrombocytopenia occurring one week post-transfusion, usually in a female patient who is Pl^{A1} negative (98 per cent of population are Pl^{A1} positive). Iso-antibody is bound to the Pl^{A1} antigen administered with the initial transfusion and immune complexes are formed which attach to the patient's own Pl^{A1}-negative platelets.

Treatment. Homologous platelets are usually ineffective. Exchange transfusion or plasmapheresis may be needed in severe cases.

Drug-induced Immune Thrombocytopenia

Aetiology. Drugs may produce thrombocytopenia in 2 main ways:

1. Drugs acting as haptens bind to plasma proteins and stimulate antibody formation. The immune complex attaches to platelets which are damaged as 'innocent bystanders' e.g. quinidine.

2. Drug combines with platelet-specific protein to stimulate production of antibodies which are drug and platelet specific, e.g. Sedormid.

Clinical Features. Onset of symptoms of thrombocytopenia commonly occurs 5–10 days after commencing the drug or much more rapidly if the patient has had prior exposure to the drug. The following drugs are amongst those most commonly implicated: sulphonamides, PAS, rifampicin, anticonvulsants, penicillins, heparin, quinine, quinidine, aspirin, thiazides, spironolactone, propylthiouracil.

Laboratory Features. In vitro assays are available for the detection of drug-induced antiplatelet antibody in some centres.

Treatment. Withdrawal of the drug is usually adequate. In severe cases, steroids, platelet transfusions or even exchange transfusion may be of value.

MICROANGIOPATHIC PLATELET DESTRUCTION

Haemolytic Uraemic Syndrome

See Chapter 11.

Thrombotic Thrombocytopenic Purpura

See Chapter 11.

Disseminated Intravascular Coagulation

See Chapter 22.

THROMBOCYTOSIS AND THROMBOCYTHAEMIA

A persistently elevated platelet count above the normal range (200–400×10^9/l) is commonly called thrombocythaemia when associated with a primary myeloproliferative disorder and thrombocytosis when due to any other cause.

Aetiology

Primary
1. Essential thrombocythaemia
2. Myelofibrosis
3. Polycythaemia vera
4. Chronic granulocytic leukaemia

Secondary or Reactive
1. Inflammatory disorders—infections; rheumatic disorders; ulcerative colitis and Crohn's disease; sarcoidosis
2. Drug-induced—vinca alkaloids
3. Immune disorders—SLE; GVH

4. Haematological disorders—bleeding; iron deficiency; haemolysis; post-splenectomy
5. Stress—postoperatively; post-exercise
6. Neoplasms—carcinoma (especially of the gut); Hodgkin's disease; non-Hodgkin's lymphoma

Clinical Features

Patients with thrombocytosis can present with bleeding or clotting problems; in thrombocythaemia there are qualitative abnormalities in platelet function. The differential diagnosis between primary and secondary thrombocytosis is based on careful clinical as well as laboratory evaluation. Hepatosplenomegaly in particular is frequent in primary thrombocythaemia though does occur in some secondary causes.

Laboratory Features

Platelet counts are often over $2000 \times 10^9/l$ in primary thrombocythaemia though this is uncommon in secondary thrombocytosis. In primary thrombocythaemia the platelets are often bizarre and frequently show abnormalities of aggregation. Poor aggregation response to adrenaline is the commonest defect and at least in some cases is due to deficient adrenaline receptors. A storage pool defect is common. Other features of a myeloproliferative disorder are also common on examination of the blood and marrow.

Treatment

With the reactive thrombocytosis treatment is for the underlying disorder. Treatment for the high platelet count itself may include attempts to prevent clotting, e.g. heparin and antiplatelet aggregating agents (*see* Chapter 24). In thrombocythaemia the marrow is suppressed with either P^{32} or busulphan. Occasionally it is of benefit to thrombopherese patients with very high counts.

QUALITATIVE PLATELET DISORDERS

Following injury to vessels platelets adhere to the vessel wall and subsequently degranulate and release their contents. This is the 'basic platelet reaction' and abnormalities have been described of platelet adhesion, aggregation and subsequent release of the pool of storage material.

Classification

Congenital
1. Defect of adhesion
   a. Bernard–Soulier syndrome
   b. von Willebrand's disease
2. Defect of primary aggregation—Glanzmann's thrombasthenia

3. Defect of platelet release reactions
  a. Storage pool disease
  b. Aspirin-like defects
4. Miscellaneous inherited qualitative defects of ill-defined aetiology
  a. Ehlers–Danlos syndrome
  b. Pseudoxanthoma elasticum
  c. Marfan's syndrome

Acquired
1. Uraemia
2. Liver disease
3. Myeloproliferative disorders
4. Paraproteinaemias
5. Collagen diseases
6. Drug-induced

CONGENITAL QUALITATIVE PLATELET ABNORMALITIES

Bernard–Soulier Syndrome

Severe bleeding disorder transmitted as autosomal recessive with the bleeding pattern characteristic of a platelet defect. The glycoprotein I complex on the surface of the platelets is abnormal. The platelets have low sialic acid content and probably lack a receptor site vital to factor VIII (RiCoF) binding and platelet aggregation with ristocetin.

Laboratory Evaluation
1. *FBC:* platelet count normal or *low*; many platelets are giant size.
2. *Clotting studies*

    2.1 Bleeding time—markedly prolonged.

    2.2 *Abnormal* platelet aggregation with ristocetin and bovine fibrinogen; both aggregating agonists require the presence of Factor VIII. The lack of response to ristocetin is not corrected by normal plasma or cryoprecipitate. There is normal aggregation with ADP.

    2.3 Clot retraction is *normal.*

    2.4 Platelet factor III is *normal.*

3. *Platelet Ultrastructure.* Abnormally vacuolized and dilated platelet open canalicular system—'Swiss cheese platelets'.

von Willebrand's Disease

von Willebrand's disease is described in greater detail in Chapter 21.
Clinical. Bleeding disorder of varying severity typical of a mild Factor VIII deficiency combined with the mucosal bleeding seen in a platelet disorder.
Haematology. FBC normal. Platelet numbers and ultrastructural morphology normal.

Clotting Studies
1. Bleeding time—variable, but usually prolonged.
2. Abnormal platelet aggregation to ristocetin as in the Bernard–Soulier syndrome, but unlike the Bernard–Soulier syndrome this is corrected by addition of normal plasma or cryoprecipitate (i.e. the platelets in von Willebrand's disease are not intrinsically abnormal). Defects in von Willebrand platelets are secondary to an abnormality of the plasma factor VIII molecule.

Glanzmann's Thrombasthenia

An autosomal recessive disorder.
Pathogenesis. There is an abnormal glycoprotein pattern in the membranes of thrombasthenic platelets with much reduced glycoproteins, IIb and III and this seems directly related to defects in ADP aggregation. The platelet A1 antigen is absent.
Clinical. Bleeding usually less severe than in the Bernard–Soulier syndrome.
Haematology. FBC normal. Platelet numbers normal. Platelet ultrastructure normal.
Clotting Studies
1. Bleeding time prolonged and clot retraction absent or defective.
2. Platelets adhere normally to subendothelium and aggregate normally with ristocetin.
3. Platelets fail to aggregate with ADP, epinephrine, collagen, thrombin, 5-HT and serotonin, arachidonic acid and PGE_2. This is the opposite of what happens in the Bernard–Soulier syndrome.
Treatment. Menorrhagia is helped by the contraceptive pill. Epistaxis usually responds to topical treatment. Platelet transfusions must be given if bleeding cannot otherwise be controlled but resistance develops due to antibody formation.

Storage Pool Disease

This represents a group of conditions in which there is a defective storage pool of platelet nucleotides resulting in an impairment of platelet aggregation at sites of vascular endothelial injury in vivo.
This is an extremely heterogeneous group of disorders occurring as a primary disorder, but also in association with:
1. Hermansky–Pudlak syndrome (oculocutaneous albinism with accumulation of ceroid pigment in marrow macrophages).
2. Wiskott–Aldrich syndrome.
3. Thrombocytopenia with absent radii.
4. Chediak–Higashi syndrome.
Clinical Features. In general, the bleeding tendency is mild.
Haematology. FBC and platelets normal. No platelet abnormalities with light microscopy. With electron microscopy the number of dense granules is markedly diminished.
Clotting Studies
1. Bleeding time prolonged.
2. Glass bead retention is reduced.
3. Primary aggregation with ADP is normal but secondary aggregation is reduced. Collagen aggregation is abnormal. Ristocetin aggregation tends to be

normal though there may be diminution of the secondary wave (ADP dependent).
    4. There is a decrease in the level of storage ADP; therefore the ATP : ADP ratio is markedly increased. Prostaglandin endoperoxidases are synthesized normally.
Management. Control bleeding episodes with local measures. Steroids may be helpful. Platelet transfusions are usually not necessary.

Aspirin-like Defects

A small number of patients have been described who have a congenital abnormality of platelet dysfunction resembling that produced by aspirin. They may have a congenital deficiency of platelet cyclo-oxygenase or other enzymes involved in prostaglandin and thromboxane formation.
Clinical. These patients have a mild bleeding tendency.
Haematology. FBC normal. With electron microscopy the platelets are normal.
Clotting Studies
    1. Bleeding time prolonged.
    2. Retention to glass beads normal.
    3. Secondary ADP aggregation absent. Collagen-induced platelet aggregation absent.

ACQUIRED QUALITATIVE PLATELET ABNORMALITIES

Uraemia

These patients bleed for many reasons including thrombocytopenia, decreased clotting factors and qualitative platelet abnormalities, the latter being most common. There may also be increased vascular prostacyclin production which exacerbates the bleeding tendency.
Platelet Abnormalities. There is impairment of glass bead retention, adhesion, and defective aggregation to ADP and collagen.

Liver Disease

Many different factors contribute to the bleeding tendency including liver-dependent coagulation factor deficiencies, coagulation inhibitors, thrombocytopenia, qualitative platelet defects, enhanced fibrinolysis and disseminated intravascular coagulation.
Qualitative Platelet Abnormalities. These include decreased adhesion, decreased aggregation (FDPs may contribute) and reduction of platelet Factor III availability.

Myeloproliferative Disorders

In many of these conditions there is a bleeding tendency in the presence of a normal or even raised platelet count. There is evidence that abnormalities of platelet function may be secondary to a storage-pool defect related to both defective platelet production by an abnormal stem cell, and a low-grade disseminated intravascular coagulation.

Platelet Abnormalities. These include defective primary and secondary aggregation, abnormal production of prostaglandin endoperoxides, decreased platelet serotonin and decreased platelet Factor III.

Paraproteinaemia

The haemorrhagic manifestation in these conditions may be due in part to protein coating the platelets and inhibiting platelet adhesion and aggregation.

Collagen Disorders

In ITP and SLE impairment of PF3 availability and platelet aggregation have been described.

Drug-induced Qualitative Platelet Abnormalities

Drugs can affect platelet function in a variety of ways, but frequently they do so by inhibitory steps in the biochemical pathway of platelet prostaglandin synthesis from arachidonic acid. Platelet function is affected by many drugs and this has been utilized in the treatment of thrombotic disorders (*see* Chapter 24).

Selected Further Reading

Harker L. A., Hoffbrand A. V., Brain M. C. et al. (1977) Platelets. In: *Recent Advances in Haematology*, 2nd ed. Edinburgh, Churchill Livingstone.

Malpass T. W. and Hooker L. A. (1980) Acquired disorders of platelet function. *Semin. Hematol.* **17**, 4.

Nichols W. L., Didishein P. and Gerrard J. M. (1981) Qualitative platelet disorders. In: *Recent Advances in Blood Coagulation*, 3rd ed Edinburgh, Churchill Livingstone.

21 Hereditary Coagulation Disorders

The congenital coagulation disorders are an uncommon group of disorders of which haemophilia A, Christmas disease and von Willebrand's disease are clinically the most important.

HAEMOPHILIA A—HEREDITARY FACTOR VIII DEFICIENCY

Classic haemophilia A is inherited as an X-linked recessive disorder affecting males and transmitted by female carriers. If less than 1 per cent of the factor is present the disease is usually severe; 1–5 per cent moderately severe; and if greater than 5 per cent the disease is mild.

Molecular Defect. The molecular defect in haemophilia A is an absence or low level of plasma factor VIII clotting activity (Factor VIII C). Factor VIII RAG and Factor VIII RiCoF are normal (*see* Chapter 19).

Clinical Features. Excessive bleeding may occur following circumcision, but is often not apparent in the first year of life. Severely affected boys show easy bruising and signs of haemarthrosis from the time of beginning to crawl. Later, soft tissue, muscle bleeding and haemarthroses dominate the clinical course with progressive deformity. Spontaneous haematuria, retroperitoneal bleeding imitating an acute abdomen and spontaneous epistaxis may also occur; spontaneous intracranial haemorrhage is rare.

Additional complications include:

1. Haemophilia pseudotumours in long bones or pelvis secondary to recurrent subperiosteal haemorrhage with bone destruction and new bone formation.

2. Chronic hepatitis due to hepatitis virus B or non A non B. This may follow repeated infusions of blood products.

3. Psychosocial and psychiatric complications including addiction to the powerful analgesics often required for pain relief.

4. Development of inhibitory antibodies to Factor VIII occur in approximately 10 per cent of haemophiliacs and may be related to exposure to extrinsic Factor VIII. Patients with inhibitors do not bleed more frequently than other haemophiliacs, but bleeding episodes can no longer be controlled with conventional Factor VIII therapy.

Diagnosis. From clinical history and laboratory screening tests (*see Table* 21.1) followed by a specific Factor VIII C assay.

Treatment. The essence of managing bleeding episodes is early treatment. The level of the Factor VIII is raised with cryoprecipitate or freeze-dried Factor VIII concentrate. For spontaneous joint bleeding, levels above 20 per cent Factor VIII following therapy are usually satisfactory, whilst for major surgery the Factor VIII

Table 21.1. Characteristics of the hereditary coagulation factor deficiencies

	Inheritance	Clinical picture	Coagulation screening tests
Fletcher factor (prekallikrein factor)	Autosomal recessive	No abnormal bleeding	PTT abnormal but shortens on incubation
Factor XII deficiency (Hageman factor)	Autosomal recessive	Most individuals do not have abnormal bleeding	PT normal PTT abnormal TT normal
Factor XI deficency	Autosomal recessive, most common in Jews	Mild mucosal bleeding. Haemarthrosis rare	PT normal PTT abnormal TT normal
Christmas disease (Factor IX deficiency)	Sex-linked	Severe joint and soft tissue bleeding.	PT normal PTT abnormal TT normal
Classic haemophilia	Sex-linked	Severe joint and soft tissue bleeding	PT normal PTT abnormal TT normal
von Willebrand's disease	Autosomal dominant	Combination of mucosal bleeding and mild joint bleeding	PT normal PTT abnormal TT normal
Factor VII deficiency	Autosomal recessive	Mucous membrane bleeding	PT abnormal PTT normal TT normal
Factor X deficiency	Autosomal recessive	Variable, may be severe joint and soft tissue bleeding	PT abnormal PTT abnormal TT normal
Factor V deficiency	Autosomal recessive	Mild mucous membrane bleeding. Menorrhagia	PT abnormal PTT abnormal TT normal
Afibrinogenaemia	Autosomal recessive	Haematemesis, melaena. Mucosal bleeding	PT abnormal PTT abnormal TT abnormal
Factor XIII deficiency	Variable	Delayed bleeding after initial coagulation	Routine tests normal

Comments on Screening Tests
1. In haemophilia and Christmas disease the clinical picture and screening tests are identical.
2. von Willebrand's disease has a prolonged bleeding time whilst haemophilia and Christmas disease do not.
3. Factors VIII, IX, XI and XII give identical screening tests, but patients with Factor XII deficiency do not usually bleed.
4. With an isolated prolonged PTT, normal assays for Factors VIII, IX, XI and XII consider Fletcher factor deficiency and look for shortening of PTT on incubation.
5. Factor XIII deficiency gives normal screening tests and must be tested for separately.
6. If there is poor or absent clot formation in all screening tests, suspect a qualitative or quantitative abnormality of fibrinogen.

level should be raised to 100 per cent and kept above 60 per cent until healing is completed. If the patient is aware of a 'funny feeling' in a joint a dose of 250 u may be the only treatment required to prevent a serious bleed. For established bleeds the dose is calculated thus:

0·5 u/kg per percentage rise required.

A blood sample should be taken immediately before and 30 min after the injection of Factor VIII for an VIII C assay. The assay of the 30-min sample is important for though an inhibitor may not be detectable the level of Factor VIII may fall rapidly and in these patients subsequent doses must be increased.

Cryoprecipitate requires to be kept at $-30\,^{\circ}$C and varies in potency from 70 u to 120 u per bag. Loss of potency occurs during the thawing process. It is essential to 'wash out' the bag with 5 ml normal saline. Cryoprecipitate contains considerable amounts of fibrinogen. Factor VIII concentrate is preferable for home use and when considerable quantities require to be given. The incidence of hepatitis (non A non B as well as hepatitis B) is much greater with Factor VIII concentrate than cryoprecipitate and the long-term risk of progressive hepatic disease exists.

Home Treatment and Prophylactic Therapy. If treatment is carried out at home then it can be given at the earliest sign of any bleeding, either by the patient himself or by a relative. This has revolutionized the treatment of many patients and contrary to the prediction of some has not resulted in an increased use of Factor VIII. Severe haemophilia can be treated prophylactically by infusion of 25 u/kg of Factor VIII twice a week; this may markedly reduce the frequency of haemorrhagic incidents.

Supplementary Treatment of Factor VIII Deficiency

Oral antifibrinolytics such as episilon aminocaproic acid (EACA) or tranexamic acid can assist haemostasis in haemophiliacs with spontaneous oral cavity bleeding or following dental extraction and may obviate the requirement for Factor VIII.

EACA inhibits the conversion of plasminogen to plasmin. The dose in adults is 3 g 4–6 times per day. The dose of tranexamic acid is 250–500 mg 3–4 times per day in adults. Ideally these drugs should be given 24 hours before dental procedures. *DDAVP* (1-deamino-8-D-arginine-vasopressin) results in a 4–6 fold rise in autologous, haemostatically effective Factor VIII and when used with EACA can provide effective haemostasis for dental procedure in haemophiliacs. Further experience with the compound is necessary, but it may replace Factor VIII replacement therapy in mild haemophiliacs.

Patients with Factor VIII Inhibitors. The following have been tried to affect haemostasis in patients with inhibitors:

1. Extremely high dose Factor VIII ($>20\,000$ u/day) for 5–7 days or more.

2. Use of highly purified porcine Factor VIII to which there may initially be little cross-reactivity. The development of anti-porcine antibodies may limit subsequent use.

3. Removal of antibody by plasmapheresis.

4. Attempted eradication of the inhibitor by immunosuppression (this usually proves unsuccessful).

5. Bypassing the need for Factor VIII in the coagulation process by the use of activated prothrombin complexes. This is potentially hazardous.

Testing for Haemophilia Carriers. All the daughters of a haemophiliac are obligate carriers. The ratio of VIII C : VIII RAG has been used as a determinant of the carrier state and low ratios; <0.65 are found in 70–90 per cent of obligate carriers. The use of the ratio has allowed better identification of carriers than the assay of VIII C alone which recognizes only 25 per cent of carriers.

Antenatal Diagnosis of Haemophilia. Known female carriers can be offered antenatal diagnostic procedures. The fetus can be sexed from an amniotic fluid sample and all males can be aborted though only half of these males will be affected. Precise diagnosis is now available in some centres; a fetal blood sample is obtained at fetoscopy during the early part of the second trimester and the plasma is assayed for Factor VIII C and immunological Factor VIII C (Factor VIII CAG).

VON WILLEBRAND'S DISEASE

Clinical Features. An autosomal dominant bleeding disorder characterized by superficial skin and mucous membrane bleeding. Bleeding after dental extraction is common as is menorrhagia; post-surgical bleeding and haemarthrosis are uncommon. Bleeding may start in childhood, but becomes less of a problem with increasing age. The disorder tends to improve during the progress of a pregnancy.
Molecular Defect. The disorder is heterogeneous at the molecular level, but most patients have a deficiency of Factor VIII RAG and Factor RiCoF with relatively normal Factor VIII C. Within individuals the Factor VIII C is variable.
Diagnosis. The bleeding time is abnormal and is the best indication of clinical severity. Factor VIII RAG and Factor VIII-RiCoF are most consistently abnormal and reduced to the same degree. Factor VIII C may be normal. Diagnostic tests may be unreliable in late pregnancy. Transfusion of normal or even haemophiliac plasma causes a delayed rise in VIII C, which may not be maximal until the following day, and is markedly in excess of the predicted level from the quantity infused.
Treatment. Fresh or fresh frozen plasma or cryoprecipitate corrects the haemostatic abnormality. Dose 10–15 ml/kg of plasma or 10–20 u of cryoprecipitate per kg body weight, though lesser doses are often sufficient. Factor VIII concentrates are of less value. The VIII C level immediately following treatment is of little value in evaluating the efficacy of treatment since the level of Factor VIII will continue to rise for many hours. The bleeding time may be the most reliable guide of the efficacy of treatment in von Willebrand's disease and levels of VIII RAG and VIII RiCoF correlate well with correction of the bleeding time.

FACTOR IX DEFICIENCY— CHRISTMAS DISEASE— HAEMOPHILIA B

The clinical picture is identical to haemophilia A though it is 8 times less common. About one-third of patients have a functionally abnormal Factor IX molecule and in other cases little Factor IX is present.
Treatment. Fresh frozen plasma is an adequate source of Factor IX for the treatment of minor bleeding episodes. Dried human Factor IX fraction is available for severely affected patients. It also contains significant quantities of Factors II and X. One unit of Factor IX per kg is necessary to raise the level by 1 per cent. The level required to arrest bleeding tends to be less than in Factor VIII deficiency.

FIBRINOGEN ABNORMALITIES

The hereditary fibrinogen abnormalities are quantitative (afibrinogenaemia) or qualitative (dysfibrinogenaemia).

Congenital Afibrinogenaemia

Clinical Features. Widespread bleeding often apparent in the first few days of life followed by a lifelong tendency to bleed though, despite complete lack of fibrinogen, the bleeding tendency may be relatively mild. The disorder probably represents the homozygous state of hypofibrinogenaemia which is usually asymptomatic in the parents.

Laboratory Features. All coagulation tests based on fibrin formation, such as PT, PTT and TT, are abnormal, but correctable by the addition of normal plasma. The diagnosis is confirmed by the complete absence or finding of only trace amounts of fibrinogen by precipitation, coagulation or immunological assay techniques.

Treatment. A fibrinogen level greater than 0·5–1·0 g/l usually produces adequate haemostasis and this can be achieved by whole blood, plasma or cryoprecipitate infusion, the long half-life of fibrinogen allowing 4–5 day intervals between infusions.

Congenital Dysfibrinogenaemia

These rare qualitative structural abnormalities of fibrinogen present with easy bruising or prolonged bleeding after minor trauma and are transmitted as autosomal dominants.

Laboratory Features. Fibrinogen as assessed by precipitation or immunological methods is normal, but coagulation assays suggest a deficiency.

Treatment. Most patients do not require treatment, but plasma or cryoprecipitate is useful for uncontrolled bleeding.

OTHER CONGENITAL COAGULATION FACTOR DEFICIENCIES

Factor V Deficiency

This is a mild bleeding disorder with mucous membrane or skin bleeding.

Laboratory Features (*see Table* 21.1). Deficiency confirmed by specific assay for Factor V.

Treatment. Fresh plasma or fresh frozen plasma should be given in a dose of 10–20 ml/kg but daily infusions are often required because of the instability of the factor.

Factor VII Deficiency

This is rare and inherited as an autosomal recessive. Serious bleeding can occur including intracranial haemorrhage in the newborn.

Laboratory Features. The finding of an abnormal PT with a normal PTT is a unique combination found only in Factor VII deficiency. The diagnosis is confirmed by specific Factor VII assay.

Treatment. Fresh frozen plasma can be given, but prothrombin complex is better because the short half-life of Factor VII (4–6 h) requires frequent infusions to cover surgery or injury.

Factor XI Deficiency

Homozygotes have Factor XI levels less than 20 per cent. The disorder is relatively mild with epistaxis, dental bleeding and bleeding after surgery. Haemarthrosis is rare.

Laboratory Features (*see Table* 21.1). Tests should be performed on very fresh plasma since Factor XI can become activated on storage.

Treatment. Fresh frozen plasma in a dose of 10–15 ml/kg once or twice daily should be given for bleeding episodes. Some batches of Factor IX concentrate contain high levels of Factor XI.

Factor XII Deficiency (Hageman Factor)

Most patients do not have abnormal bleeding and some have undergone tonsillectomy and adenoidectomy without incident. Rarely, patients do bleed and a single dose of FFP is usually sufficient treatment since the half-life of Factor XII is 50–70 hours.

Fletcher Factor Deficiency

None of the patients so far recognized have had any bleeding at all and surgery has been carried out without complication.

Laboratory Features. PT normal. PTT prolonged, but after a 10–15 min incubation the PTT is shortened. This does not occur with other coagulation factor deficiencies. The plasma of these patients lacks prekallikrein with resulting abnormalities of bradykinin generation and fibrinolysis.

Factor XIII Deficiency

Factor XIII is necessary for stabilization of the normal clot and with deficiency bleeding manifestations commence early in life with delayed bleeding from the umbilical cord being a very common presentation. Later, easy bruising and haematoma formation are common.

Laboratory Features. Routine coagulation tests normal. To confirm the diagnosis, the solubility of patient's clot in 0–5 M urea must be examined. Normal clots remain insoluble for 24 hours.

Treatment. Bleeding, if significant, can be treated with fresh frozen plasma 5–10 ml/kg. The half-life of Factor XIII is 6 days and a single infusion is usually all that is required.

Selected Further Reading

Bloom A. L. (1980) The von Willebrand syndrome. *Semin. Hematol.* **17**, 215.
Bloom A. L. and Pearce J. R. (1977) Factor VIII and its inherited disorders. *Br. Med. Bull.* **33**, 219.
Rizza C. R. (1979) Congenital coagulation disorders. *Clin. Haematol.* **8**, 1.

Chapter 22

Acquired Coagulation Disorders

Acquired haemorrhagic disorders due to coagulation abnormalities can be classified as shown in *Table* 22.1.

Table 22.1. Acquired coagulation disorders

Abnormalities of coagulation factor production	Liver disease. Vitamin K deficiency/oral anticoagulants
Consumption of coagulation factors	Disseminated intravascular coagulation. Fibrinolysis
Dilution of coagulation factors	Massive transfusion with stored blood
Loss of coagulation factors	Nephrotic syndrome. Amyloidosis
Inhibitors to coagulation	

LIVER DISEASE

Aetiology

1. Lack of production of clotting factors due to parenchymal damage. The vitamin K-dependent Factors II, VII, IX and X as well as Factor V are most commonly deficient.

2. If there is biliary tract disease, malabsorption of vitamin K may be present.

3. Abnormal fibrin polymerization due to Factor XIII deficiency and occasionally synthesis of fibrinogen with abnormal polymerization capacity. Fibrinogen levels may fall in severe liver disease.

4. Increased fibrinolysis occurs due to decreased clearance of plasmin and decreased synthesis of fibrinolytic inhibitors.

5. Thrombocytopenia occurs in liver disease especially in the presence of splenomegaly.

6. Disseminated intravascular coagulation.

Antithrombin III levels are also reduced, but this is not of clinical significance.

Clinical Features. Bleeding is seldom severe except from local lesions such as peptic ulcers, varices, following liver biopsies and surgery; bleeding may then be uncontrollable.

Laboratory Features. There is prolongation of the PT and PTT. The TT is not usually prolonged unless there are reduced fibrinogen levels or disseminated intravascular coagulation. The PT is an excellent test of hepatic function. The platelet count may be low.

Management of Bleeding in Liver Disease
1. Local management of lesions such as oesophageal, gastric or duodenal ulcers and bleeding varices.
2. Management of clotting defect:

2.2 Vitamin K_1 (10 mg i.v. daily for up to 5 days) may produce some response, but many patients will not improve due to inability of the liver to synthesize the clotting factors.

2.2 Blood transfusion. Freshly donated blood should be administered, as stored blood is deficient in labile clotting factors.

2.3 Fresh frozen plasma. This is a useful way of providing appropriate clotting factors, but volume overload must be avoided. Complete correction of the clotting defect is seldom attained.

2.4 Platelet concentrates may be required in those patients with severe thrombocytopenia.

2.5 Prothrombin complex concentrates. These may have some value, but must be used with extreme caution. Even in small volumes defibrination and thrombosis may occur.

2.6 Fibrinolytic inhibitors should only be used when excess fibrinolysis can be clearly demonstrated.

VITAMIN K DEFICIENCY

Factors II, VII, IX and X fail to develop essential calcium binding sites in the absence of adequate vitamin K (*see* Chapter 19).

Aetiology
1. Haemorrhagic disease of the newborn due to lack of bacterial synthesis of the vitamin and due to low stores of the vitamin. The liver has low synthetic capacity for coagulation factors, especially in premature infants.
2. Impaired absorption due to:

2.1 Biliary obstruction or fistulae.
2.2 Pancreatic disease.
2.3 Steatorrhoea of other causes.

3. Secondary to oral anticoagulants (Chapter 24).
4. Prolonged treatment with broad-spectrum antibiotics in association with low dietary intake in severely ill patients.

Clinical Features. Bruising ecchymoses and mucous membrane bleeding may occur.

Laboratory Features. PT↑, PTT↑, TT normal, with correction of PT and PTT following vitamin K administration.

Management. Vitamin K_1 i.v. (10–20 mg in adults); the drug should be given very slowly, no faster than 5 mg/min. In neonates 1–2 mg should be given i.v. very slowly, every 6 hours. Vitamin K_1 may cause haemolysis and even kernicterus. A few hours are required before maximum benefit is obtained in adults and longer in neonates. Fresh frozen plasma (2 units for an adult) or prothrombin complex will correct the coagulation abnormality immediately.

DISSEMINATED INTRAVASCULAR COAGULATION (DIC)

This is a process triggered by a wide variety of stimuli, including procoagulant factors released from leucocytes and damaged endothelial cells, activated Hageman factor, and activated complement. There is widespread deposition in the microcirculation of altered fibrinogen and platelets, with consumption of coagulation factors and platelets.

Aetiology

1. Bacterial toxins, e.g. gram-negative septicaemia, meningococcal septicaemia. Other infections, e.g. falciparum malaria.

2. Hypovolaemic shock.

3. Obstetric complications, e.g. amniotic fluid embolism, abruptio placentae and intrauterine death.

4. Tissue factor release as occurs in:

        4.1 Trauma, especially cardiothoracic surgery.

        4.2 Burns and heat stroke.

        4.3 Leukaemia (especially promyelocytic).

        4.4 Other malignancies.

5. Vascular.

        5.1 Giant haemangioma.

        5.2 Pulmonary embolism.

        5.3 Aortic aneurysm.

6. Immunological.

        6.1 Anaphylaxis.

        6.2 Haemolytic transfusion reactions (also tissue factor release).

7. Acute pancreatitis.

8. Snake venoms, e.g. Malayan pit viper.

Clinical Features. These are extremely variable and dependent upon the combination of decreased clotting factors, thrombocytopenia and the presence of FDPs. Easy bruising and oozing from venepuncture sites are often the initial manifestations, going on to massive mucous membrane bleeding. The syndrome is sometimes seen with thrombotic manifestations in addition to haemorrhagic ones.

Laboratory Features

1. The platelet count is very low—a diagnosis of DIC should not readily be made with a platelet count over $100 \times 10^9/l$.

2. The blood film may show evidence of red cell fragmentation but this is not essential.

3. The prothrombin time is prolonged because Factor V is depleted, fibrinogen is low and FDPs are present.

4. The PTT (K) is prolonged because Factor VIII is depleted, fibrinogen is low and FDPs are present.

5. The thrombin time is prolonged because fibrinogen is low and FDPs are present.

6. Fibrinogen level is low, hence thrombin and reptilase times are prolonged.

7. FDPs and fibrin monomers are present.

The screening tests are usually not corrected by the addition of normal plasma because an inhibitor (FDPs) is present.

Treatment
1. Treat the underlying cause.
2. General supportive measures, e.g. treatment of hypoxia and shock.
3. Treatment of haemorrhage with:
    3.1 Fresh blood.
    3.2 Fresh plasma, fresh frozen plasma and cryoprecipitate to replace clotting factors. Very rarely fibrinogen concentrate is required.
    3.3 Platelet concentrates.
4. *Heparin.* Heparin has been given in DIC in an attempt to 'switch off' or inhibit whatever process is activating intravascular coagulation though its use remains controversial.

ABNORMAL FIBRINOLYSIS

Aetiology
1. Excessive liberation of plasminogen activators:
    1.1 Carcinoma of the prostate.
    1.2 Extensive surgery, especially decortication of the lung and cardiac bypass surgery.
2. Impaired fibrinolytic inhibition, as occurs in liver disease, especially during surgery to perform portacaval anastomoses.
3. Streptokinase or urokinase therapy.
4. Some snake venoms.
5. Accompanying DIC.
Clinical. Fibrinolysis without DIC is a very rare, but serious cause of bleeding.
Investigations. The PT, PTT and TT are prolonged due to fibrinogenolysis with production of vast quantities of FDPs. Factors V and VIII levels may be normal or moderately reduced in contrast to the marked reduction that occurs in DIC. The euglobulin lysis time is very rapid in primary fibrinolysis, unless the plasminogen levels become depleted, in which case the lysis time lengthens.
Treatment
1. Treatment of any underlying disorder.
2. In life-threatening situations epsilon aminocaproic acid can be given. If there is any evidence of coexisting DIC, heparin may also be required.

MASSIVE TRANSFUSION WITH STORED BLOOD

See Chapter 27.

NEPHROTIC SYNDROME

Factor IX or Factor XII deficiency may develop. The deficiencies are usually diagnosed from abnormal laboratory tests rather than from a clinical bleeding tendency. The coagulation factors are lost along with other proteins in the urine. A more common problem is thrombosis related to acquired AT III deficiency.

AMYLOIDOSIS

Factor X deficiency occurs in amyloidosis due to rapid plasma clearance and binding to body tissues.

ACQUIRED INHIBITORS TO CLOTTING FACTORS

These are antibodies to coagulation factors. Factor VIII inhibitors are the most common.

Aetiology

1. Associated with exogenous factor administration in haemophilia and related deficiency states.

2. Idiopathic.

3. Collagen vascular diseases, including inflammatory bowel disease.

4. Malignant diseases.

5. Pregnancy and postpartum.

6. Chronic skin diseases.

7. Penicillin-induced.

In systemic lupus erythematosus specific Factor VIII antibodies may occur. More commonly there is a non-specific 'lupus anticoagulant' with prolongation of both the PT and PTT. In some of these cases there is also an inhibitor of prostacyclin production.

Treatment. Therapy may not be required. If necessary, high dose steroids (1 mg/kg) and/or immunosuppressives, such as azathioprine or cyclophosphamide, can be given, though the inhibitor may be refractory to therapy. In acute situations plasmapheresis may be of value. Attempts to 'swamp' the antibody with massive infusions of the appropriate factor may be indicated in an emergency.

Selected Further Reading

Sharp A. A. (1977) Diagnosis and management of disseminated intravascular coagulation. *Br. Med. Bull.* **33**, 265.

23

The term 'hypercoagulable' has been applied to a group of individuals with a predisposition to thrombosis. The thrombotic tendency may be due to an abnormality of the platelet/vessel wall interaction or of fibrinolysis rather than of coagulation and the term 'prothrombotic state' is preferable.

Possible Causes of a Prothrombotic State

Coagulation Abnormalities
  Increased concentration of clotting factors
  Increased concentration of activated clotting factors
  Decreased concentration of coagulation inhibitors (especially antithrombin III deficiency)
Fibrinolysis Abnormalities
  Decreased plasminogen
  Decreased plasminogen activators
  Inhibitors of plasminogen activation
  Increased concentrations of antiplasmins
Abnormalities of the Platelet/Vessel Wall Interaction
  Thrombocytosis
  Increased platelet adhesion/aggregation
  Decreased prostacyclin production
Circulatory Stasis
  Mechanical
  Hyperviscosity

COAGULATION ABNORMALITIES

1. *Increased Concentration of Clotting Factors*

Many factors may be raised in thrombosis, but there is limited evidence for a pathogenic relationship.

1.1 Families with a thrombotic tendency and increased Factor VC or Factor VIIIC have been described.

1.2 One prospective study has shown that high levels of fibrinogen, Factor VIIIC and Factor VIIC are associated with a higher risk of coronary death.

1.3 Studies of acute thrombosis show increased fibrinogen and Factors VIIIC and VC, all of which are acute phase reactants and rise in most illnesses. Factor VIIC is also raised in thrombosis.

213

214 A Synopsis of Haematology

1.4 Many known risk factors for thrombosis are associated with increased clotting factors (*Table* 23.1).

2. *Increased Concentration of Activated Clotting Factors*

These are probably more thrombogenic than non-activated factors, especially if there is blood stasis. Increased activation could be due to an abnormality of the clotting factor rendering it more susceptible to activation, due to increased activators (e.g. collagen, endotoxin, prosthetic valves, procoagulants in pro-myelocytic leukaemias, mucin from adenocarcinomas), or due to decreased clearance of activated clotting factors. The latter occurs in liver disease.

3. *Coagulation Inhibitor Deficiency*

The most important coagulation inhibitor is antithrombin III (AT III); its mechanism of action is discussed in Chapter 19. Antithrombin III deficiency occurs in several conditions.

Hereditary AT III Deficiency. This is an autosomal dominant condition, probably more common than haemophilia. In most cases there is decreased synthesis of normal AT III, but cases have been described in which there is normal or decreased synthesis of an electrophoretically abnormal AT III together with normal AT III. The normal range is between about 70 and 130 per cent and functional levels of 40–70 per cent are found in hereditary AT III deficiency.

Clinical Features. Over half the affected individuals have more than one thrombotic episode. Thrombosis is rare before puberty and is particularly common after surgery, during pregnancy and with the contraceptive pill. Venous thromboses occur in the usual sites and also in the mesenteric veins (rare in idiopathic thrombosis). There is no increase of arterial thromboses.

Treatment. Heparin is used to treat thromboses but control is difficult. Heparin is less effective than usual with the low levels of its co factor, and the levels of AT III tend to fall further with heparin therapy. AT III is now available for infusion with heparin, but in an emergency fresh frozen plasma is of value.

Oral anticoagulants are effective in preventing thromboses and in some individuals result in a rise of AT III levels.

Special attention must be paid to surgery and pregnancy, and the whole family should be screened and given appropriate advice. The contraceptive pill is contraindicated.

Acquired AT III deficiency. This occurs in the nephrotic syndrome and may contribute to thrombosis. AT III levels also fall with pregnancy, the pill and after major surgery, as well as with DIC and severe burns. AT III levels are also reduced in liver disease due to decreased synthesis but there is no increased risk of thrombosis.

ABNORMALITIES OF FIBRINOLYSIS

1. Decreased plasminogen levels are a theoretical cause of hypercoagulability but in fact increased plasminogen levels have been reported to be associated with coronary artery disease.

2. Decreased plasminogen activators can be measured crudely by the euglobulin lysis test. Decreased plasminogen activators have been associated with many conditions with a known increased risk of thrombosis.

3. Inhibitors of plasminogen activation have been described in venous thrombosis and in Behçet's syndrome.

4. Increased antiplasmins have been reported in diabetes, hypercholesterolaemia, idiopathic pulmonary hypertension, recurrent DVTs and with pregnancy, the pill, obesity, malignancy and following surgery. The major antiplasmins are α_1-antiplasmin and α_2-macroglobulin.

In general, fibrinolysis is poorer in the lower than upper extremities and this is perhaps one reason why DVTs are more common in the legs.

ABNORMALITIES OF THE PLATELET/VESSEL WALL INTERACTION

1. *Thrombocytosis*

An increased platelet count in myeloproliferative disorders may be associated with microvascular ischaemia though not usually arterial or venous thrombosis. A bleeding diathesis is more common. Opinions differ whether secondary thrombocytosis, as occurs after splenectomy, increases the risks of thrombosis.

2. *Increased Platelet Adhesion/Aggregation*

2.1 Platelet adhesion is often increased in acute venous thrombosis, but is usually normal between attacks in patients with recurrent DVTs and in patients with arterial disease. Adhesion is influenced by the haematocrit, flow rate and Factor VIII RiCoF.

2.2 Platelet aggregation is increased in hyperlipoproteinaemia Type II and in diabetes, especially in those with vascular or neuropathic complications; the mechanism is obscure. There may also be increased ADP-induced aggregation in patients with coronary artery disease; this may be reversed with β-blockers.

2.3 Spontaneous aggregation may occur in myeloproliferative disorders and be associated with digital ischaemia reversible with aspirin. The spontaneous aggregation may indicate extreme sensitivity to ADP. Spontaneous aggregation also occurs in diabetes.

3. *Decreased Prostacyclin Production*

This may be due to:

3.1 Decrease of plasma prostacyclin stimulating factor, as is thought to occur in some cases of haemolytic uraemic syndrome and thrombotic thrombocytopenic purpura.

3.2 Inhibitors of prostacyclin synthesis or release. Some cases of systemic lupus erythematosus with recurrent thromboses have such inhibitors.

3.3 Primary endothelial cell abnormality.

Prostacyclin synthesis, as determined by 6oxo $PGF_{1\alpha}$ levels, is reduced in some diabetics. Atherosclerotic arteries have been shown to secrete less prostacyclin than normal, but it is not clear whether this is primary or secondary.

CIRCULATORY STASIS

1. A sluggish circulation as occurs when a limb is immobilized.

2. Hyperviscosity. A raised haematocrit is probably the commonest cause of hyperviscosity. A massive increase in plasma proteins (e.g. myeloma) or of white cells (e.g. chronic granulocytic leukaemia) can also cause hyperviscosity and predispose to thrombosis.

LABORATORY INVESTIGATIONS IN PROTHROMBOTIC STATES

There are broadly two types of tests; those that indicate that thrombosis has or is occurring even if subclinical, and those designed to delineate the cause of the thrombosis. Progress in this area is hampered by the difficulty in diagnosing many thromboses and in determining whether changes in laboratory parameters are a cause or effect of thrombosis.

Table 23.1. Conditions with increased risk of thrombosis

Condition	Type of thrombosis Arterial	Venous	Haemostatic changes
Age	+	+	↑ Factors VC, VIIC, VIIIC and IXC Fibrinogen ↓ Plasminogen activators in women ↓ ATIII
Family history	+	+/−	
Blood group A	+	+	
Male sex	+		
Haematocrit	+		
Obesity	+	+	
Pregnancy and puerperium		+	↑ Factors VIII RAG, VIIIC, VII and X ↑ Fibrinogen ↓ Fibrinolysis
Oral contraceptives	+	+	↑ Factors II, VII, IX, X and XII ↑ Fibrinogen ↑ Plasminogen ↓ ATIII (controversial)
Smoking	+	−	↓ Factor VIIIC ↑ Fibrinogen ↓ Fibrinolysis ↑ Viscosity

Table 23.1 (Cont.)

Condition	Type of thrombosis Arterial	Venous	Haemostatic changes
Diabetes	+		↑ Factors VIIIC, XC ↑ Antiplasmins (controversial) ↓ ATIII ↑ Blood viscosity ↑ Mean platelet volume ↑ Platelet aggregation ↓ Prostacyclin
Hyperlipoproteinaemia	+		↑ Plasminogen ↑ Antiplasmins ↑ Platelet aggregation
Heart failure	+		
Immobilization		+	
Nephrotic syndrome		+	↓ ATIII
Homocysteinuria	+	+	↑ Platelet adhesiveness ↑ Platelet aggregation to ADP Damage to vascular endothelium
Infection		+	↑ Factors VC and VIIIC ↑ Fibrinogen

Malignancy		+	↑ Factors VC and VIIIC
			↑ Fibrinogen
			Activation of clotting factors esp.
			    Factor X
			Production of tissue thromboplastins
			    e.g. acute promyelocytic leukaemia
			↑ Antiplasmins

Behçet's disease	+	+	↑ Factor VIIIC ↑ Fibrinogen ↑ Plasminogen activation inhibitors ↓ Spontaneous fibrinolytic activity ↓ ATIII ↑ Platelet adhesion ↑ Platelet aggregation with ADP
Trauma and surgery		+	↑ Factors VIIIC and XC ↑ Fibrinogen ↓ Plasminogen activators (after initial rise) ↑ Plasminogen clearance ↑ Plasmin inhibitors ↓ ATIII ↑ Viscosity ↓ Flow rate due to hypovolaemia and immobilization ↑ Platelet count ↑ Platelet adhesiveness

Investigations Primarily used to detect Thrombosis or Prothrombotic States

Identification of Activated Coagulation Factors. A rise in the Factor VIII RAG : VIIIC ratio may indicate ongoing factor activation. Other tests are also available but none can be confidently used to diagnose or predict thrombosis.

Measurement of Fibrinogen and Fibrin Breakdown Products. Fibrinopeptides A and B are formed during the conversion of fibrinogen to fibrin and their presence may indicate thrombosis or a prothrombotic state; they are also increased in infective conditions. Circulating fibrin monomer complexes often complexed with fibrinogen or FDPs, are found in most cases of proven DVT or pulmonary embolism. The protamine sulphate precipitation technique is too insensitive to detect subclinical thrombosis but 'gel exclusion chromatographic techniques' may be of value. Raised FDPs are usually found after pulmonary embolism but the results are inconsistent in DVTs.

Platelet Survival. Platelet survival may be reduced in subclinical thromboses and prothrombotic states. It is difficult to measure directly though isotope labelling techniques are available. The presence of megathrombocytes may suggest platelet consumption. The most convenient means of assessing platelet life span is to measure the malondialdehyde (MDA) level, give aspirin which blocks MDA synthesis for the life span of the platelets and then observe the time taken for the MDA level to return to baseline values. Shortened life spans have been demonstrated in peripheral arterial disease.

Platelet release. Measurement of PF4 and β-thromboglobulin may indicate platelet consumption. Increased levels have been reported in myocardial infarction, diabetes, hyperlipoproteinaemia, venous thrombosis, chronic arterial disease and with diseased and prosthetic heart valves.

Platelet Prostaglandin Synthesis. This can be determined by measurement of thromboxane B_2 or MDA. Reduced levels found after myocardial infarction may indicate 'exhausted platelets'.

Investigations primarily intended to delineate the Cause of a Prothrombotic State

Such investigations should not be performed during acute thromboses and investigations must follow careful clinical evaluation. It must be emphasized that with few exceptions the available tests are difficult to interpret precisely.

Full Blood Count. This is the most important test in the investigation of hypercoagulable states in that polycythaemia and thrombocythaemia are amenable to treatment.

Serum Proteins. Estimation of the serum proteins is performed; markedly raised γ globulins may suggest an immunoproliferative disorder with hyperviscosity; a very low albumin should raise the suspicion of nephrotic syndrome with associated AT III deficiency.

Routine Clotting Tests. A slight shortening of the PTT or an increase in Factors V, VII, VIII and X or fibrinogen may be found in some prothrombotic conditions, but these changes are so non-specific that they are generally of little value.

Antithrombin III Estimation. This can be determined in a heparin co-factor assay or by an immunological assay.

Euglobulin Lysis Time. Determination of the euglobulin clot lysis time reflects the level of plasminogen activators. The test may be more informative if performed before and after a challenge such as exercise or tourniquet occlusion of a limb, to measure 'reserve'. The euglobulin clot lysis time was found to have predictive value in a study of postoperative DVTs after gynaecological surgery.

Measurement of Fibrinolytic Inhibitors. Antiplasmin can be measured in both functional and immunological assays.

Platelet Function Tests. Platelet adhesion and aggregation with a variety of agonists are most readily measured.

Prostacyclin Levels. In vivo prostacyclin synthesis assessed by 6oxo $PGF_{1\alpha}$ levels.

Serum Factors influencing Prostacyclin Synthesis. Factors influencing the secretion of prostacyclin-like substances from endothelium can be assessed by using fine rings of rabbit aorta incubated with different sera and measuring anti-aggregatory activity in the supernatant. Both deficiency of serum-promoting factor and an inhibitor of prostacyclin release can be detected.

Selection of Patients

The above tests represent only a fraction of the possible investigations in the study of hypercoagulability and it is apparent that few laboratories can offer such extensive facilities. Many cases must be referred to centres with a special interest, and it is only cost effective to study carefully selected patients. Possible indications for investigation of patients who have had a DVT are shown below.
1. Family history of DVT, pulmonary embolus or mesenteric thrombosis.
2. DVT before the age of 35 years.
3. DVT in early pregnancy.
4. Recurrence of DVT, especially if during heparin therapy.
5. Severe proteinuria (to exclude AT III deficiency).
6. Known myeloproliferative disorder.

Preoperative screening, or screening for arterial disease risk factors is not at present justifiable in a routine laboratory. Emphasis must be placed on detecting abnormalities that are amenable to treatment, and these are mainly hyperviscosity, spontaneous platelet aggregation in the myeloproliferative disorders, and AT III deficiency. Recurrent DVTs and pulmonary embolism often necessitate long-term oral anticoagulation and extensive investigation is unlikely to modify therapy.

Selected Further Reading

Prentice C. R. M. (ed.) (1981) Thrombosis. *Clin. Haematol.* **10**, 2.

Chapter 24 — Anticoagulants and Antithrombotic Drugs

Heparin

Structure

Heparins are a group of a negatively-charged sulphated polysaccharides (glycosaminoglycuronan sulphate esters). They have a helical structure with variable mol. wt averaging 15 000.

Mode of Action

The antithrombotic action of heparin appears to require a plasma cofactor which is an α_2-globulin, antithrombin III, which combines with and inhibits activated clotting factors (serine proteases); these include thrombin, Factors XI, IXa, Xa and XIIIa.

Heparin may bind to lysyl residues on antithrombin III rendering a conformational change which accelerates the inhibitory activity of the antithrombin III. Heparin also binds to thrombin and it is likely that the most efficient inhibition of thrombin takes place when both AT III and thrombin bind to the same heparin molecule. Heparin also has effects on platelets, but the significance of this is controversial. It may enchance primary aggregation directly, but may also inhibit platelet aggregation indirectly by neutralization of the aggregating agent thrombin.

Effect on Coagulation Tests

Heparin has a multisite effect on the coagulation cascade and on platelets, thus many laboratory tests are affected by heparin administration. These include: whole blood clotting time, activated partial thromboplastin time, prothrombin time and the thrombin time. The reptilase time is normal, which can be useful in determining whether abnormalities of the above tests are due to heparin. No completely satisfactory test has been devised for the control of heparin therapy.

Indications for Use

Heparin is considered for use in the following circumstances:
1. Treatment of venous thrombosis and pulmonary embolism.
2. Prophylaxis of venous thrombosis and pulmonary embolism.
3. Treatment of acute arterial occlusion.
4. Maintenance of blood fluidity in extracorporeal circulations such as heart–lung machines.
5. Treatment of disseminated intravascular coagulation.

Treatment of Venous Thrombo-embolism. Heparin is of benefit in deep venous thrombosis and pulmonary embolism, both in the prevention of death and the reduction of non-fatal recurrence.

All patients with popliteal, femoral or iliac vein thrombosis should be treated since these carry a high risk of pulmonary embolism. Treatment of asymptomatic calf vein thrombosis is controversial, but symptomatic calf vein thrombosis is usually treated. Heparin is chosen for initial treatment because its action is immediate. It is usually given for 7–10 days (it takes approximately that time for an experimental thrombus to become adherent to a vessel wall). Risk of recurrent venous thrombo-embolism is greatest in the few weeks after the event and diminishes over the following 6 months or so. Oral anticoagulant therapy is therefore usually continued after 7 days of heparin, the two drugs being overlapped for 2–3 days after the oral anticoagulants are started. Heparin is likely to be as active in saline dextrose though controversy remains. Continuous infusion of heparin is preferred to intermittent intravenous injection as this reduces the incidence of significant short-term over-anticoagulation with consequent bleeding, and ensures a reasonably constant level of anticoagulant not seen with intermittent injection since the half-life of heparin is only 3–8 hours.

Continuous Infusion of Heparin. Give i.v. bolus loading dose of 5000–10 000 u (anticoagulant potency of heparin is standardized so that 100 i.u. of heparin = 1 mg) and then a continuous maintenance infusion of about 25 000–40 000 u/24 hours. The higher doses are recommended in acute pulmonary embolism, to neutralize the preformed thrombin and because the high levels of platelet factor 4 circulating in this situation tend to neutralize the heparin. The dosage is adjusted to keep the PTT or TT 2–3 × normal. If monitoring by a heparin assay the heparin level is kept between 0·3–0·5 u/ml. Lower loading and maintenance doses should be given immediately postoperatively and in liver and renal disease.

Intermittent i.v. Injection of Heparin. Heparin can be given by intermittent i.v. injection either 4- or 6-hourly. If dose monitoring is carried out the PTT or TT is kept to approximately 2 × normal in the period immediately preceding the next injection. 25 000–40 000 units/24 hours are usually given.

The Prophylaxis of Venous Thrombo-embolism. Low-dose heparin probably inhibits the serine proteases early in the clotting cascade; the higher doses necessary to neutralize thrombin are not necessary in this context. One of the most attractive aspects of the low-dose regime is the relative infrequency of haemorrhagic complications. A number of low-dose heparin regimes have been reported to prevent calf popliteal and femoral venous thrombosis with subsequent pulmonary embolism after elective gynaecological and abdominothoracic surgery. Results have been less encouraging after hip surgery and prostatic surgery. Low-dose heparin is also used in pregnancy for prophylaxis in high-risk patients already having suffered a DVT in pregnancy. Heparin does not cross the placenta and therefore does not cause bleeding or teratogenic hazard to the fetus. It may also be useful in preventing DVT in the leg in patients after myocardial infarction.

It is usually given as 5000 u s.c. shortly before surgery and then 5000 u b.d. or t.d.s starting 12 hours postoperatively and continuing for 7–14 days. Much lower doses may, however, be equally effective. Injections are given through a fine gauge needle into subcutaneous fat in the anterior abdominal wall or thigh, and pressure is applied for 5 min after the injection. Low-dose heparin therapy is rarely complicated by haemorrhage.

Heparin in Acute Arterial Occlusion. Heparin is used almost routinely in patients who have had acute peripheral arterial occlusion; it is also frequently used to maintain the patency of vascular grafts and arteriovenous shunts.

Extracorporeal Circulations. High-dose heparin is used.

Heparin in Disseminated Intravascular Coagulation. There is a great conflict of evidence and no good controlled trials of the use of heparin in DIC. In obstetric complications, fulminant infection and malignant disease there is no convincing evidence for the use of heparin. Heparin may (in DIC) be useful in the following circumstances:

1. In renal disease with DIC.
2. Haemolytic uraemic syndrome.
3. Thrombotic thrombocytopenic purpura.
4. Postpartum renal failure.
5. Acute promyelocyte leukaemia.

The dosage of heparin used in DIC is controversial: full convential heparinization is usually not used and low dose i.v. or s.c. heparin is preferred.

Side Effects of Heparin

The most important effect is bleeding. This is not usually seen whilst laboratory tests are in the therapeutic range. Less common complications include osteoporosis, alopecia, hypersensitivity reactions and thrombocytopenia.

Heparin Reversal

Overdose can be immediately neutralized by a strongly basic substance, protamine sulphate—1 mg of protamine neutralizing 1 mg heparin. To neutralize heparin 60 min after a heparin injection give 50 per cent of the neutralizing dose and only 25 per cent at 2 hours. Neutralization is assessed by PTT or TT immediately after the protamine.

ORAL ANTICOAGULANTS

Warfarin or bishydroxycoumarin acts by interfering with the metabolism of vitamin K. Vitamin K is converted in the liver to phylloquinone epoxide by an epoxidase and may be reconverted by a reductase; treatment with warfarin leads to an accumulation of phylloquinone epoxide. This prevents carboxylation of the glutamic acid residues on prothrombin and Factors VII, IX and X. The 'acarboxy' clotting factors do not bind to calcium or phospholipids and are thus unable to undergo the usually rapid activation in the clotting cascade.

Warfarin is given by mouth and rapidly absorbed. The half-life is 30–60 hours and the daily dose is usually 2–15 mg. Warfarin is carried in the plasma bound to albumin and it is the free warfarin which has the anticoagulant effect. More than 95 per cent is protein bound and displacement of only 1–2 per cent from albumin can cause a considerable increase in the anticoagulant activity.

Dindevan (phenindione) acts in the same way as warfarin but the depression of the coagulation factors is slightly slower and is delayed for 36–48 hours following the administration of the initial dose. The half-life of Dindevan is about 5 hours. Its metabolites may colour the urine pink.

Oral Anticoagulants and Laboratory Tests

The dosage of these drugs is monitored by tests of the extrinsic system such as the prothrombin time (PT) or the thrombotest. The PT detects deficiencies of Factors II, V, VII and X whereas the vitamin K antagonists affect Factors II, VII, IX and X. Therefore the PT does not measure Factor IX deficiency, one of the factors affected by oral anticoagulants. The rate of development of a long PT is influenced by the half-lives of the factors involved. Factor VII falls most rapidly (half-life 5–7 hours) and Factor II most slowly (half-life 60–120 hours). The maximum depressant effects of a given dose of warfarin occur after at least 2–3 days. Since Factors II, IX and X are affected by warfarin the PTT is also prolonged. The full antithrombotic effect of warfarin is not seen for about 5 days.

Indications for the Use of Oral Anticoagulants

Although these drugs have been in use as antithrombotic agents for over 30 years a great deal of controversy still surrounds their use. The following are situations in which oral anticoagulants appear to be of use:

1. Deep vein thrombosis.
   a. Prophylaxis in high-risk patients, such as trauma cases, burns, gynaecological surgery, immobilized patients, old patients with fractured lower limbs and selected puerperal and postoperative patients.
   b. In established venous thrombosis following heparin therapy.
   c. In established pulmonary embolism, following heparin therapy. At least 6 months' oral anticoagulants are usually given.
2. Cerebrovascular disease. Anticoagulants may be beneficial in transient ischaemic attacks.
3. Following myocardial infarction. Short-term oral anticoagulants may prevent the thrombo-embolic complications of bed rest. Long-term therapy may reduce the death rate and number of reinfarctions in men under 55 years.
4. Rheumatic heart disease. Oral anticoagulant therapy may reduce the incidence of emboli to the cerebral and peripheral arteries, especially in patients with atrial fibrillation.
5. Prosthetic heart valves.

Dosage and Monitoring of Oral Anticoagulant Therapy

Warfarin is preferable to Dindevan and may be advantageous in patients taking oral hypoglycaemic agents or phenytoin. Therapy with warfarin may be initiated with a loading dose of 30 mg followed by a PT on the third day but initiation with a daily dosage of 8–18 mg/day followed by a PT on the third day is preferable. The onset of the anticoagulant effect is similar but precipitous Factor VII deficiency and bleeding is less likely. Warfarin tablets are colour-coded in the UK:

   1 mg brown
   3 mg blue
   5 mg pink
   10 mg yellow

   Maintenance warfarin varies between about 2 and 15 mg/day. A loading dose of Dindevan may be 150–200 mg with a maintenance dose of usually 50–150 mg but a sensitive patient may need less than 50 mg/day. Using a standard thromboplastin (the British Comparative Thromboplastin of Poller) the patient's PT is compared to a normal control, the therapeutic range being between 2·0 and 4·0 (patient's PT in sec/control in sec). Smaller doses may be necessary in the aged, in liver disease, renal disease and hypermetabolic states, such as fever and thyrotoxicosis; obesity and myxoedema increase requirements. Foreign travel to warm climates is frequently associated with a decreased requirement; close monitoring is advised. Heparin is usually given to initiate anticoagulant therapy and is usually continued for a few days after the oral anticoagulant has been started. Heparin therapy is discontinued after 3 days on oral anticoagulation and a prothrombin time is determined after a further 8 hours.

Drug Interactions in Patients on Oral Anticoagulants

Many drugs interact with oral anticoagulants in a variety of ways (*Tables* 24.1; 24.2; 24.3).

Table 24.1. Oral anticoagulants: mechanism of drug interactions

Mechanism	Result
Displacement of albumin binding	Potentiation
Inhibition of coumarin metabolism	Potentiation
Interference with vitamin K production and metabolism	Potentiation
Acceleration of coumarin metabolism	Decreased activity
Enhanced synthesis of clotting factors	Decreased

Table 24.2. Drugs which potentiate oral anticoagulants

	Mechanism
Alcohol	Enzyme inhibition
Salicylates	Competition for protein receptor sites plus inhibition of platelet function. Also cause gastric erosions
Broad-spectrum antibiotics	Inhibit intestinal flora and bio-synthesis of vitamin K
Chloramphenicol	Enzyme inhibition
Chlorpromazine	Inhibition of enzymes metabolizing oral anticoagulants
Clofibrate	Decreased triglyceride lessens availability of vitamin K
Co-trimoxazole	Competitive affinity for receptor sites and displacement
Mefenamic acid	Competitive affinity for receptor sites and displacement
Phenformin	Additive effect since it increases fibrinolysis
Phenylbutazone	Displacement from binding sites
Probenecid	Displacement from binding sites
Sulphonamides	Displacement from binding sites
Tolbutamide	Displacement from binding sites

Table 24.3. Drugs which decrease the activity of oral anticoagulants

	Mechanism
Barbiturates	Stimulation of liver enzymes metabolizing anticoagulants
Cholestyramine	Reduced absorption of anticoagulant
Dichloralphenazone (Welldorm)	Enzyme induction
Oral contraceptives	Increase clotting factor levels and increase requirement for anticoagulant
Rifampicin	Increase metabolic activity in liver
Vitamin K-containing preparations	Competitive inhibition

Contraindications to Anticoagulation

1. *Absolute* contraindications include active bleeding, blood dyscrasias with haemorrhage, subacute bacterial endocarditis, dissecting aneurysms, CNS and eye surgery and recent non-embolic strokes.

2. *Relative* contraindications include patients with insufficient co-operation or intelligence, lack of adequate laboratory control facilities, severe hypertension, pregnancy, hepatic or renal insufficiency, alcoholism, and advanced age.

Side Effects of Oral Anticoagulants

Warfarin side effects include alopecia, skin rashes, skin necrosis, diarrhoea and jaundice. These are all rare. Haemorrhage from overdosage is the most common and most serious complication. *Dindevan* side effects are manifestations of hypersensitivity and exfoliative dermatitis, fever, leucopenia and agranulocytosis, diarrhoea, hepatitis and renal tubular necrosis. Warfarin is usually tolerated by patients sensitive to Dindevan and vice versa.

Nicoumalone (Sinthrome) may be useful in patients sensitive to both warfarin and Dindevan.

Reversal of Oral Anticoagulant Effect

1. Stop anticoagulant.
2. Fresh frozen plasma or even prothrombin complex may need to be given for immediate reversal.
3. If bleeding, consider vitamin K 1 or 2 mg i.v., though this takes some hours to act and may block adequate anticoagulation for some days afterwards.

Resistance to Oral Anticoagulants

Patients may become resistant to one type of oral anticoagulant but usually not the others. If resistance is suspected, check the following:
1. Is the patient taking his correct dose?
2. Stop any possible interfering drug, e.g. barbiturate.
3. Change to the other main oral agent or consider heparin.
4. Give tetracycline for 4–7 days to alter gut flora.

FIBRINOLYTIC AGENTS

There are two major groups of fibrinolytic agents.

1. Naturally-occurring compounds which convert plasminogen to plasmin, e.g. streptokinase and urokinase. The aim of therapy with these agents is to activate plasminogen absorbed on to thrombus, promoting local fibrinolysis, without excessive systemic action. Plasmin digests fibrin, fibrinogen, Factors II, V and VIII and also activates Factor XII.

2. Synthetic agents which produce only a moderate increase in fibrinolytic activity, and may be of value in preventing venous and arterial thrombosis. Such agents are still experimental and include:

> 2.1 Biguanides such as metformin and phenformin. These agents will increase fibrinolytic activity for several months when resistance develops.
>
> 2,2 Anabolic steroids such as ethyloestrenol and stanozolol which maintain increased fibrinolytic activity for many months. These drugs may cause masculinization and cholestatic jaundice.

Streptokinase

Streptokinase is a water-soluble protein obtained from a filtrate of β-haemolytic streptococci. It has a mol. wt of 47 000. It combines with plasminogen to form an active complex which converts other plasminogen molecules to plasmin.

$$\text{Streptokinase} + \text{Plasminogen (equimolar)} \rightarrow \text{Active complex}$$
$$\downarrow$$
$$\text{Plasminogen} \rightarrow \text{Plasmin}$$

Possible Indications for Streptokinase Therapy

1. Deep venous thrombosis.

Streptokinase given early to phlebographically-proven venous thrombosis is probably superior to heparin in terms of reducing clot extension and preserving venous valves. The risks of streptokinase are much greater than with heparin.

2. Pulmonary Embolism

Streptokinase has been used as first-line treatment in life-threatening pulmonary embolism though most centres prefer emergency surgery and reserve streptokinase for major embolism that is not immediately life-threatening. Pulmonary angiography should be performed and streptokinase can be given into a pulmonary artery catheter.

3. Acute arterial thrombosis or embolism in a limb.

The occlusion most suitable for treatment is that below the origin of the superficial and deep femoral artery. Most of these cases show resolution if the occlusion is less than 12 hours old. The value of streptokinase in more severe occlusions is uncertain.

4. Streptokinase may reduce the mortality in myocardial infarction.

5. Clearing arteriovenous shunts.

6. Central retinal vein thrombosis.

7. Priapism.

Dosage and Monitoring. There is little agreement on optimum dosages.

Streptokinase is antigenic and naturally-occurring antibodies (probably due to previous streptococcal infections) must first be neutralized; a loading dose of 250 000–600 000 u is usually given, followed by maintenance therapy of 100 000 u/hour for 3–7 days. Steroids are usually given to counteract possible febrile and allergic reactions, and diuretics are also often given. Measurement of the thrombin time, fibrinogen level and degradation products give some indication of the therapeutic efficacy but the data is difficult to interpret; many centres do not consider laboratory control necessary. A full blood count, clotting screen and blood group should be performed before starting thrombolytic therapy.

Complications of Streptokinase Therapy. Bleeding is common especially from drip sites and areas of trauma. Fever and allergic reactions such as hoarseness, bronchospasm and stridor are not uncommon.

Contraindication to Fibrinolytic Therapy.
1. Major surgery within the previous week.
2. Postpartum.
3. Peptic ulcer.
4. Recent stroke.
5. Severe hypertension.
6. Known coagulation defect.
7. Streptokinase therapy in the previous 6 months.

Urokinase

Urokinase is isolated from human male urine and is non-toxic and non-antigenic. It is presently very expensive.

Uses

As for streptokinase.

The dose used is very variable but one possible regime is to give a loading dose of 150 000 i.u. followed by 2500 i.u./kg/hr.

Urokinase may be especially useful in closed situations where the cost is not so prohibitive, e.g. hyphaema and vitreous haemorrhage when urokinase is injected into the eye.

DEFIBRINATION THERAPY

Ancrod

Ancrod is a snake venom which converts fibrinogen to soluble fibrin by cleavage of fibrinopeptide A; fibrinogen levels fall and the levels of FDPs rise. Other clotting factors are unaffected.

Ancrod is as effective as heparin in the treatment of DVTs but it is expensive and potentially very hazardous which limits its usefulness.

ANTIPLATELET AGENTS

Many drugs inhibit various aspects of platelet function, but the clinically most important are aspirin, dipyridamole and sulphinpyrazone. They have been used in many conditions though there is a paucity of well-designed clinical trials.

Aspirin

Mechanism of Action. The major effect of aspirin is the irreversible acetylation of platelet cyclo-oxygenase (*see Fig.* 19.4) with the inhibition of platelet prostaglandin production. Aspirin also inhibits prostacyclin production and there is some evidence that this effect on vessel walls requires a higher dose. The effect on prostacyclin is short-lived as, unlike platelets, nucleated endothelial cells can synthesize further cyclo-oxygenase. In theory, therefore, low-dose aspirin (e.g. 300 mg twice a week) may be superior to high-dose aspirin as an antithrombotic agent. In high doses aspirin also reduces the concentration of Factors II, V, VII and X; this effect is reversed by vitamin K.

The bleeding time and platelet aggregation tests are all affected by aspirin.

Possible Uses

1. Cerebrovascular Transient ischaemic attacks (TIAs)
2. Valvular disease of the heart.

Aspirin added to oral anticoagulants (e.g. warfarin) decreases the thrombo-embolic problems seen with prosthetic valves, but complicates the anticoagulant management.

3. Coronary artery disease and myocardial infarction.

Several studies show a favourable trend with aspirin therapy but the differences are not significant.

4. Venous thromboses.

Aspirin apparently reduces the frequency of DVTs after hip surgery but not general surgery.

5. Maintenance of arteriovenous shunts.
6. Hypercoagulable conditions.

Aspirin is often given in conditions such as the myeloproliferative disorders with high platelet counts. Good data are lacking.

In many of the above situations aspirin is used in combination with dipyridamole and sulphinpyrazone.

Dipyridamole (Persantin)

Mechanism of Action. A pyrimido-pyrimidine compound initially introduced as a vasodilator. Its major effect on platelets is inhibition of platelet phosphodiesterase with a consequent increase in cyclic AMP and a fall in cytoplasmic Ca^{2+}. Platelet adhesion and aggregation are thus reduced.

Uses. As for aspirin with which it is usually given in combination. The dose is 100–200 mg t.d.s.

Sulphinpyrazone (Anturan)

Mode of Action. The mode of action is poorly understood; it is probably a competitive inhibitor of cyclo-oxygenase. One of its metabolites is probably also an active anti-platelet agent. Sulphinpyrazone inhibits in vitro aggregation but has little effect on the bleeding time.

Uses

1. Myocardial Infarction

A large study showed a decreased early mortality after myocardial infarction in those patients given sulphinpyrazone. The design of this study has been questioned.

2. Maintenance of arteriovenous shunts.
3. TIAs—not shown to be as effective as aspirin. The usual dose is up to 200 mg qds after commencing at 25–50 mg tds and increasing over 2–3 weeks.

Selected Further Reading

Fuster V. and Cheseboro J. H. (1981) Antithrombotic drugs: Role of platelet inhibitor drugs. *Mayo Clin. Proc.* **56**, 102.
Kakhar V. V. and Scully M. F. (1978) Thrombolytic therapy. *Br. Med. Bull.* **34**, 191.
Prentice C. R. M. (ed.) (1981) Thrombosis. *Clin. Haematol.* **10**, 2.

Chapter 25

Blood Groups, Antibodies and Compatibility Testing

RED CELL ANTIGENS

Chemical Structure

The ABO, Lewis, Ii and P systems have antigen specificity determined by glycosphingolipids; most of the other systems are proteins.

Inheritance

All red cell antigens and serum groups (except the Xg system) are autosomally inherited. The incidence of the ABO blood groups in Europeans is shown in *Table 25.1*.

Table 25.1. Incidence of ABO blood groups in the UK

Blood group	Incidence in UK
A	36%
B	14%
AB	3%
O	47%

The ABO System

There are three alternative genes A, B and O which act on the product of an early gene H. O leaves the H antigen unchanged; A causes the addition of an N-acetyl-galactosamine sugar group and B leads to the addition of a D-galactose group. The phenotypes and genotypes of the ABO system are given in *Table 25.2*.

Table 25.2. The ABO blood group system

Phenotype	Genotype	Antibodies present
A	AA or AO	anti-B
B	BB or BO	anti-A
AB	AB	Nil
O	OO	anti-A and anti-B

Subgroups of A are recognized; approximately 80 per cent of Europeans being designated A_1 and 20 per cent A_2. A_2 is like a weak form of A_1, but there must also be a qualitative difference as some A_2 patients form anti-A_1. Rare weak expressions of the A antigen occur and include A_3, A_X, A_M and A_{el}. Weaker expressions of the B antigen are less important than those of the A antigen, but do occur, e.g. B_3, B_X, B_{el}.

Rarely, the amount of A, B, H antigens decrease in acute leukaemia. Rarely, a B-like antigen is acquired on the red cells of elderly patients with carcinoma.

The Lewis System (Table 25.3)

The antigens are soluble antigens present in the serum which are passively absorbed on to the red cell membranes. The Le^a antigen depends on the Le gene (Le a$^+$). The Le^b antigen depends on both the Le gene and the presence of the secretor gene Se. In adults only small amounts of the Le a$^+$ substance remain and the phenotype is designated Le (a$^-$b$^+$). At birth there is poor expression of Le a$^+$ and cord blood groups as (Le a$^-$b$^-$). The b$^+$ antigen develops more slowly than the a$^+$ antigen and young children who later group as Le (a$^-$b$^+$) express both the a$^+$ and b$^+$ substance.

Antibodies to Lewis antigens occur in 1 per cent of the population and are one of the commonest causes of incompatibility in ABO matched blood though rarely causing severe haemolytic transfusion reactions. If in these patients Le (a$^-$b$^-$) blood cannot be obtained the antibodies can be neutralized by the prior administration of plasma containing the Lewis antigens.

Table 25.3. The Lewis blood group system

Genotypes	Red cell antigens	Adult incidence in UK
Le Le Se Se Le le Se se Le Le Se Se Le le Se se	Le (a$^-$b$^+$)	73%
Le Le se se Le le se se	Le (a$^+$b$^-$)	22%
le le Se Se le le Se se le le se se	Le (a$^-$b$^-$)	5%

Ii System

Red cells of the newborn react strongly with anti-i, but weakly with anti-I, whereas in adults the converse usually occurs. In some haematological disorders there is an increase in i substance, e.g. situations of marrow stress, congenital dyserythropoietic anaemia Type II, some hypoplastic anaemias and leukaemias. After mycoplasma infection, there may be a temporary rise in the titre of anti-I and this can cause haemolysis. In cold haemagglutinin disease the antibody present often has anti-I specificity. Anti-i may occur after infectious mononucleosis and occasionally in cold haemagglutin disease.

P System

In Europe 75 per cent are P_1 and 25 per cent P_2. Most P_2 adults have anti-P_1 which is a cold antibody rarely active above 20 °C and is not of consequence in transfusions.

Scolices of *Taenia echinococcus* contain a P-like substance and patients with hydatid disease have high titres of anti-P in the serum.

The Donath–Landsteiner test in paroxysmal cold haemoglobinuria recognizes an IgG antibody with anti-P specificity.

Rhesus (Rh) Group System

The original classification of individuals into Rh positive (85 per cent in Europeans) was due to the presence or absence of the D antigen. The system is known to be composed basically of three closely-linked allelic genes, C or c, D or d, E or e, one set being inherited from each parent. Certain genetic combinations are more common and are listed in *Table 25.4*.

Table 25.4. Incidence (approximate) of commonest Rhesus genotypes

CDe/cde (R_1r)	31%
CDe/CDe (R_1R_1)	16%
cDE/cde (R_2r)	13%
CDe/cDE (R_1R_2)	13%
cde/cde (rr)	15%

By using specific type sera (all are available except anti-d), the most likely pair of genotype sets can be determined. The D antigen is most important; 85 per cent of the population are D positive. For the purposes of blood transfusion a recipient is called rhesus negative if he is d/d. For donors more stringent criteria are usually applied and a rhesus-negative donor must be cde/cde so as to prevent antibodies developing to C or E.

D Subgroups (D^u). Some D^u subjects possess the D type antigen, but there are fewer antigen sites on the red cell surface. Other D^u subjects have some component fraction of D absent and the subject may make antibodies to the missing fraction. There is a spectrum of the number of fractions missing. As the type of D^u cannot be identified it is safer for such patients to receive D negative (d/d) blood, though the risk of such patients developing anti-D is very remote.

Kell (K) System

In Europe 9 per cent of the population are Kell positive (KK or Kk). Next in frequency to the ABO and Rh systems, Kell antibodies are the most frequent in clinical practice. About 1 in 1000 pregnancies are affected and haemolytic disease of the newborn sometimes is severe.

Duffy (Fy) System

In Europe 66 per cent of the population have the phenotype Fy (a^+b^-) or Fy (a^+b^+), 34 per cent are Fy (a^-b^+). In West Africa there is a high incidence (over 90 per cent) of Fy (a⁻b⁻). It is associated with resistance to infection with *Plasmodium vivax* as the Duffy antigens are involved in the plasmodium binding site.

Haemolytic disease of the newborn may occur due to Duffy antibodies.

Kidd (Jk) System

In Europe 76 per cent of the population possess Jkᵃ, 50 per cent have the phenotype Jk (a⁺b⁺) and 26 per cent Jk (a⁺b⁻). Haemolytic disease of the newborn is very rare. It may be a cause of delayed transfusion reaction.

MNS System

The MN system is very rarely of clinical significance. The SS locus is very close to the MN locus hence inheritance of both systems is closely associated.

Lutheran (Lu) System

In Europe 8 per cent of the population have the phenotype Lu (a⁺b⁺) and 92 per cent have (Lu a⁻b⁺). The phenotypes Lu (a⁺b⁻) and Lu (a⁻b⁻) are very rare. Anti-Luᵃ has not been responsible for either transfusion reactions or haemolytic disease of the newborn. Anti Luᵇ is a rare cause of delayed transfusion reactions.

BLOOD GROUP ANTIBODIES

A primary antibody response leads to the slow development of low titres of IgM.

A secondary antibody response is brisker and gives higher levels of antibody, mainly of the IgG class.

Antibodies to the absent AB antigens appear by 6 months of age and are called 'naturally-occurring antibodies'. Antibodies to the Rhesus system occur after transfusion or pregnancy and are called 'immune antibodies'.

Cold antibodies cause optimal agglutination at 0–4 °C and react weakly or not at all at 37 °C. Warm antibodies react at both temperatures but cause agglutination more rapidly at 37 °C. A complete antibody will agglutinate erythrocytes bearing the appropriate antigens. An incomplete antibody only causes agglutination if the red cell negative charge is reduced by enzyme treatment or by coating in albumin. Incomplete antibodies can still activate complement. (*Table 25.5.*)

Table 25.5. Classification of red cell antibodies

Naturally-occurring antibodies	—	Cold	—	Complete	—	IgM
Immune antibodies	—	Warm	—	Complete	—	IgM
			—	Incomplete	—	IgG

BLOOD GROUPING AND COMPATIBILITY TESTING

Sample Collection and Preparation

A sample taken into 3 per cent sodium citrate is suitable for immediate red cell grouping; the sample should be taken into ACD and stored at 4 °C if red cell grouping is undertaken the next day. A clotted sample may be taken to provide a serum sample; after centrifugation, normal saline may be added to the clot to elute red cells which are washed by recentrifugation and resuspended to form a 20 per cent concentration for rapid slide grouping techniques or 3 and 5 per cent concentrations for tube techniques. The antigenic status decreases more rapidly in red cells obtained from a clot than in a citrated sample. P and K antigens especially are less detectable after storage.

Complement deteriorates rapidly in unseparated blood at room temperature, thus samples should be separated as soon as possible. Complement deteriorates less rapidly in citrated plasma stored at 4 °C than in serum, but serum stored at −20 °C usually shows little deterioration of complement after several weeks but some sera may become anticomplementary and antibodies such as anti-Le may be undetected in such samples. Heparin is anticomplementary and is unsuitable as an anticoagulant for blood grouping or compatibility testing samples. Red cells must be washed prior to testing, otherwise (1) rouleaux may be increased; (2) albumin agglutinins may produce false results; (3) anticoagulant present may be anti-complementary; (4) soluble antigens of ABO, Le and Ii systems may inhibit agglutination.

Sterility of Grouping Sera

To preserve sterility vials of 2 ml or 5 ml should be stored at −20 °C until required. When being used storage at 4 °C is satisfactory but a bacteriostatic agent such as 0·01 per cent sodium azide should be added. Care should be taken not to use azide in laboratories with metallic waste plumbing as explosive compounds such as copper azide or lead azide may be formed. Neomycin, gentamicin and chloramphenicol may be used to reduce the risk of bacterial contamination if sodium azide cannot be used.

Various bacteria (as well as some enzymes) will activate the latent T receptors of red cells. Some 'normal' sera contain anti-T and if the T receptors are exposed the cells are polyagglutinable, thus false positive results are obtained with anti-A, anti-B and other specific grouping sera.

Routine Red Cell Typing

Rapid ABO typing may be carried out at room temperature by adding an equal volume of a 20 per cent cell suspension to a slide containing one or two drops of anti-A and a slide containing one or two drops of anti-B, mixing and noting the presence or absence of agglutination after 2 min of gently 'rocking' the slide.

Tube agglutination typing techniques are carried out by adding an equal volume of a 3 per cent cell suspension to the grouping serum and left for 90 min at room temperature for ABO typing and at 37 °C for Rh typing.

For ABO typing, using the tube technique red cells are tested with anti-A, anti-B and also anti-A plus anti-B. The serum is tested for the presence of the complementary antibody to act as a check to the cell typing.

Results of the standard ABO typing are shown on *Table 25.6*.

Table 25.6. ABO typing

Group of individual tested	Reaction with cells by specific antisera			Results of agglutination with sera of individuals		
	Anti-A	Anti-B	Anti-A+B	A_1 cells	B cells	O cells
A_1	+	Neg	+	Neg	+	Neg
B	Neg	+	+	+	Neg	Neg
AB	+	+	+	Neg	Neg	Neg
O	Neg	Neg	Neg	+	+	Neg

Some Group A_2 and some Group A_2B individuals have anti-A_1 in their sera and therefore may react thus:

A_2	+	Neg	+	+	+	Neg
A_2B	+	+	+	+	Neg	Neg
Ax (containing anti-A_1)	Neg	Neg	+	+	+	Neg

The use of serum from a Group O individual (containing anti-A, anti-A_1 and anti-B) will detect the rare subtypes of A not detected by anti-A and -A_1 present in serum from a Group B individual.

Rhesus Typing

Testing with anti-D may be carried out in four ways: (1) To a 5 per cent red cell suspension incomplete anti-D in the presence of 20 per cent bovine albumin is added, incubated at 37 °C and the presence or absence of agglutination noted after 90 min; (2) The indirect antiglobulin (Coombs) technique is used whereby cells are incubated with incomplete anti-D at 37 °C for 1 hour, washed three times with normal saline, anti-human globulin (AHG) added. Cells which have been coated by anti-D (Rhesus positive) agglutinate; (3) The rapid screening test involves the use of a reagent which causes agglutination of rhesus positive cells directly. The reagents contain an enzyme (such as trypsin, papain or ficin) sometimes with the addition of a rouleaux-enhancing agent (such as dextran) which facilitates agglutination of rhesus-positive cells by the otherwise incomplete anti-D; (4) A saline-reacting complete anti-D, which is an IgM antibody (cf. the incomplete IgG antibody) sometimes is produced as an initial response by D-negative subjects to the D antigen. Cells may thus be tested in a tube by incubating directly with the saline-reacting antibody. For urgent cases the cells may be centrifuged lightly after 15 min incubation and evidence of agglutination determined microscopically.

Rhesus Grouping of Blood Donors

Blood donors who are Rh-D negative are further screened with anti-C and anti-E so that 'Rhesus-negative' donors' blood is of the genotype cde/cde (r/r).

Provision of Blood for Patients

While the ABO and Rhesus groups are being determined it is helpful for the patient's serum to be tested against a panel of Group O cells, with differing combinations of other blood groups, so that the presence of atypical antibodies may be determined prior to the compatibility testing.

Compatibility Testing using Normal Ionic Strength Saline (NISS)

The term 'cross-matching' is a misnomer, for only the major cross-match—donor cells with recipient serum—is tested; the minor cross-match, recipient cells with donor serum, is not normally performed.

In the standard compatibility tests, donor red cells of the appropriate ABO and Rh groups are selected and tested by the following techniques.

Saline Technique. An equal volume of 2 per cent washed donor red cells is added to the patient's serum, mixed, and incubated at 20 °C and also at 37 °C and evidence of agglutination determined microscopically by aspirating the sedimented red cells, after 90 min incubation, and laying gently on a slide. These procedures act as a check for ABO compatibility, the presence of atypical IgM antibodies including 'cold agglutinins' which have a high thermal amplitude. A control test using the patient's own red cells and serum should be included to determine whether autoagglutinins are present.

Albumin Technique. An equal volume of 2 per cent washed donor red cells is added to 1 volume of the patient's serum and 1 volume of 20 per cent bovine albumin. After incubation for 90 min the results are determined in like manner to the saline technique. This procedure will demonstrate the presence of immune antibodies, including 'incomplete' types.

Indirect Antiglobulin Test. A unit volume of 3 or 5 per cent washed donor red cells is added to 2 volumes of the patient's serum, mixed, and incubated at 37 °C for 90 min. The red cells are then washed three times with normal saline and a unit volume of a broad-spectrum anti-human globulin (containing anti-IgG, anti-IgM and also anti-complement) are added. The red cells are lightly centrifuged and examined microscopically for evidence of agglutination. A control of the patient's red cells incubated with the patient's serum should be used to determine the possible presence of auto-antibodies.

Compatibility Testing using Low Ionic Strength Saline (LISS). In recent years many laboratories have introduced the use of LISS in place of normal ionic strength saline (NISS) in compatibility testing to increase sensitivity and reduce incubation time. LISS contains approximately 0·2 per cent sodium chloride either in a glucose solution or in buffered sodium glycinate. Donor red cells are washed in LISS and resuspended to form a 5 per cent solution.

Principle. At low ionic strengths erythrocytes have less repulsive negative charge and agglutinate more readily.

Saline Technique. The tests are carried out at 20 °C and 37 °C and read microscopically as described previously except that the incubation time is only 20 min instead of 90 min.

LISS is more sensitive than normal saline for detecting 'cold antibodies', thus weak reactions may be disregarded provided the results at 37 °C are negative.

Albumin Technique. A unit volume of 5 per cent red cells is added to 1 volume of serum, mixed and incubated at 37 °C for 20 min. One volume of bovine albumin is added and the mixture reincubated for a further 10 min, then read.

Indirect Antiglobulin Test. This is carried out as described previously except that the cells are washed after only 10 min incubation.

Selected Further Reading

Mollison P. L. (1979) *Blood Transfusion in Clinical Medicine,* 6th ed. Oxford, Blackwell Scientific Publications.

Chapter 26 Use of Blood Products

Most blood products in the UK are obtained from healthy volunteers between the ages of 16 and 65 years. The blood is screened for Australia antigen and syphilis. Transmission of non-A non-B hepatitis remains a major problem with many products.

USE OF WHOLE BLOOD

1. To restore the intravascular volume as well as increasing the oxygen-carrying capacity of the blood, e.g. acute blood loss.

2. Hypovolaemia without loss of oxygen-carrying capacity, as in the early stages of burns or peritonitis, requires red-cell-free volume expanders. In the later stages whole blood is also necessary.

Initially, saline, plasma protein fraction or plasma expanders such as low molecular weight dextran may be used until whole blood is available. In previously healthy patients a 500-ml loss is well compensated; quantities greater than this require volume replacement though 1000 ml are often well tolerated and up to 1500 ml may be lost before shock develops. In patients with pre-existing disorders, especially cardiac, serious consequences may develop with smaller volumes of blood loss. Quantitation of blood loss may be assessed by:

2.1 Direct estimation of blood loss.

2.2 Increase of pulse rate.

2.3 Fall in blood pressure (previously known levels in hypertensive patients are very important).

2.4 Symptoms of hypovolaemia such as pallor and cold skin due to vasoconstriction, sweating, thirst, restlessness and air hunger.

2.5. Monitoring the central venous pressure, also a valuable aid to management.

The haemoglobin level is not helpful in acute blood loss; without replacement therapy the haemoglobin level does not change significantly for 3–6 hours. If a massive transfusion is required, at least 1 in 4 units administered should be fresh blood. If in an emergency, fresh blood is not available, labile coagulation factors should be provided by the administration of 2 units of fresh frozen plasma with every 5 units of stored blood. Although the platelet count falls, platelet concentrates are rarely required (*see* Chapter 27 for hazards of massive blood transfusion).

3. Exchange transfusion in neonates suffering from haemolytic disease of the newborn to remove sensitized red cells and lower bilirubin levels; blood less than 48 hours old must be used to avoid hyperkalaemia as well as to supply labile clotting components.

4. Sickle-cell disease to raise haemoglobin level, suppress erythropoiesis and reduce incidence of crises. Whole blood, being less viscous than red cell concentrate is preferable.

5. In priming heart–lung machines and some renal dialysis equipment; heparinized blood is used in heart–lung machines to avoid de-ionization of calcium.

RED CELL CONCENTRATES

Plasma-reduced blood with a haematocrit of 70 per cent is especially suitable for transfusion to severely anaemic patients. Anaemic patients should not be transfused until adequate blood examination has been performed and samples taken for further investigations; nor should they receive transfusion if the anaemia will respond to haematinics unless: (i) the patient is seriously ill from anaemia; (ii) requires preparation for acute surgery; (iii) severe anaemia is present late in pregnancy.

ADMINISTRATION OF WHOLE BLOOD AND RED CELL CONCENTRATES

It is advisable to give the first 50–100 ml of every unit slowly so that untoward reactions can be observed and, if necessary, the transfusion stopped. In otherwise healthy adults 6 ml of whole blood or 4 ml of red cell concentrate/kg of body weight/hour may be given; in anaemic patients 3 ml/kg of body weight/hour is recommended. The calculation of the rate of infusion for infants and children is similar to adults. As an approximation, 6 ml of whole blood/kg of body weight will raise the haemoglobin level 1 g/dl.

WASHED RED CELLS

The red cells are washed three times in saline; the cells should be administered within 12 hours of washing. The preparation contains few white cells and few platelets, consequently antibodies to these cells are less likely to be produced and reactions due to pre-existing antibodies are less. Plasma is also removed, so reactions due to IgA antibodies are avoided.

FROZEN STORAGE OF RED CELLS

Red cells are kept at $-80\,°C$ or lower. Two basic procedures are used: (i) slow freezing with a 4M glycerol concentration; (ii) rapid freezing with 2·25M glycerol concentration. The glycerol must be removed prior to transfusion, using a blood processor such as Fenwall, Hemonetics or IBM machine, for 'washing' cells prior to transfusion. Because of risk of bacterial contamination the washed red cells are administered within 12 hours of thawing and 'washing' procedures.

This preparation benefits from indefinite storage of red cells, hence is used for red cells of rare phenotypes. There is less contamination by white cells and platelets than any other preparation and frozen red cells can be used to minimize transfusion reactions in the multiple transfused patient. In some centres frozen blood is used for potential organ-transplant recipients to reduce sensitization to HLA antigens.

GRANULOCYTE CONCENTRATES

Granulocyte preparations may be obtained by (i) continuous flow cell separator such as Aminco or IBM centrifuge machines. Heparinized or citrated blood is centrifuged and the granulocyte fraction separated, the depleted blood returned to the donor; (ii) intermittent-flow separator designed by Hemonetics which requires the addition of a rouleaux-forming agent such as hydroxyethyl starch, Plasmagel (a modified liquid gelatine) or Dextran 150; (iii) by filtration leucophoresis in which blood from a donor is heparinized and pumped through nylon filters and returned to the donor via a vein in the other arm. The granulocytes are subsequently eluted from the filters with an ACD–plasma–saline mixture.

Administration of etiocholanolone or steroids to the donor enhances the yield of granulocytes. It is believed that granulocytes obtained by filtration are physiologically and kinetically inferior to those obtained by centrifugation. Side effects in the recipient such as cough, dyspnoea, cyanosis, fever and rigors are more common with granulocyte preparations prepared by filtration.

Indications for Administration

1. Infections unresponsive after 24 hours treatment with broad-spectrum antibiotics in patients with severe neutropenia (some centres recommend earlier administration).

2. Prophylaxis in patients with severe transient neutropenia due to drugs, chemicals or radiation. This is controversial.

The daily dose of granulocytes should exceed 1×10^{10} if obtained by continuous flow separation and 5×10^{10} if by filtration. The value of granulocyte transfusions is difficult to assess.

PLATELET CONCENTRATES

Preparations

These may be obtained by use of continuous-flow or intermittent-flow cell separators as used for harvesting granulocytes or by separating off red cells from normal donated blood packs by centrifugation at 4000 g for 3 min or 400 g for 15 min, transferring the plasma to a satellite bag containing additional ACD, then spinning the satellite bag. It is important to avoid transferring any of the 'buffy coat' to avoid contamination with leucocytes. Ideally, donor's HLA matched with the recipient are used, a cell separator being required.

There may be contamination of routine platelet preparations with leucocytes and red cells may also present in the preparations. For this latter reason ABO and rhesus compatibility is observed.

Indications for Administration

1. Thrombocytopenia associated with bleeding.
2. Prophylaxis in severe thrombocytopenia (platelets $< 20 \times 10^9/l$) or moderate thrombocytopenia ($< 80 \times 10^9/l$) if surgery is anticipated. The indications for use of platelets in these situations are poorly defined but depend on the rate of fall of the platelet count as well as the absolute value. Sensitization to platelet antigens may reduce the efficacy of future platelet transfusions. In immune thrombocytopenia, platelets are usually only given for life-threatening haemorrhage. The half-life of the platelets in these patients is very short.
3. Bleeding associated with qualitative platelet defects.

Platelet Storage

Platelets stored at 22 °C with constant agitation give better survival figures than storage at 4 °C but the latter temperature storage provides better activity as demonstrated by ADP aggregation. It is recommended that for management of bleeding, platelets stored at 4 °C are used, but for prophylactic support therapy platelets stored at 22 °C (which will survive for 3–4 days in vivo) should be used. Platelets frozen in 5 per cent dimethyl sulphoxide (DMSO), in liquid nitrogen have no initial haemostatic defect when prepared for administration but recover function within 3 hours; survival times are good.

Platelet Transfusions

An attempt should be made to maintain the platelet level above $20 \times 10^9/l$ during therapy though in association with thrombasthenia levels above $50 \times 10^9/l$ may be required. Following transfusion, up to 80 per cent of the platelets become temporarily sequestrated in the spleen but re-enter the circulation over the next few hours. The success of platelet transfusions should be assessed by arrest of bleeding and reduction in bruising rather than by the recorded platelet count.

Reactions occurring with platelet transfusions may be due to:
1. Contamination of leucocytes in previously sensitized patients producing symptoms of mild fever though occasionally rigors occur.
2. Pulmonary sequestration of platelet aggregates producing dyspnoea and cyanosis.
3. Sensitization to platelet antigens.

DRIED PLASMA

Use has diminished owing to the increased risk of hepatitis associated with pooling of plasma from several donors during preparation.

FRESH PLASMA

Preparation

Plasma is separated from freshly donated whole blood by centrifugation and transferred into a satellite pack or by use of a cell-separator for plasmapheresis of a donor.

Indications for Use

Identical with those described under FFP *below*.

FRESH FROZEN PLASMA (FFP)

Separated within 6 hours of donation and stored at $-30\,°C$ or less. It contains about 60 per cent of the original Factor VIII C, 90 per cent of original Factor IX and 80 per cent of Factor XI.

Indications for Administration

1. Transfusion of large amounts of stored blood which are deficient in the labile Factors V and VIII; 20 per cent of infused plasma should be either in fresh whole blood or FFP.
2. Acquired coagulation disorders:
       2.1 Due to liver impairment.
       2.2 Caused by oral anticoagulants, such as warfarin or phen-indione. 500 ml–1 litre of FFP are usually sufficient to correct the abnormal prothrombin and partial thromboplastin time.
3. Von Willebrand's disease—minor haemorrhages can often be treated with FFP though cryoprecipitate is the preparation of choice.
4. Factor XI deficiency: mild bleeds respond to 500 ml, but major bleeds and preoperative management require 1 litre. The half-life of Factor XI is about $2\frac{1}{2}$ days.
5. Angioneureotic oedema—C1 esterase inhibitor deficiency corrected.
6. Hyaline membrane disease may be associated with a low plasminogen level which may be corrected by fresh frozen plasma.
7. Fluid replacement in hypovolaemia without blood loss.

PLASMA PROTEIN FRACTION (PPF)

Plasma protein fraction (PPF) is a 4–5 g per cent protein solution presented in 400 ml volume exerting the same colloid osmotic pressure as an equal volume of reconstituted dried plasma. Over 90 per cent of the protein has the electrophoretic mobility of albumin and it contains 130–160 mmol/l of sodium and less than 2 mmol/l of potassium. It can be given without regard to the blood group of the recipient. PPF contains no fibrinogen or clotting factors and should not be used to treat coagulation disorders, unlike FFP.

Indications for Use

1. As a plasma volume expander when red cells are not required, or before red cells are available, e.g. in burns, crush injury, oligaemic shock.
2. Replacement fluid during plasmapheresis.

DRIED ALBUMIN (LOW SALT CONTENT)

Preparation is reconstituted with sterile pyrogen-free distilled water. Compared with PPF there is less sodium and less potassium.

Indications for Use

1. Shock without blood loss, e.g. burns, peritonitis. If clotting is normal PPF is preferable to FFP, but use is limited by its price and availability.
2. Shock with blood loss until blood is available.
3. Replacement fluid during plasmapheresis.

CRYOPRECIPITATE

Preparation

Plasma is frozen and then just thawed, the remaining protein precipitate contains about 50 per cent of the original Factor VIII present, that is between 50 and 100 i.u. of Factor VIII C. It also contains a high concentration of fibrinogen (250 mg/u) and the so-called 'stimulating factor' (Factor VIII VW). Cryoprecipitate can be stored at $-20\,°C$ for 2 years without significant deterioration.

Indication for Administration

1. Management of haemophilia.
2. Management of von Willebrand's disease.
3. Replacement therapy in disseminated intravascular coagulation.

FACTOR VIII CONCENTRATE

Preparation

This preparation is less bulky than cryoprecipitate and can be stored at $4\,°C$. It is particularly suitable for home therapy. Contains only low levels of fibrinogen.

FACTOR VIII CONCENTRATES— ANIMAL ORIGIN

Both porcine and bovine preparations are available. Suitable only for use in patients who have developed inhibitors to human Factor VIII. Antigenic and therefore liable to produce severe reactions in previously sensitized patients. Not usually effective after initial 10 days of use due to antibody neutralization of Factor VIII. May induce specific anti-animal Factor VIII which does not cross-react with human Factor VIII.

FACTOR IX FRACTION CONCENTRATES

Contain Factors II, IX, and X to approximately the same degree. Factor VII may or may not be present, depending on mode of preparation.

Indications for Use

1. Christmas disease.
2. Liver disease.
3. Correcting anticoagulant deficiencies.
4. Congenital defect of Factor V (*note*: congenital Factors V and VIII deficiency may occur together).
5. Factor VII deficiency.

Use in liver disease should be with great caution because the Factor IX concentrate may contain activated factors and patients with liver disease have decreased ability to clear activated factors so that intravascular coagulation may occur.

FACTOR IX, PURIFIED PREPARATION

Preparation

This may contain some amounts of Factors II and X. Initial recovery after administration is often low, about 30–50 per cent due to diffusion into extra-vascular space. Hence levels decline biphasically, the half-life is about 24 hours.

DRIED FIBRINOGEN

Preparations

Contain 1·5–2·0 g fibrinogen reconstituted with 200 ml sterile pyrogen-free distilled water.

Indications

Congenital fibrinogen deficiency, low fibrinogen levels (<1 g/l), and dysfibrino-genaemia.

Selected Further Reading

Cash J. D. (1976) Blood transfusion and blood products. *Clin. Haematol.* **5**, 1.

Chapter 27

Hazards and Complications of Blood Transfusion

DETERIORATION OF STORED BLOOD

Anticoagulants
1. Citrate–phosphate–dextrose, CPD.
2. Acid–citrate–dextrose, ACD.
3. Heparin.

CPD is less acidic than ACD and survival of red cells is longer in storage with CPD, the level of 2,3-diphosphoglycerate being better maintained. Blood stored in CPD or ACD can be used for up to 3 weeks. Heparinized blood is used without a red cell preservative and must be administered within 48 hours.

Cellular Components

1. Red Cells. Deterioration is about 1 per cent per day. Blood should not be transfused after 3 weeks' storage when about 20 per cent of the red cells are lost within 24 hours. Patients with impaired liver function are especially likely to become markedly jaundiced following transfusion with long-stored blood. During storage lactic acid is produced by glycolysis, and the pH falls, interfering with the glycolytic enzymes, hexokinase and phosphofructokinase. After 3 weeks' storage in CPD the pH falls from about 7·1 to 6·4. 2,3-Diphosphoglycerate levels fall in stored blood with consequent shift of the oxygen dissociation to the left. This may contribute to the raised mixed venous oxygen tension in patients receiving massive transfusions. Following transfusion 2,3-DPG levels return to 50 per cent of normal within 24 hours. There is a progressive fall in intracellular ATP levels resulting in: (*a*) red cells becoming spherical; (*b*) depletion of membrane lipid; (*c*) increased rigidity of cell wall; (*d*) potassium loss from cells into surrounding plasma and influx of sodium ions into cells. The extracellular potassium concentration rises by about 1 mmol/l (mEq/l) day. Following transfusion, the original electrolyte balance is restored; sodium within one day, though potassium may take up to 6 days.

2. White Cells. Granulocytes lose viability in stored blood rapidly; by 24 hours the phagocytic activity is reduced and viability is one-third of that of fresh granulocytes. Lymphocytes survive well in stored blood and viability of some of these cells can be demonstrated after 3 weeks' storage. To avoid graft versus host disease in patients with immune deficiency it is recommended that blood be irradiated with 1·5 Gy (1500 rads).

3. Platelets. At 3 days, recovery in vitro is about 45 per cent. The quantity present in the whole blood is not of much therapeutic significance.

Plasma Components

After 10 days the plasma potassium concentration reaches about 15 mmol/l (15 mEq/l) and rises to 25 mmol/l (25 mEq/l) after 3 weeks. It is essential that blood used for exchange transfusion in infants is less than 4 days (preferably less than 48 hours) old. Citrate increases the risk of potassium intoxication. The toxic risk of hyperkalaemia is increased with massive rapid transfusions and in patients whose plasma potassium level is already high. The ammonia concentration also rises in stored blood (9 fold in 3 weeks) and old blood should be avoided in neonates and in hepatic failure.

Coagulation Factors

1. Fibrinogen gradually becomes denatured during storage.
2. Factors II, V and VIII are very labile and are not present in therapeutic levels after 48 hours of storage.
3. Factors VII, IX, X, XI, XII and XIII are relatively well preserved.

Massive transfusions cause dilutional decrease of labile factors; it is recommended that 1 unit of FFP and 2 units of cryoprecipitate be given with every 4 units of stored blood transfusion.

COMPLICATIONS OF BLOOD TRANSFUSION

1. Haemolytic reactions—serological; mechanical; thermal.
2. Circulatory overload.
3. Febrile reactions.
4. Allergic reactions.
5. Infections.
6. Potassium and citrate toxicity.
7. Air embolism.
8. Thrombophlebitis.
9. Transfusion siderosis.
10. Immunological sensitization.
11. Untoward effects of drugs added to blood.
12. Complications of massive transfusion.

HAEMOLYTIC REACTIONS

1. Serological

1.1 Destruction of donor cells by antibodies in recipient's plasma.

1.1.1 Immediate. This is due to antibodies present before transfusion and should be detected in the cross-match. It is usually due to ABO incompatibility, occasionally Rhesus incompatibility and rarely other antibodies such as anti-K, anti-Fy^a and anti-Jk^a. Anti-Jk^a is notable in that it causes greater in vivo destruction than in vitro tests often indicate (it is complement-dependent and complement levels fall rapidly in vitro). With the immediate cell lysis there is activation of complement with liberation of $C3_a$ and $C5_a$ which contract smooth muscle and produce liberation of histamine from mast cells. Such incompatible blood transfusions are most frequently due to clerical error rather than errors of laboratory techniques.

1.1.2 Delayed. Delayed reactions occur when an antibody that was not present at the time of transfusion develops rapidly. Haemolysis occurs between 1 and 2 weeks. These rapid antibody responses are 'secondary responses' and thus usually occur in those who have been previously transfused.

1.2 Destruction of recipient's cells by haemolytic antibodies present in the donor plasma is a rare occurrence. Group O used as a 'universal donor' and administered to a Group A or Group B recipient may produce severe haemolysis if the donor plasma contains a high titre of the specific haemolytic antibody (usually IgG). Vaccines may be a potent source of sensitization with A and B substances.

2. Mechanical

Mechanical lysis of donor red cells may occur: (*a*) if blood is forced through a small-calibre needle under pressure—a rare occurrence; (*b*) blood is obtained by powerful suction from the heart during open heart surgery and returned to the circulation.

3. Thermal

Thermal damage to red cells: (*a*) blood stored under incorrect refrigeration especially likely if there is lack of air circulation and blood is in proximity to the cooling coils (blood freezes at $-3\,°C$); (*b*) heating to $50\,°C$ causes lysis; liable to occur if water-bath technique is used for blood warming without critical maintenance of water temperature or if ultrasonic equipment is used with packed cells when intended only to be used with whole blood.

Clinical Features

Symptoms of complement-mediated transfusion reactions, as occur with ABO incompatibility, may be very severe and often present within a few minutes though may be delayed for 1 or 2 hours. It is advisable to give the first 50–100 ml of any blood unit slowly if clinically possible. The symptoms may include: (1) restlessness; (2) breathlessness; (3) retrosternal pressure or angina pain (due to coronary artery spasm); (4) abdominal discomfort (associated with hyperperistalsis) producing vomiting and/or urgency of defaecation; (5) aching in the lumbar region; (6) a throbbing headache; (7) rigors associated with a rise in temperature; (8) bruising and haemorrhage, associated with disseminated intravascular coagulation due to: (*a*) thromboplastic substances liberated from damaged red cells; (*b*) initiation of clotting process by activated complement factors; (9) renal failure due principally to the consequences of complement activation rather than damage from haemoglobin.

Physical Findings

(1) Rapid pulse and respiration with a fall in blood pressure. (2) Initial pallor followed by flushing. (3) Shock. (4) Renal failure, featured by: (*a*) initially oliguria which usually occurs within 24 hours and may last several days; (*b*) the diuretic phase which is associated with electrolyte loss.

Laboratory Investigations

After transfusion has been *stopped* and saline substituted to preserve venous access the following investigations are required: (1) Carefully check the identity and blood group of patient and donors. (2) Collect (with care to avoid mechanical haemolysis) heparinized, citrated, sequestrene and clotted samples from the other arm, then: (*a*) centrifuge heparinized sample and examine supernatant for (i) free haemoglobin, and (ii) methaemalbumin; (*b*) citrated sample is used to check: (i) prothrombin time; (ii) partial thromboplastin time; (iii) thrombin time; these tests are to determine whether disseminated intravascular coagulation has occurred, and if so, its severity; (*c*) sequestrene sample is used to determine total haemoglobin level and platelet count; (*d*) clotted sample is used for rechecking blood group, for direct antiglobulin test and for detecting and identifying atypical antibodies, though this sample is not as good as the pretransfusion sample because antibodies may have been absorbed by the donor cells. (3) Urinary output is maintained and samples examined for haemoglobin content.

Treatment

Initial (1) The transfusion must be stopped immediately and the unit of blood returned to the laboratory for serological tests and bacterial culture. (2) Hydrocortisone 100 mg and chlorphenyramine maleate 10 mg given i.v. and repeated if necessary. (3) Saline, or, if necessary, plasma or whole blood, must be transfused to maintain the venous return and systolic blood pressure. (4) Renal output should be maintained by giving a diuretic provided adequate venous return has been established. Mannitol, 100 ml 20 per cent solution, can be given over 5 min, the dose may be repeated if a diuresis has not been obtained. Alternatively, frusemide may be given, 80–120 mg i.v. and this dose may be repeated if a urinary output of less than 50 ml/hour is not maintained. (5) I.v. administrations of alkalis such as sodium bicarbonate or sodium lactate have been given on the theoretical basis that haemoglobin is more soluble in alkaline than acid urine. Oliguria is not due to tubular precipitation of haemoglobin but to impaired glomerular filtration. (6) Oliguric and polyuric renal failure, if it occurs, is managed in the standard way. **Disseminated Intravascular Coagulation**
Management of this complication is described in Chapter 17.

CIRCULATORY OVERLOAD

Next to haemolytic reactions, circulatory overload is the most common cause of death following transfusion.

Clinical Features

Most commonly the clinical presentation is that of acute pulmonary oedema. Premonitory symptoms of headache, lightness in the chest and a dry cough may occur. It is essential that the jugular venous pressure be monitored during a transfusion. Avoidance of circulatory overload may be achieved by: (1) administration of blood slowly; (2) use of plasma-reduced red cell concentrations, a haematocrit of 70 per cent being suitable (further reduction of plasma concentration causes problems of administration due to viscosity); (3) keeping the patient warm to increase peripheral vasodilatation; (4) not exceeding 2 units at a time in adults in the treatment of longstanding anaemia; (5) administration of a diuretic, e.g. frusemide 40–80 mg i.v.

Treatment

(1) Stop transfusion and if necessary even venesect patient; (2) patient maintained in the sitting position which minimizes cardiac venous return; (3) oxygen—100 per cent by mask to compensate for reduced oxygen diffusion; (4) give i.v. frusemide; (5) morphine which reduces anxiety and consequently sympathetic activity; (6) digitalization may be of value in acute cardiac failure; (7) aminophylline may be useful, particularly if there is significant bronchial spasm; (8) in very severe cases, endotracheal intubation and positive-pressure ventilation may be necessary.

FEBRILE REACTIONS

Aetiology

Febrile reactions are commoner in persons who have received many previous transfusions; sensitization may have resulted from pregnancies. Platelet antibodies (although responsible for reducing the effectiveness of platelet transfusions) contribute only slightly to febrile reactions which are mostly due to leuco-agglutinins or leukocytotoxins.

Clinical Features

Usually the fever does not start until after half an hour from commencement of the transfusion and may be delayed for an hour. The fever may continue to rise for 2–6 hours and may persist for 12 hours. Occasionally there may be associated symptoms of nausea, vomiting, diarrhoea, and pains in the chest and back and very occasionally hypotension and cyanosis. Leucoagglutination in the pulmonary capillaries associated with rigors, dyspnoea, cough and tachycardia is a rare complication; symptoms improve within a few hours but the infiltrates may persist for a day or two.

Treatment

If symptoms are mild, slowing the rate of transfusion, administration of para-cetamol and an antihistamine, such as chlorpheniramine maleate, is usually the only treatment required but occasionally hydrocortisone requires to be given. If reactions are a regular occurrence, or if any symptoms are severe, leucocytes and platelets should be removed from blood either by filtration or by washing the red cells.

ALLERGIC REACTIONS

Aetiology

1. Sensitivity to some, but not all IgA idiotypes usually follows previous transfusions or pregnancies. The reactions are frequently mild.

2. Antibodies to all IgA types developing in IgA-deficient subjects, the antibody titre is usually high as reactions may be severe.

Clinical Features

Mild symptoms consist of an erythematous rash, urticaria and headache; fever is unusual. Severe anaphylactic reactions in IgA-deficient subjects include profound hypotension, retrosternal pain, dyspnoea (occasionally associated with laryngeal spasm), cyanosis, abdominal cramps, vomiting and diarrhoea.

Diagnosis

Demonstration of the absence of IgA, together with anti-IgA in the patient confirms the absence of this immunoglobulin fraction.

Treatment

If the reaction is mild, slowing the rate of transfusion and administration of an antihistamine is all that is required. If severe, the administration of the blood product must be stopped, hydrocortisone and an antihistamine (such as chlorpheniramine maleate) given intravenously; adrenaline subcutaneously may also be required.

Prevention of future reactions is by use of washed red cells. Albumin and PPF should not be administered as they may contain sufficient IgA to produce reactions. If blood products such as white cells, platelets or protein fractions are essential, IgA deficient donors must be used.

INFECTED BLOOD PRODUCING BACTERAEMIC SHOCK

Aetiology

Pseudomonas, coliform and achromobacter groups of bacteria will multiply at 4 °C and utilize citrate as a primary source of carbon without producing necessarily visual evidence of deterioration of the blood until citrate depletion produces clotting; sometimes slight haemolysis has been observed when the blood unit has been re-examined following a transfusion disaster.

Physical Findings

Immediate collapse with severe shock, tachycardia and peripheral circulatory failure may follow the administration of only a few ml of infected blood. Other symptoms include rigors, vomiting, diarrhoea; malaena, purpura and other manifestations of disseminated intravascular coagulation.

Laboratory Investigations

The unit of blood must be returned immediately for microbiological examination; direct gram staining, anaerobic and aerobic (in the presence of carbon dioxide) cultures must be performed. Blood cultures should be taken from the patient.

Treatment

(1) The transfusion of blood should be discontinued; (2) plasma expanders are given to maintain adequate venous return immediately; (3) chlorpheniramine maleate 10 mg and hydrocortisone 200 mg should be given i.v.; if life-threatening shock persists 1 g of methyl prednisolone should be given i.v.; (4) broad-spectrum antibiotics with particular attention to gram-negative organisms should be given i.v.

INFECTIONS TRANSMITTED BY BLOOD

1. Hepatitis B (HBV)

Screening of the donors for the surface antigen (HBsAg) has reduced very significantly the incidence of this disease caused by transfusion. Incubation period 30–150 days.

2. Hepatitis A (HAV)

HAV is a rare cause of post-transfusion hepatitis. The incubation period is 15–60 days. Diagnosis is made by detection of specific antibodies or by identification of the virus particles in stool samples.

3. Hepatitis Non A Non B (NANB)

NANB is still a major cause of clinical and subclinical hepatitis following blood transfusion and especially with blood products such as Factor VIII concentrate (because of the pooling sera from many donors). Hepatic biopsies in patients receiving blood products have revealed a high incidence of chronic active hepatitis in patients who frequently receive blood products.

4. Cytomegalo virus (CMV) Infection

About 6 per cent of donors have antibodies to CMV and possibly about 10 per cent of donors have subclinical viraemia. The incidence of infection in patients receiving transfusions depend on three factors: (*a*) if the patient has complement-fixing CMV antibodies to a titre of 1 in 28, infection is almost unknown; (*b*) the fresher the blood administered the greater the risk of infection; (*c*) immune-suppressed patients are prone to infection. Atypical lymphocytes present in the peripheral blood 3–6 weeks following a transfusion, associated with symptoms similar to infectious mononucleosis, strongly suggest CMV infection.

5. Infectious Mononucleosis

Infectious mononucleosis due to the EB virus has a post-transfusion incubation period of 2–4 weeks. Diagnosis is made by the presence of atypical cells in the peripheral blood, the presence of a positive Paul–Bunnell test often associated with biochemical evidence of subclinical hepatitis.

6. Brucellosis

Brucellosis may be transmitted by blood products. It is very much a chronic infection, thus persons with a history of this infection should not be considered suitable as blood donors.

7. Tropical Infections

Malaria, South American trypanosomiasis (Chagas' disease), African trypano-somiasis (sleeping sickness), leishmaniasis and filariasis have all been transmitted by blood transfusion. Malaria can be prevented by giving a prophylactic antimalarial drug prior to the donation.

8. Syphilis

The risk of transmission is now very rare due to routine serological screening of donors. *T. pallidum* is unlikely to survive after blood has been stored at 4 °C for more than 4 days.

POTASSIUM AND CITRATE TOXICITY

Potassium toxicity is rare but must be considered in: (1) exchange transfusion in infants; (2) massive transfusions; (3) transfusions to patients with pretransfusion raised potassium levels (renal failure and especially if associated with massive muscle injury). Citrate is rapidly metabolized in the liver, and toxicity only usually arises in infants, patients with advanced liver disease, those undergoing hibernation anaesthesia, or during very rapid massive transfusion. The major problem is of tetany and cardiac dysrhythmias.

AIR EMBOLISM

This is a very rare complication since the introduction of plastic bags in place of bottles. Small air emboli may result if air is not expelled from transfusion tubing before commencing an infusion. The symptoms are cough, dyspnoea and collapse. The presence of a septal defect increases the risk of cerebral complications due to paradoxical air embolism.

THROMBOPHLEBITIS

Predisposing causes of thrombophlebitis are: (1) cut-downs; (2) administration of high concentrations of glucose; (3) prolonged intravenous administration, especially longer than 12 hours; (4) certain drip sites; the long saphenous vein and the medial aspect of the ankle are more prone to thrombosis than arm veins.

TRANSFUSION SIDEROSIS

Aetiology

Each blood unit of 500 ml contains approximately 250 mg of iron. Frequent transfusions over very many months or years results in an iron overload similar to that found in haemochromatosis.

Prevention

The administration of subcutaneous desferrioxamine (by a pump so that the chelating drug is injected over an 8-hour period to increase the urinary excretion of iron) should be considered in any patient likely to receive multiple transfusions over a prolonged period. These include patients suffering from thalassaemia major, aplastic anaemia or red cell aplasia, chronic haemolytic anaemia and sideroblastic anaemia.

IMMUNOLOGICAL SENSITIZATION

This potential consequence of transfusion must always be borne in mind. If patients are to receive multiple transfusions it is important that the red cell phenotype for the rhesus group and also Kell and Duffy be determined, for in the presence of transfused cells the patient's red cell phenotype cannot be determined. Appropriate donor phenotypes should be selected to reduce the risk of antibody formation.

The untoward effects of immunological sensitization are: (1) the possibility of haemolytic disease of the newborn occurring in future pregnancies; (2) difficulties with the provision of compatible blood; (3) the rapid development of detectable antibodies with subsequent transfusions producing lysis of transfused cells.

UNTOWARD EFFECTS OF DRUGS ADDED TO BLOOD

Drugs should not be added to blood for the following reasons: (1) Increase of infection being introduced to the blood; (2) Some drugs cause red cell lysis, e.g. ethacrynic acid; (3) Some drugs may be unsuitable in the aqueous solution of blood products; (4) The altered pH may affect the stability of the drug; (5) Effectiveness of the drug may be impaired compared with a bolus injection prior to the transfusion.

COMPLICATIONS OF MASSIVE TRANSFUSIONS

Most of the complications have been covered in the preceding sections. They include: (1) hypothermia due to the transfusion of blood at 4 °C; local venous spasm may prevent entry, especially in infants—sonic blood warmers are available; (2) acidosis; (3) hyperkalaemia; (4) citrate toxicity; (5) decreased oxygen availability to the tissue due to 2,3-DPG depletion; (6) lack of labile coagulation factors; (7) thrombocytopenia. It should be noted that the greatest hazard of massive transfusion is that it was not great enough.

Selected Further Reading

Cash J. D. (ed.) (1976) Blood transfusion and blood products. *Clin. Haematol.* 5, No. 1. London, Saunders.
Conrad M. E. (ed.) (1981) Transfusion problems in haematology. In: *Semin. Hematol.* 18, 2.
Mollison P. L. (1979) *Blood Transfusion in Clinical Medicine*, 6th ed. Oxford, Blackwell Scientific Publications.

Chapter 28 / Useful Investigations

STAINS

May–Grünwald–Giemsa (MGG)

Freshly-made films, dried as quickly as possible to avoid cell distortion due to osmosis, are fixed in methanol for 10 min. After 5 min in diluted May–Grünwald stain the slides are transferred without washing to diluted Giemsa stain for 10 min, washed three times with buffered water to differentiate, then allowed to drain and dry. In general, cell proteins stain pink and nucleic acids blue.

Reticulocyte Stain

Two drops of fresh EDTA blood are added to 4 drops of new methylene blue in a test-tube, mixed and incubated for 20 min at 37 °C. The red cells are gently mixed prior to a film being made. The film is dried and can be examined without counterstaining (counterstains are only used if permanent preparations are required). Reticulocytes contain stained strand remnants of RNA.

Sudan Black

Dried films are fixed with a formol/ethanol mixture, rinsed in water and dried before staining with Sudan black B solution for 30 min at 37 °C. The stain is drained off and the slides counterstained with MGG. Sudan black stains the phospholipid component of the granulocytic granules.

Peroxidase Stain

The dried film is fixed in a formaldehyde-methanol mixture for 1 min, rinsed in tap water and stained with the peroxidase agent, containing o-toluidine and hydrogen peroxide, for 30 sec. It is then rinsed in tap water and counterstained with Giemsa. Its staining pattern is similar to Sudan black.

Periodic Acid–Schiff (PAS)

Dried films are fixed in methanol for 10 min, then placed in periodic acid for 10 min followed by immersion in Schiff's reagent (leucobasic fuchsin) for 30 min. The slides are washed once with tap water, left in distilled water for 5 min before counterstaining with haematoxylin. PAS stains glycogen, polysaccharides, muco-polysaccharides, glycoproteins and mucoproteins. Neutrophils stain strongly and early granulocytic cells weakly; monocytes stain very weakly; mature lymphocytes have occasional fine granules whereas lymphoblasts may show block positivity;

255

normal red cell precursors are unstained, but normoblasts may be positive in a variety of dyserythropoietic states, especially thalassaemia and erythroleukaemia. In the latter the staining is often in clumps.

Non-specific Esterase (NSE)

Two dried films are fixed in formalin vapour for 20 min and washed gently in distilled water for 2 min. One slide is immersed in 1 per cent sodium fluoride solution for 2 min, the other remains as a control. Both slides are immersed in buffered substrate (Naphthol AS Acetate and Fast Blue RR) for 90 min, then rinsed in distilled water and counterstained with neutral red. Myeloid cells have fluoride-resistant esterase, monocytes have fluoride-sensitive esterase.

Chloracetate Esterase

Naphthol AS-D chloracetate is used as a substrate with Fast Blue RR. The reaction is positive for myeloid cells (including late myeloblasts). Auer rods are positive. Little or no activity is found with monocytes.

Iron (Prussian Blue Reaction)

The dried film is fixed in methanol for 20 min, allowed to dry and submersed in acidified (with hydrochloric acid) potassium ferrocyanide solution. The slide is then washed in running tap water for 20 min, rinsed in distilled water and counterstained with eosin for 10 sec.

Neutrophil Alkaline Phosphatase (NAP)

Fresh dried films are fixed in a formalin/methanol mixture for 30 sec at 4 °C, rinsed in tap water, drained and dried. The slides are flooded with freshly prepared substrate (containing Naphthol AS phosphate and Fast Blue BB) at room temperature for 15 min. After washing with tap water, the slides are counterstained with neutral red for 5 min.

One hundred neutrophils are counted, each cell being graded according to its staining intensity from 0 to 4. The normal range varies between laboratories, but is approximately 30–120.

SURFACE MARKER STUDIES

Low-density leucocytes are prepared on a discontinuous ficoll hypaque gradient (sp.gr. 1·077) by centrifugation at 1200 g for 20 min. The interfacial band contains leucocytes with the exception of granulocytes and some metamyelocytes which are pelleted with the red cells at the bottom of the tube.

Rosetting Techniques

The following are mixed in tissue culture medium to give approximately the concentrations shown. Leucocytes to be tested (5×10^6) ml, indicator red cells (1–2 per cent v/v), fetal serum 10 per cent. The cells are pelleted at 200 g for 10 min and then incubated on ice for 1 hour. The cells are very gently resuspended and a drop of the cells is mixed with a drop of acridine orange solution. The cells are placed under a coverslip and examined with a ultraviolet microscope. Viable leucocytes are stained green, and those cells with 3 or more red cells attached are scored as rosette-forming cells.

Various indicator cells can be used to detect different leucocyte subpopulations (*Table 28.1*).

Table 28.1. Leucocyte subsets defined by rosetting techniques

Indicator cells	Cells rosetting
Sheep red blood cells	T lymphocytes (E$^+$)
AET or neuraminidase-treated sheep red blood cells	Increased rosetting by T lymphocytes (plus some cells of uncertain origin with natural killer activity)
Mouse red blood cells	Some B cells; CLL but not B-prolymphocytic leukaemia
IgG coupled to ox cells	Cells bearing the Fc receptor for IgG A minority of T cells and most myeloid cells
IgM coupled to ox cells	Cells bearing the Fc receptor for IgM Majority of T cells
Anti-immunoglobulin coupled to ox cells. (Antisera to different immunoglobulin classes or light chain types can be used)	Cells bearing surface immunoglobulin; most B cells (not plasma cells) and also cells with strong Fc receptors, such as monocytes, with bound antibody not synthesized by those cells

Immunofluorescent Techniques

Single Layer Method. Leucocytes are incubated for 30 min on ice with fluorescein or rhodamine-labelled antibody specific for a membrane component of interest. The incubation is performed in the presence of excess non-immune serum to reduce non-specific binding of labelled antibody to Fc receptors. The cells are then washed thoroughly and examined with an ultraviolet microscope. This method is commonly used with sheep or goat anti-human Ig to detect cells with surface immunoglobulin.

Double Layer Method. Leucocytes are incubated for 30 min on ice with specific unlabelled antisera, frequently a mouse monoclonal antibody. The cells are washed and then incubated for a further 30 min on ice with fluorescein or rhodamine-labelled sheep or goat anti-mouse immunoglobulin. This sandwich technique increases the sensitivity of the method and also allows for appropriate negative controls, e.g. irrelevant first-layer antibody plus second-layer antibody, which are not possible with a direct staining method.

The most useful antisera in haematological practice are:
anti-human Igs (IgG, IgA, IgM, IgD, IgE, κ and λ chains)
antithymocyte and pan T cell antisera

antisera against 'suppressor T cells'
antisera against 'helper T cells'
Ia (HLA-Dr) antisera
'common ALL' antisera (cALL)
anti-Tdt antisera

Double staining with Tdt and T cell antisera is particularly useful in the diagnosis of bone marrow relapse in T cell ALL. Cells can be stained with two antibodies providing the antibodies are derived from different species or are of different antibody class or subclass if mouse monoclonal antibodies. One antibody is stained with a fluorescein-conjugated second layer and the other with a rhodamine conjugate.

Terminal Deoxynucleotidyl Transferase (Tdt)

This nuclear enzyme is present in lymphocytic precursor cells and their leukaemic counterparts. It may also be a pluripotential stem cell marker and is present in some myeloid leukaemias. The activity of the enzyme in leukaemic cells can be determined biochemically or its presence can be detected by immunofluorescent techniques with anti-Tdt antisera. As the enzyme is not expressed on the cell surface, fixed cells (usually cytocentrifuge preparations) must be used.

CYTOGENETICS

Investigations usually are carried out on bone marrow aspirates by direct examination because of the high mitotic activity. However, studies on the peripheral blood may be used if bone marrow cells are present in the circulation or by the use of mitotic stimulants to examine lymphocytes in haematologically normal or leukaemic patients.

Technique

Bone marrow aspirates should be added to tissue culture medium containing heparin; colchicine is added and the sample centrifuged after 90 min. Sterile heparinized peripheral blood is diluted with tissue culture medium and calf serum (to which phytohaemagglutinin has been added if a stimulant is required) and incubated for up to 72 hours prior to the addition of colchicine.

The supernatant having been removed the cells are resuspended in hypotonic potassium chloride solution for 15 min to swell the cells and are then fixed with a methanol/acetic acid mixture, centrifuged and, following removal of excess fixative, the cells are resuspended and left for 12 hours at 4 °C. After the addition of 60 per cent acetic acid, slide preparations are made, flamed quickly and dried. Slides are left for a further 48 hours prior to staining procedure. Various staining techniques are available to demonstrate chromosome bandings. G banding with heat denaturation prior to Giemsa staining is the most common.

Recently, cells have been cultured in the presence of methotrexate for 72 hours prior to making chromosome preparations. A large proportion of prometaphases are obtained in which some 850 bands can be recognized compared with some 300 bands seen in metaphase with the standard technique.

Terminology

Of the 46 chromosomes there are 22 pairs of autosomes which are numbered in decreasing size from No. 1 to No. 22. Morphologically similar chromosomes are allocated letters; there are seven groups from A to G. The X chromosome morphologically resembles the C group and the Y resembles the G group. The point of attachment of the four arms of the chromosome is the centromere, short arms are designated p and long arms q (*Fig. 28.1*). Plus and minus signs designate additional or absent chromosomes, if used as a prefix, e.g. $+8$ represents trisomy 8 and -7 represents monosomy 7; if used as a suffix the signs represent an increase or decrease in length.

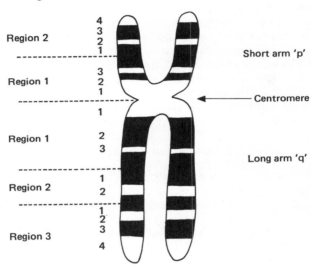

Fig. 28.1. Chromosomal banding.

Chromosome bands are numbered from the centromere, thus the Philadelphia chromosome is identified at $(9+:22-)$ (q34 q11) showing that the break point for the translocation is at band 34 on No. 9 chromosome and at band 11 on the No. 22 chromosome.

HAEMOGLOBIN STUDIES

Sickle-cell Screening Test

Principle of Test. An aliquot of red cells is added to a buffered solution (pH 7·1) containing a haemolysing agent. Sickle haemoglobin (HbS) is precipitated and therefore the solution appears cloudy whereas HbA and most other haemoglobin variants remain in solution.

Haemoglobin Electrophoresis

Principle. Cells from a blood sample taken into anticoagulant are washed three times with normal saline, lysed by water and the lysate centrifuged to remove red cell stroma. Electrophoresis may be carried out on paper, cellulose acetate, agar or starch gels. The usual pH is 8·6, but a different pH must be used for haemoglobins which do not separate at that pH, e.g. HbS and HbD. The identification of haemoglobin variants is determined by their varying mobilities, appropriate markers being run in parallel (*see Fig. 9.3*, p. 76).

Technique for Cellulose Acetate. Cellulose acetate strips are soaked in a Tris-EDTA-borate buffer (pH 8·9) and are placed in a specifically-designed electrophoresis apparatus with each end of the strip secured and attached to a trough of buffer. The haemoglobin lysate is applied at the origin and a potential of 220 v at 5 mA is applied across the strip for about 2 hours. The anode is behind the origin; most haemoglobins migrating to the cathode.

Quantitation is carried out by cutting out the band which has been separated on cellulose acetate, eluting the haemoglobin and measuring photometrically.

Globins may be prepared by adding the lysate to an acid-acetone mixture. The globin chains are separated by either electrophoresis or column chromatography.

Normal Values. After the age of 1 year, HbA_2 comprises $1·8 - 3·2$ per cent and HbF is less than 1 per cent; the remainder is HbA. HbA contains subfractions HbA_{1A}, HbA_{1B}, HbA_{1C}; these fast-flowing fractions comprise less than 5 per cent of the total HbA. At birth HbF comprises 55–98 per cent of the circulating haemoglobin.

Globin Chain Synthesis

Principle. Erythrocytes or marrow are incubated with high specific activity tritiated leucine to label newly-synthesized globin. Globin is prepared and separated by column chromatography and the activity in the eluate fractions is quantified.

Uses

1. Antenatal diagnosis of thalassaemia major.
2. Definitive diagnosis of obscure thalassaemic syndromes.

Determination of Haemoglobin F

Principle. HbF is more resistant to acid and alkali than HbA. Red cell lysate is treated with sodium hydroxide and after a time interval the reaction is stopped with ammonium sulphate. The mixture is filtered and the concentration of HbF in the filtrate is determined spectrophotometrically.

Pathological Variation. Increased levels of HbF are found in β-thalassaemia, hereditary persistence of fetal haemoglobin, sickle-cell disease and in a variety of acquired haematological disorders (*see* Chapter 9).

Kleihauer Acid Elution Test for HbF-containing Cells

Principle. Red cells containing HbF resist acid elution to a greater extent than cells containing HbA. Smears are fixed in ethanol, dipped in the acid buffer, washed and stained with eosin. Red cells which contained HbA appear as ghosts and fetal cells an intense pink. Reticulocytes are more resistant to acid elution than normal cells and may appear as varying shades of pink.

Physiological Variation. Hereditary persistence of fetal haemoglobin (HPFH) shows an evenly distributed slightly pink appearance of all cells in the heterozygote and a deeper pink in the homozygote. In the other disorders associated with the presence of HbF (listed *above*) only some of the red cells show the intense pink.

Detection of HbF-containing Cells by Immunofluorescence

Fixed (acetone/methanol) red cells are stained with a fluorescein conjugated anti-HbF antisera to detect 'F cells'.

Detection of Unstable Haemoglobins

Heat Instability. A red cell lysate is prepared and heated at 50 °C for up to 1 hour. A precipitate is performed by unstable haemoglobins. This precipitate can be quantified colorimetrically after conversion to cyanmethaemoglobin.
Isopropanol Instability. The lysate is treated with an isopropanol buffer at 37 °C for up to 40 min to look for precipitation. Haemoglobin F is also precipitated by this method.

It is essential to test concurrent normal controls by these methods.

Oxygen Dissociation Curves

A dilute suspension of red cells or haemoglobin lysate in phosphate or bis-Tris buffer is fully deoxygenated by vacuum extraction and the absorption spectrum of the deoxy-Hb is determined. Measured volumes of air are added to the suspension in a tonometer of known volume. The spectra are determined at the different Po_2s calculated from the known volumes indicated above. From the absorbance readings at 560 and 578 nm (*Fig. 28.2*) the percentage oxygen saturation at each

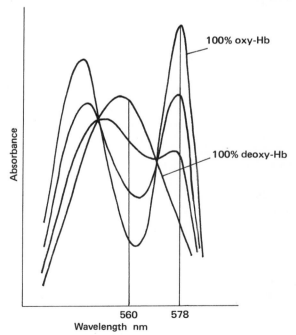

Fig. 28.2. Absorption spectra of haemoglobin.

100% oxy-Hb

100% deoxy-Hb

Absorbance

560   578
Wavelength nm

Po_2 is determined and an oxygen dissociation curve plotted. A normal and high affinity haemoglobin is shown in *Fig. 10.2*, p. 9.

2,3-DPG Estimations

2,3-DPG levels are essential in the correct interpretation of abnormal oxygen dissociation curves. A low 2,3-DPG moves the curve to the left. It is also of value in determining the site of enzyme defects affecting glucose metabolism (*see* Chapter 11).

The enzyme activity is measured in a trichloroacetic acid deproteinized solution, by a spectrophotometric technique using a commercially available reagent kit.

Methaemoglobin (Hi) Detection and Quantitation

1. The presence of methaemoglobin may be suspected by the brown discoloration of the haemolysate.
2. Methaemoglobin may be detected on a starch gel running just behind HbA. The separation is poor and this method of detection is unreliable.

If a methaemoglobin band is present, a further sample should be run after treatment with cyanide. If there is methaemoglobin A, the band will disappear, but not if there is HbM.

3. Methaemoglobin may be detected with a reversion spectrophotometer, though this method is not very reliable.
4. The method of choice for detecting methaemoglobin is by difference spectra between 600 and 700 nm, of the haemoglobin in the presence of carbon monoxide with and without dithionate. The methaemoglobin gives an absorption peak at 632 nm which disappears to baseline after reduction by dithionate if there is methaemoglobin A, or moves to about 600 nm if there is HbM (*Fig. 28.3*).

INVESTIGATION OF HAEMOLYSIS

Serum Haptoglobins

Normal Value. 0·3–2·0 g of haemoglobin binding per litre.

Principle of Test. Haptoglobins are mucoproteins which bind with haemoglobin to form complexes which can be isolated by electrophoresis or by Sephadex column.

Technique. The serum sample is incubated for 30 min at 20 °C with known concentrations of haemoglobin prior to electrophoresis. By scanning the peroxidase-stained electrophoretic strip the quantities of free and haptoglobin complexed haemoglobin can be determined and the haptoglobin concentration expressed in g Hb binding capacity/litre.

Physiological Variation. Levels slightly higher in men than women. Levels vary during menstrual cycle.

Pathological Variation. Low levels or absent with haemolysis, congenital ahaptoglobulinaemia and liver disease. Raised levels may be found in malignancy (especially secondary carcinoma of bone and Hodgkin's disease), collagen diseases, trauma, steroid therapy and biliary cirrhosis. In these conditions a 'normal' haptoglobin level does not exclude haemolysis.

Serum Haemopexin

Normal Value. For adults, 0·5–1·0 g/l. At birth, low levels, even lower in premature infants; adult levels attained at end of first year.

Principle and Significance of Bindings. This β-globulin is measured by starch-gel electrophoresis or by radial immunodiffusion. Like haptoglobin, haemopexin is a binding protein. In mild haemolysis, although haptoglobin may be absent, the haemopexin level may be normal or only slightly reduced and therefore may be a better indication of the degree of haemolysis.

Fig. 28.3. (a) Absorption spectra of methaemoglobin.

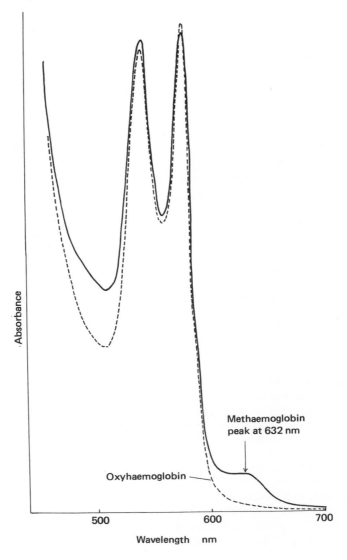

Fig. 28.3 (b) Absorption spectra of methaemoglobin before and after treatment with dithionate.

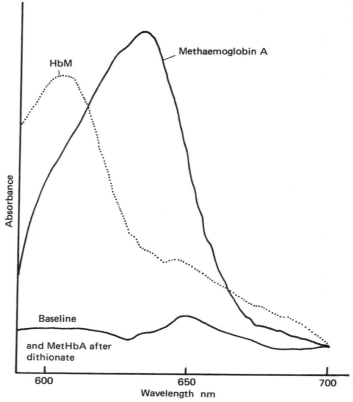

Physiological Variation. Below the age of 1 year, levels are lower; at birth the level is about 0·3 g/l.

Pathological Variation. Low or absent levels with haemolysis. Disproportionately low levels are present in thalassaemia, renal and hepatic diseases. Increased levels in diabetes mellitus, carcinoma and infections.

Plasma Haemoglobin

Normal Value. Less than 20 mg/l.

Principle and Significance of Findings. It is very important to avoid haemolysis during collection. A wide bore needle must be used and the syringe rinsed before use with sterile saline. The amount of haemoglobin in the plasma is determined (after light centrifugation of a citrated or heparinized sample) by colour development with *o*-toluidine. Free haemoglobin reflects severe haemolysis (after haptoglobins and haemopexins have been fully bound). The renal threshold is approximately 1·5 g/l.

Pathological Increase. Slightly raised levels occur in sickle-thalassaemia and haemoglobin C disease. Moderate increases occur in acquired autoimmune haemolytic anaemia, mechanical intravascular haemolysis (such as with prosthetic heart valves), thalassaemia major and sickle-cell anaemia. High levels occur with severe intravascular haemolysis as with incompatible blood transfusion, black-water fever, paroxysmal nocturnal haemoglobinuria, paroxysmal cold haemoglobinuria and march haemoglobinuria.

Methaemalbumin

Normal Value. Nil.
Principle and Significance of Findings. In severe intravascular haemolysis, free haem becomes oxidized to methaem and binds to albumin. The methaemalbumin complex remains in the plasma until free haemopexin becomes available to bind the methaem.
Technique. The presence of methaemalbumin may be detected by the Schumm's test. Plasma or serum is covered by a layer of ether, ammonium sulphide added which converts the pigment to ammonium haemochromogen which has an absorption band at 558 nm. The quantitative determination uses a spectrophotometric technique.
Pathological increase occurs with intravascular haemolysis and acute haemorrhagic pancreatitis.

Lactic Acid Dehydrogenase (LDH) Level

Normal Value. Less than 240 iu/l.
Principle and Significance of Findings. LDH catalyses the interconversion of lactate and pyruvate. It is present in high concentrations in red cells, heart, skeletal muscle, liver, kidneys and brain. Levels are assayed by a spectrophotometric technique. Five iso-enzymes can be isolated by electrophoresis, termed LD_1 to LD_5. LD_1 is present in red cells, blast cells, heart muscle and kidney; this enzyme is active against hydroxybutyrate as substrate (HBD).
Pathological Variation. Levels raised in haemolytic anaemia; very high levels occur in megaloblastic anaemia, acute leukaemia and also in cardiac, hepatic and renal diseases.

Haemosiderin in Urine

Principle and Significance of Findings. Centrifuged urine, deposit stained with potassium ferrocyanide (Prussian blue reaction) demonstrates haemosiderin—present in chronic intravascular haemolysis. Result reflects iron of renal tubular origin. N.B. A negative result is common in haemochromatosis.

Estimation of Iron Absorption, Plasma Iron Clearance and Iron Turnover Studies

See section on radio-isotopes.

Osmotic Fragility

Normal Range. Shown in *Fig. 28.4.*
Principle and Significance. The amount of red cell lysis expressed as a percentage in varying concentrations of buffered saline is plotted. Heparinized or defibrinated blood may be used; the test should be carried out within 2 hours of collection

Fig. 28.4. Osmotic fragility curves.

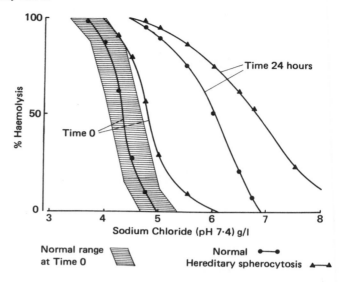

unless stored at 4 °C (permissible up to 6 hours). Lysis is complete after 30 min. The incubated fragility is performed after sterile heparinized or defibrinated blood has been incubated at 37 °C for 24 hours. Normal red cells, being biconcave discs, can increase in volume by 70 per cent. Spherocytes (irrespective of aetiology) have increased susceptibility to hypotonic saline, whereas abnormally thin cells have increased resistance. Reticulocytes (because of increased membrane available for expansion) have increased osmotic resistance.

Aetiology of Increased Osmotic Fragility
1. Hereditary spherocytosis.
2. Acquired.

2.1 Autoimmune haemolytic anaemia (including drug-induced).
2.2 Associated with thermal injury.

Autohaemolysis Test

Normal Range. Lysis at 48 hours without glucose 0·2–2·0 per cent and with glucose 0–1·0 per cent.

Principle and Significance. The amount of haemolysis depends upon the metabolic competence of the cells and the integrity of the red cell membranes.

Abnormal Results

1. Type I. Membrane disorders, such as hereditary spherocytosis, show increased haemolysis without glucose and are usually within the normal range with glucose. Impairment of the pentose phosphate pathway (G-6-PD deficiency) may produce normal results or Type I haemolysis.

2. Type II. Impairment of the glycolytic pathway (such as pyruvate kinase deficiency) results in increased autohaemolysis at 48 hours which may be more severe with added glucose. The autohaemolysis test is normal with PNH.

Glucose-6-phosphate Dehydrogenase (G-6-PD) Deficiency Screening Test with Brilliant Cresyl Blue

Normal Result. Decolorization time is between 35 and 55 min.

Principle and Significance. Haemolysates are incubated with substrate glucose-6-phosphate (G-6-P) and nicotinamide adenine dinucleotide phosphate (NADP) as a coenzyme in the presence of brilliant cresyl blue. Reticulocytes possess relatively high enzyme activity and thus false 'normal' results may occur with the reticulocytosis which follows a haemolytic episode. Correction requires to be made for anaemia by adjusting the haematocrit by the removal of plasma before cells are added to the substrate. Results with female heterozygotes vary.

Glucose-6-phosphate Dehydrogenase and 6-phosphogluconate Dehydrogenase Assay

Normal Range. 0·5–1·7 iu/ml red cells at 25 °C for G-6-PD; 0·5–2·0 iu/ml red cells at 25 °C for 6-PGD.

Principle and Significance. A fresh sample of any anticoagulated blood is required for red cell lysate preparation. Reaction of lysate with substrates in temperature-controlled spectrophotometer measures: (1) 6-PGD; and (2) 6-PGD + G-6-PD activities. Hence individual enzyme activities can be calculated. Different forms of G-6-PD deficiency may be demonstrated by electrophoretic techniques.

Acidified Serum Test (Ham's Test)

Normal Findings. No haemolysis.

Principle and Significance. Patient's red cells obtained from heparinized, citrated, EDTA or defibrinated samples are added to acidified ABO compatible serum, known to lyse PNH cells. Controls include acidified patient's serum and sera in which the complement has been inactivated by heating. The degree of haemolysis is measured after 1 hour's incubation at 37 °C. Maximum haemolysis occurs when the pH is between 6·5 and 7·0. In PNH 5–30 per cent lysis occurs in acidified sera, but very little in the inactivated sera; reticulocytes and young red cells (which may be obtained by differential centrifugation) are the most sensitive. In HEMPAS some of the cells undergo marked lysis with normal acidifed sera, but less with the patient's acidified serum. In congenital and acquired spherocytosis haemolysis may occur with inactivated and fresh acidified sera.

Donath–Landsteiner Test

Principle and Significance. The antibody causing paroxysmal cold haemoglobinuria is an IgG, of anti-P specificity, which is lytic to normal cells. Blood is placed in two glass tubes warmed to 37 °C. One tube is placed in crushed ice, the other kept at 37 °C. After 1 hour the tube kept ice-cold is incubated at 37 °C. When the clots have retracted the supernatant serum is examined for haemolysis which with a positive result should be present only in the tube which has been placed initially in the ice.

Autoagglutinin Tests at 4°, 20°, and 37°C

Normal Values. Harmless cold agglutinins found in all subjects have a thermal range up to about 15 °C; occasionally, harmless antibodies will agglutinate cells up to 25 °C. The normal titre is less than 1 in 32 at 4 °C. Harmless autoantibodies are usually either anti-I (very occasionally accompanied by anti-i) or anti-H specificity. **Principle and Significance of Findings.** The clotted blood sample must be taken in a syringe warmed to 37 °C and the sample kept at that temperature until the serum has been separated. The serum is diluted and cells from the patient, group O adult cells (containing I antigen) and group O cord cells (containing i antigen) are added to dilutions of serum and incubated at 4°, 20° and 37 °C. The maximum titre causing agglutination is determined after 2 hours.

SERUM PROTEIN INVESTIGATIONS

Protein Electrophoresis

This is usually performed by zone electrophoresis on cellulose acetate strips followed by staining with Ponceau-s. Apart from separating various protein components as shown in *Fig. 28.5*, this technique will also demonstrate the

Fig. 28.5. Serum protein electrophoresis.

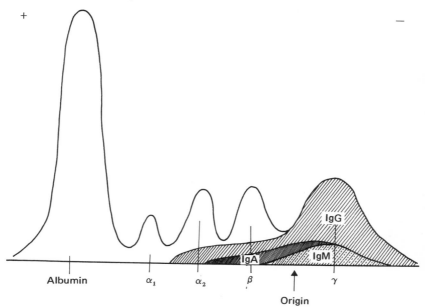

presence of a paraprotein. The protein fractions can be quantified by photometric scanning, but this usually adds little to visual inspection.

Serum should always be used as fibrinogen present in plasma gives a marked peak between the β and γ regions which may be mistaken for a paraprotein and also may mask the presence of true paraproteins.

Immunoglobulin Detection and Quantitation

1. *Immunoelectrophoresis.* Following electrophoresis in agar in the first dimension immune precipitation is carried out by diffusion in the second dimension using broad-spectrum, or class-specific, antihuman immunoglobulins or anti-light chain antisera. A concurrent normal control is run in parallel for comparison. This technique is used to define serum M Bands and to look for urinary light chains.

2. Immunoglobulin levels can be quantitated by an immunoprecipitation technique with subsequent measurement by nephelometry or by radio-immunoassay.

Bence Jones Protein (Free immunoglobulin light chains and fragments

1. Filtered urine is acidified ($\rightleftharpoons$pH 5) and gently heated in a water bath. If Bence Jones protein is present a precipitate is formed below 60 °C which redissolves on further heating. If a precipitate does not redissolve the urine is filtered while hot and then allowed to cool; any Bence Jones protein masked by other protein precipitation will re-precipitate.

2. A more accurate method is to perform electrophoresis on a concentrated (100–200 ×) urine sample looking for a monoclonal band. Using immunoelectro-phoresis these can be identified as κ and λ chains.

Plasma Viscosity

Normal Value. Using the Harkness viscometer the ratio of the rate of flow of plasma to water is 1·4 : 1·8, and is expressed in centipoises (cP).

Principle. The sample of plasma is introduced into a capillary tube and the progress along the tube, governed by a mercury manometer, is timed electronically.

Pathological Variation. The plasma viscosity usually parallels the ESR, but is of especial benefit in hyperviscosity syndromes, especially IgA myeloma and macro-globulinaemia. Symptoms of hyperviscosity tend to occur with a viscosity over 4·0 cP.

The Sedimentation Rate

Normal Value. The range is 1–5 mm for males and 1–8 mm for women, but higher rates occur in the elderly due to lower plasma albumin levels.

Principle of Test. The formation of red cell rouleaux increases the rate of red cell fall. The negative charge on the surface of the red cell (zeta potential) will be reduced if the dielectric constant of the plasma increases, thus increasing rouleaux formation. An increased rate may be produced by a raised fibrinogen level, increase of α and β globulin levels, decrease of albumin level, or an increase of some lipid components.

Technique. Westergren method. This test is performed by diluting blood (4 parts) with 3·12 per cent trisodium citrate solution (1 part), mixing well and performing the test within 4 hours. Sequestrene blood samples may be kept overnight and the dilution in citrate made the following day. A column of blood is drawn up in a 200-mm Westergren tube and the amount of plasma above the red cells is measured in mm after 1 hour.

Physiological Variation

1. Increased in pregnancy, especially in the last trimester, due to a lower haematocrit associated with increased plasma volume, an increase in fibrinogen level and an increased globulin level.

2. It is decreased in the newborn because of the high haematocrit and low globulin levels.

Pathological Variation

1. Decrease responsible for 'normal' values when otherwise a 'raised' value would be obtained.

      1.1 Raised haematocrit.

      1.2 Sickle cells—do not form rouleaux.

      1.3 Cryoglobulins—may precipitate at room temperature preventing red cell sedimentation.

      1.4 Blood clotted.

2. Increase.

    Very high sedimentation rates (often > 100 mm):

      2.1 Severe bacterial infections, especially endocarditis.

      2.2 Collagen diseases.

      2.3 Multiple myeloma.

      2.4 Malignant neoplasma, especially when associated with widespread secondary deposits.

      2.5 Cold agglutinin disease and other disorders with auto-red cell antibodies.

    Moderately raised rates:

      2.1 Anaemia (low haematocrit).

      2.2 Tissue injury (following surgery).

      2.3 Inflammation.

Use of the ESR. Very high levels may be of diagnostic value as indicated above. Moderately raised values occasionally help in differentiating disorders such as myocardial infarction and ischaemia, and rheumatoid arthritis and osteoarthrosis, but better tests are available and the ESR is frequently misleading. Elderly patients should not be extensively investigated just to find the cause of a moderately raised ESR. The ESR can be of considerable use in monitoring disease in individual patients, e.g. in Hodgkin's disease, SLE, rheumatoid arthritis and tuberculosis.

AUTO-ANTIBODIES

Antinuclear Factor (ANF)

Principles. In the rapid slide test ANF causes agglutination of DNA (from calf thymus)-coated polystyrene latex particles.

In the immunofluorescent technique frozen sections of rat's liver are incubated with test serum, followed by fluorescein-tagged rabbit anti-human γ globulin.

Radioimmune techniques are available and are probably the most sensitive and specific of all the techniques.

Pathological Findings. Positive ANF results occur in SLE and many other autoimmune disorders, such as rheumatoid arthritis, chronic hepatitis, thyroiditis, myasthenia gravis, ulcerative colitis, Sjögren's syndrome, pernicious anaemia and some red cell aplasias.

DNA Antibodies

Antibodies binding with DNA are usually measured in a radioimmunoassay. It is important that the test DNA antigen has not been denatured to single strands; double-stranded DNA binding is characteristic of serum from SLE, whereas antibodies to single-stranded DNA are found in many autoimmune disorders.

Latex Rheumatoid Arthritis Screening Test

Latex particles coated with IgG are agglutinated by serum of most patients with rheumatoid arthritis. For quantitative assessment of the rheumatoid factor the Rose–Waaler Test is performed.

Rose–Waaler Test Sheep Cell Agglutinating Titre (SCAT)

Principle. Rheumatoid factor, an IgM protein, acts as an anti-γ globulin and will agglutinate sheep cells sensitized with a subagglutinating titre of anti-sheep red cell antibodies. The sensitized cells are added to dilutions of human serum and incubated at 37 °C and the titre of agglutination determined.
Normal Value. A positive result is interpreted as agglutination at a 16-fold greater dilution than normal serum.
Pathological Findings. Positive results occur in about 80 per cent of patients with rheumatoid arthritis, and in about 30 per cent of patients with SLE. The results are negative in non-rheumatoid arthritis, including ankylosing spondylitis.

Organ-specific Auto-antibodies

Cryostat sections of appropriate tissues are incubated with patient's serum, washed thoroughly and then incubated with fluoresceinated-anti-human immunoglobulin. The slide is examined with an ultraviolet microscope. Tissues commonly examined include stomach (parietal cells), thyroid, liver, kidney, pancreas (islet cells) and adrenal glands.

ISOTOPE INVESTIGATIONS

Types of Radiation

α particles are helium nuclei; composed of two neutrons and two protons.
β particles are single electrons.
γ particles are high-frequency electromagnetic waves.

Measuring Equipment

α emitters and detectors are not used in haematology.
β emissions are measured in a liquid scintillation counter. The isotope is mixed with a liquid phosphor (such as β-terphenyl in xylene) at 4 °C to reduce non-specific impulses. Proteins reduce sensitivity of counting techniques by exerting a 'quenching' effect.

γ emissions are measured with a scintillation counter, a thallium-activated sodium iodide crystal which emits a photon when it absorbs a γ ray. The photon is converted to electrons by a photomultiplier. The number of pulses is proportional to the isotope activity and the height of the pulses to the energy of the individual γ rays, which vary from isotope to isotope. Pulse height analysers will select emissions from a given isotope hence these analysers possess 2 or 3 output channels to provide individual counts from a mixture of isotopes. Rate meters are used for determining rapid changes in activity over an organ; connection to a chart record allows isotope uptake tracings to be produced. Scalers determine the number of counts in a given unit of time.

Technique of Labelling Red Cells with ^{51}Cr

^{51}Cr in the form of sodium chromate, $Na_2{}^{51}CrO_4$ (half-life 27·8 days) is administered in a dose of 7·5 kBq/kg (0·2 µCi/kg) body weight for red cell mass determinations and 25–50 kBq/kg (0·7 µg—1·4 µCi) body weight for red cell survival studies, external counting and for quantitating faecal blood loss. Sodium chromate enters the red cell, the chromium becomes reduced from the anion hexavalent form to the trivalent cation, which binds preferentially to the β-chain of the haemoglobin molecule. Elution of chromium is about 1 per cent per day and correction may be made for this loss. Chromium is toxic above a concentration of 10 µg/ml for normal cells and 5 µg/ml with glutathione reductase or other enzyme deficiencies in the hexose monophosphate shunt. High specific activity is thus essential.

Determination of Red Cell Mass

Normal Values. Men 25–35 ml/kg; women 20–30 ml/kg.
Principle. An injection of the patient's own labelled red cells is given into one arm and a sample is taken from the other arm at 15 min. If red cells are being sequestrated in the spleen, three samples should be taken at 5-min intervals and the blood volume value for each is calculated. Subsequently the plot of counts against time allows extrapolation back to zero time to give the corrected count (i.e. as if instantaneous mixing had occurred). The red cell mass is calculated by the formula:

$$\text{Mass} = \frac{\text{total counts per minute injected}}{\text{counts per minute per ml of sample}} \times \text{Hct.}$$

Red Cell Survival

1. Random Labelling. Red cells are labelled with 25–50 kBq/kg (0·7–1·4 µCi/kg) body weight of ^{51}Cr as described above. An initial sample is taken from the other arm some 20 min after the initial injection. Further samples are collected daily (if a short survival is anticipated) or every 3 days (if a near-normal survival is probable).

If the activity in a unit volume of each sample is determined on the same day no allowance is required for radioactive decay. The counts are expressed as a percentage of the initial sample and plotted. The day when the activity has fallen to 50 per cent ($T\frac{1}{2}$) is determined. The normal range is 25–32 days. *Fig. 28.6* shows a normal survival curve and *Fig. 28.7* shows a survival curve composed of two populations of cells; such a double population is found in paroxysmal nocturnal

Fig. 28.6. Normal red
cell survival curve.

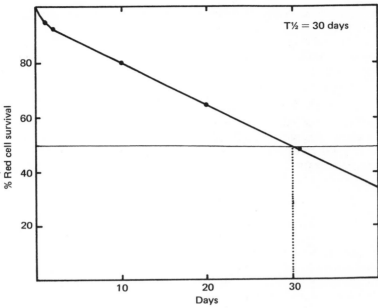

Fig. 28.7. Red cell
survival showing
double population.

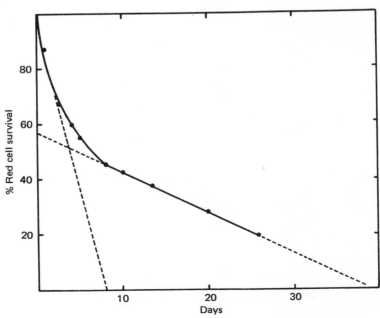

haemoglobinuria, some enzymopathies, sickle-cell disease and when labelled cells consist of a mixture of patients and transfused cells.

2. Cohort Labelling. The potential advantage of cohort labelling is the direct determination of the red cell life span. Radioactivity can be introduced into forming red cells with ^{15}N-glycine, ^{14}C-glycine or ^{59}Fe. ^{59}Fe, although technically easier to measure, is unsatisfactory because of re-utilization of ^{59}Fe from effete red cells.

Determination of Plasma Volume

Normal Value. Men and women 40–50 ml/kg.

Principle. An injection of human serum albumin (HSA) labelled with ^{125}I (half-life 60 days) is given intravenously and 15 min later a sample is taken from the other arm. If plasma leakage is a possibility, 3 samples are collected and plots made of the counts and extrapolated back to zero. The plasma volume is calculated from the formula:

$$\text{Volume} = \frac{\text{total counts per minute injected}}{\text{counts per minute per ml of sample}} \times (1 - \text{Hct}).$$

^{131}I (half-life 8 days) and ^{126}I (half-life 2·3 hours) present difficulties because of their short life, but may be used for labelling HSA. ^{51}Cr is satisfactory for labelling protein (used as ^{51}Cr Cl$_3$) but is not suitable if simultaneous red cell studies using ^{51}Cr are required. When red cell and plasma studies are performed simultaneously, ^{51}Cr and ^{125}I counts may be separated by use of a pulse height analyser, but a correction factor must be made for the Cr counts appearing on the I channel. Often the ^{126}I HSA is administered at the end of a red cell survival so that the ^{51}Cr is separated physically by centrifugation of the red cells from the plasma. When using iodine radio-isotopes, an oral dose of potassium iodide should first be given to block thyroid uptake of isotope.

Physiological Variation. Increased in pregnancy.

Pathological Variation

1. Increased

    1.1 Nephrotic syndrome
    1.2 Congestive cardiac failure
    1.3 ADH secreting tumours
    1.4 Over-transfusion with intravenous fluids

2. Decreased

    2.1 Burns
    2.2 Dehydration
    2.3 'Stress polycythaemia'
    2.4 Myxoedema (may partially mask the anaemia due to the reduced cell mass)
    2.5 Prolonged bed rest
    2.6 Altitude acclimatization

Surface Counting after the Injection of ^{51}Cr-labelled Red Cells

Normal Results. Counts made over the spleen are determined with a rate meter. Normally, equilibrium, shown by a plateau in the counts, occurs within 90 sec following the intravenous injection of labelled red cells; no significant increase in the counts should occur over the next 20 min (*Fig. 28.8*).

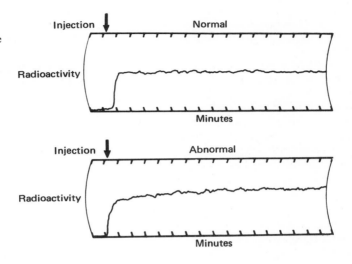

Fig. 28.8. Radioisotope rate meter recordings following the intravenous injection of ^{51}Cr-labelled red cells. (Reproduced by courtesy of the publishers of *Hospital Medicine*.)

Pathological Findings. In hypersplenism, the surface counts over the spleen after the injection of labelled red cells rise during the next 20 min; the so-called 'pooling-curve' (*Fig. 28.8*). Organ counts may be classified according to the following patterns.

1. Excess counts over the spleen but not liver occurs in hereditary spherocytosis, hereditary elliptocytosis and some autoimmune haemolytic anaemias.

2. Excess counts over liver and spleen in some cases of autoimmune haemolytic anaemia.

3. Excess counts over the liver, but not the spleen in sickle-cell disease, the spleen having atrophied because of infarcts.

4. No excess counts over liver or spleen in some hereditary non-spherocytic haemolytic anaemia and paroxysmal nocturnal haemoglobinuria.

Iron Absorption

Normal Value. Between 10 and 35 per cent of the test dose is absorbed.

Principle. $^{59}FeCl_3$, dose 50 kBq (1·4 µCi) is added to a carrier dose of 5 mg of aqueous ferrous sulphate and taken orally after an overnight fast. The amount absorbed is calculated either by determining the amount lost in the stools or by assessing the amount retained by using a whole body counter.

Physiological Variation. Absorption varies greatly with the form of iron (different foods vary widely in the availability of their iron content), its concentration and also the presence of other substances, such as ascorbic acid.

Pathological Variation. Increased absorption occurs with iron deficiency, idiopathic haemochromatosis and dyserythropoietic anaemias associated with iron overload.

Plasma Iron Clearance

Normal Value. The plasma iron turnover is taken as the period for half the dose of injected iron to be removed from the plasma; half-life = 60–140 min.
Principle. It is essential that injected iron becomes bound to transferrin otherwise it will not be transported to the bone marrow but be removed by the reticulo-endothelial system. If the patient's transferrin level is low the $^{59}FeCl_3$ in normal saline is added to 10 ml of normal heparinized plasma rather than the patient's plasma, mixed and injected intravenously. Samples are collected from the opposite arm at 20-min intervals over the next 2 hours.
Pathological Variation. Increased clearance occurs in haemolytic anaemia, iron-deficiency anaemia and polycythaemia rubra vera, and sometimes with extra-medullary erythropoiesis. Decreased clearance occurs in aplastic anaemia and in erythropoietic depression in leukaemia and other myeloproliferative disorders. Iron clearance studies do *not* differentiate between normal and abnormal erythropoiesis.

Plasma Iron Turnover

Normal Range. 0·4–0·8 mg/day.
Principle. The clearance is calculated from the plasma iron clearance and the iron content of the plasma.
Pathological Variation. Plasma iron turnover is increased in haemolytic anaemia, iron deficiency, myeloid metaplasia, and ineffective erythropoiesis, especially thalassaemia. Variable results may occur in aplastic anaemia. As with the plasma iron clearance it does not differentiate between normal and abnormal erythropoiesis.

Iron Utilization

Normal Value. 70–80 per cent of the level of injected iron reappears during the tenth to fourteenth day.
Pathological Variation. A rapid plasma clearance is usually associated with an early and high utilization. If there is severe haemolysis the utilization curve will become distorted. In ineffective erythropoiesis there is rapid plasma clearance but low utilization.

Surface Counting after Injection of ^{59}Fe (*Fig. 28.9*)

Normal Results. The normal count rises over the sacrum to reach a maximum of double the initial count at 4–6 hours. There is then a decline reaching the initial activity at about the fourth day. There is very little variation from the initial counts over the liver and spleen until the eighth to tenth day. The counts over the heart fall during the first 4 hours and gradually rise from the end of the first day until the eighth day.
Pathological Findings
  1. In iron deficiency the counts over the sacrum rise rapidly to double the initial count within 1 hour and reach approximately threefold at 4 hours.

Fig. 28.9. Surface counting after administration of ^{59}Fe.

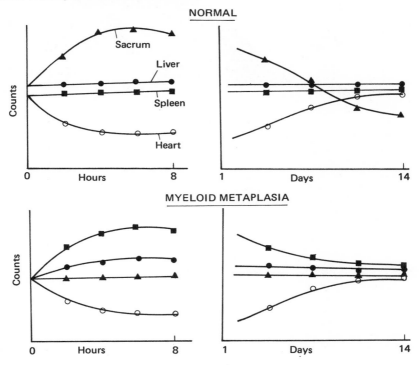

2. In aplastic anaemia there is virtually no change to the sacral counts, but counts over the liver rise.

3. In erythroid metaplasia the counts rise over the liver and spleen.

Selected Further Reading

Bowring C. S. (1981) *Radionuclide Tracer Techniques in Haematology.* London, Butterworth.

Dacie J. V. and Lewis S. M. (1975) *Practical Haematology,* 5th ed. Edinburgh, Churchill Livingstone.

Hayhoe F. G. J. and Quaglino D. (1980) *Haematological Cytochemistry.* Edinburgh, Churchill Livingstone.

Chapter 29 — Cytotoxic Drugs in Haematology

Cytotoxic drugs effective in haematological malignancy exert their action by a variety of different mechanisms, some of which are not completely known. They fall into the general categories shown in *Table 29.1*.

Table 29.1. Categories of cytotoxic drugs in haematology

Type of drug	Useful drugs in haematological diseases
Alkylating agent	Nitrogen mustard
	Cyclophosphamide
	Chlorambucil
	Melphalan
	Busulphan
	Dibromomannitol
	DTIC
	BiCNU
	CCNU
Antimetabolites	Methotrexate
	6-mercaptopurine
	Cytosine arabinoside
	5-azacytidine
Antibiotics	Daunorubicin
	Doxorubicin
	Mithramycin
	Bleomycin
Vinca alkaloids	Vincristine
	Vinblastine
	Vindesine
Hormones	Corticosteroids
Miscellaneous agents	Procarbazine
	Hydroxyurea
	L'asparaginase
	Etopside (VP16)

The normal cell cycle is shown in *Fig. 29.1*. The inner circle represents the DNA content of the normal diploid cell, the outer circle representing the double DNA content which is attained during the synthesis phase and maintained during G_2 prior to mitosis. G_0 represents the quiescent phase; cells capable of further division can re-enter the cell cycle when appropriately stimulated. Most normal marrow cells are cycling, though the majority of pluripotent stem cells may be in G_0.

Virtually all cytotoxic drugs are more active against rapidly proliferating tissues. Pharmacodynamically the drugs can be divided into two major groups:

1. Drugs whose activity rises exponentially with increasing dose to a certain

level, and then reaches a plateau. These include the vinca alkaloids, antimetabolites and procarbazine. It follows that these drugs should not be given as a large
single bolus for maximum cytotoxic effect.

2. Drugs in which the cell survival is related exponentially to the dose given,
including the alkylating agents and antibiotic cytotoxic drugs.

Fig. 29.1. The cell
cycle.

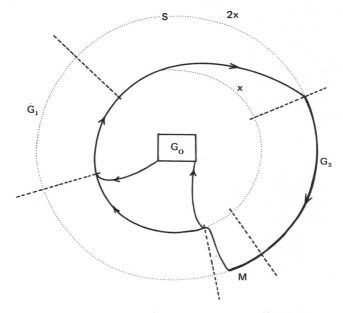

The difference between the two groups probably reflects the different sites of
action. Group 1 drugs are cell cycle phase specific and resting stem cells are
presumably protected. When two drugs given in combination act at the same phase
of the cell cycle they should be given at different times for maximal effect. Group 2
drugs have greater activity against cycling cells and often show phase preference
but they also have some activity against non-proliferating cells. Within this group
there is considerable variation in the degree to which an individual drug is active
against non- or slowly proliferating cells and this varies with a given drug from
tissue to tissue. Busulphan, melphalan and the nitrosoureas have high relative
activity against slowly proliferating tissues and this largely explains the protracted
marrow hypoplasia that can occur with these drugs. Cyclophosphamide, by
contrast, has less relative activity against quiescent cells.

Many attempts have been made to design combination chemotherapy regimes
using drugs that act by different mechanisms at different stages in the cell cycle,
given at appropriate times to obtain the maximum pharmacokinetic effects. Such
regimes have rarely been more effective than those designed empirically.

ALKYLATING AGENTS

Alkylating agents produce breaks and cross-linking of the DNA molecule. They
are not cycle specific.

Nitrogen Mustard (Mustine)

Chemical Characteristics. Bischlorethylamine.
Action. The drug is not cell-cycle specific but does have greatest effect at mitosis and the G_1/S interface. Similar effects are produced by ionizing radiation, so the drug is said to be radiomimetic.
Indications and Administration. The drug is a vesicant and is therefore administered intravenously into a rapidly running saline drip. It can also be given into a body cavity. It is used in:
  1. Hodgkin's disease in MOPP (mustine, vincristine (Oncovin), procarbazine, prednisone).
  2. Other lymphomas.
  3. Occasionally in carcinomas.
Side Effects
  1. Nausea and vomiting.
  2. Bone marrow depression with the nadir at 2–4 weeks.

Cyclophosphamide (Cytoxan; Endoxana)

Chemical Characteristics. It is a phosphonic acid derivative of nitrogen mustard.
Action. It is an alkylating agent which is inert until converted in the liver to aldophosphamide and subsequently the active phosphoramide mustard. The metabolites are primarily excreted via the kidneys. The breakdown product, acrolein, is the major cause of haemorrhagic cystitis which may occur with this drug.
Administration and Indications. It can be given either orally or intravenously. Used in:
  1. Non-Hodgkin's lymphomas, e.g. CHOP (cyclophosphamide, doxorubicin (Hydroxydaunomycin), vincristine (Oncovin) and prednisone.
  2. Sarcomas.
  3. Some carcinomas.
  4. Second-line therapy in acute chronic lymphatic leukaemia.
  5. Myeloma.
  6. Used as an immunosuppressive in transplantation and autoimmune disease.
Toxicities
  1. Nausea and vomiting, particularly when used in high dose intravenously.
  2. Haemorrhagic cystitis. This can often be avoided by maintenance of an alkaline diuresis. 2-Mercaptoethane sulphonate (MESNA) neutralizes the toxic effect of acrolein and may allow very high doses of cyclophosphamide to be given safely.
  3. Marrow suppression.
  4. Fluid retention.
  5. Sterility.
  6. Fetal damage.
  7. Delayed carcinogenesis.
  8. Cardiac damage when used in very high dosage.
  9. Alopecia.

Chlorambucil (Leukeran)

Chemical Characteristics. Phenylbutyric acid derivative of nitrogen mustard.

Action. It is a slowly acting alkylating agent.

Administration. It is given orally and is relatively less toxic than other alkylating agents.

Indications

1. Very useful in chronic lymphatic leukaemia as single agent or with prednisolone.

2. Lymphomas in second-line combination chemotherapy.

Toxicities

1. Marrow suppression.

2. Immunosuppression.

3. Mild gastrointestinal symptoms.

Melphalan (Alkeran)

Chemical Characteristics. Phenylalanine derivative of nitrogen mustard.

Action. Alkylating agent.

Administration. Given orally, usually in pulses every 4–6 weeks.

Indications

1. First-line drug for treatment of myelomatosis.

2. Also used in ovarian and breast cancer and in high dosage with autologous marrow rescue in childhood neuroblastoma.

Toxicities

1. Marrow suppression.

2. Nausea and vomiting.

3. Alopecia, though less than with cyclophosphamide.

Busulphan (Myleran)

Chemical Characteristics. It is an alkyl sulphonate.

Action. An alkylating agent with relatively high bone marrow stem cell toxicity.

Administration. Given by the oral route usually on a daily basis, but can be used in intermittent single large doses.

Indications.

1. Widely used as drug of first choice in chronic myeloid leukaemia.

2. Can be used in other myeloproliferative disorders, e.g. PRV, myelofibrosis and essential thrombocythaemia. Small doses are essential if there is significant myelofibrosis.

Toxicities

1. Can produce severe marrow depression which is sometimes irreversible.

2. Hyperpigmentation syndrome.

3. Pulmonary fibrosis.

4. Cataracts.

5. Gynaecomastia.

Dacarbazine (DTIC)

Chemical Characteristics. It is an imidazole carboxamide which is a structural analogue of certain purines.

Action. It is inactive until transformed via oxidative N-demethylation and photodegradation to active alkylating metabolites.

Administration. Given intravenously, but in selected tumours, such as melanoma, may be given intra-arterially.
Indications
 1. Second-line drug in lymphoma, i.e. in ABVD with adriamycin, bleomycin, and vinblastine used in Hodgkin's disease.
 2. Melanoma and sarcoma.
Toxicities
 1. Anorexia and vomiting.
 2. Moderate marrow suppression.
 3. Influenza-type syndrome.
 4. Alopecia.
 5. Hepatic dysfunction.

The Nitrosoureas, Carmustine (BCNU) and Lomustine (CCNU)

Chemical Characteristics. BCNU is a bis 2-chloroethyl nitrosourea. CCNU is 2-chloroethyl-3-cyclohexyl nitrosourea.
Action. They have a similar variety of actions including alkylation, carbamylation and inhibition of DNA repair and because of this multiplicity of actions they lack cross resistance with other alkylating agents. They have a broad spectrum of activity.
Administration. BCNU is given as a single i.v. injection every 6–8 weeks whilst CCNU is given as a single oral dose at the same interval.
Indications
 1. Myeloma second-line treatment.
 2. Lymphomas as second-line treatment.
 3. Other malignancies, including brain tumours, lung cancer and melanomas.
Toxicities
 1. Nausea and vomiting.
 2. Delayed toxicity to bone marrow, with nadir at 4–6 weeks.
 3. Stomatitis.
 4. Alopecia.
 5. Renal dysfunction.
 6. Pulmonary fibrosis.

ANTIMETABOLITES

Methotrexate (Amethopterin)

Chemical Characteristics. It is a folic acid antagonist in which there are two substitutions in the structure of folic acid—an NH_2 group for an OH group and a CH_3 group for an O.
Action. It competes avidly for the folate-binding site of dihydrofolate reductase and decreases synthesis in cells of thymidine and purine nucleotides. This can result in complete suppression of DNA synthesis. Methotrexate is cell-cycle specific with maximum activity in S phase. The cytotoxic action of methotrexate on normal tissues can be reversed by folinic acid (leucovorin) which bypasses the block produced by methotrexate. In some regimes asparaginase is given after methotrexate and acts as a 'rescue'.

Administration
1. Low-dose oral or parenteral therapy not requiring rescue.
2. In very high dose i.v. with folinic acid rescue.
3. Intrathecally.

Indications
1. Acute lymphoblastic leukaemia.
   1.1 Systemic (oral or parenteral) low-dose therapy in maintenance.
   1.2 High dose with folinic acid rescue in consolidation.
   1.3 Intrathecally as treatment or prophylaxis of CNS leukaemia.
2. Choriocarcinoma.
3. Carcinoma of head and neck, breast and testis.

Toxicities
1. Ulceration of rapidly proliferating tissues: stomatitis, diarrhoea.
2. Hepatic dysfunction with ultimate fibrosis.
3. Megaloblastic change in the marrow.
4. Pneumonitis.
5. Osteoporosis.
6. Teratogenic.
7. Renal failure with high-dose regimes.

6-Mercaptopurine (6-MP; Puri-Nethol)

Chemical Characteristics. Purine analogue with a mercapto group substituting in the C-6 position of the purine ring.

Action. Requires activation to its ribonucleotide for cytotoxicity and is then incorporated into RNA. It may also directly inhibit ribonucleotide conversion to inosine. It is cell-cycle S-phase-specific.

Administration. Usually given by mouth as a daily dose. Cross-resistance does not occur with other anti-cancer drugs except for the purine analogues. When given with the xanthine oxidase inhibitor, allopurinol, metabolism of 6-MP is delayed and clinical effect is increased 2–4 fold: the daily dose should therefore be reduced accordingly.

Indications
1. In maintenance therapy in acute lymphoblastic leukaemia.
2. In chronic myeloid leukaemia refractory to busulphan.
3. As an immunosuppressive in refractory immune thrombocytopenia or autoimmune haemolytic anaemia.

Toxicities
1. Marrow suppression.
2. Gastrointestinal symptoms.
3. Cholestatic jaundice.
4. Dermatitis.
5. Fever.
6. Hyperuricaemia.

Thioguanine (6-TG; Lanvis)

Chemical Characteristics. Sulph-hydryl substitution of a purine base.

Actions. Requires conversion to ribonucleotide form and is then incorporated into DNA. It is a cell-cycle S-phase-specific agent.

Administration. Usually given by mouth in divided daily doses; absorption may be erratic.

Indications

1. As part of combination chemotherapy for induction of acute myeloid leukaemia (e.g. DAT).

2. As gentle myelosuppressive therapy without anthracyclines in those cases of AML not suitable for aggressive induction therapy.

3. In maintenance therapy of acute myeloid leukaemia.

4. Myeloproliferative disorders, such as chronic granulocytic leukaemia.

Toxicities

1. Myelosuppression.

2. Nausea, vomiting, anorexia.

3. Stomatitis.

4. Liver dysfunction.

Both 6-MP and 6-TG are closely related to allopurinol, an analogue of the purine base hypoxanthine; whilst the use of allopurinol with 6-MP requires dose reduction of the latter this is not required for 6-TG. The immunosuppressive agent azathioprine (Imuran) is also structurally related to 6-MP and 6-TG.

Cytarabine (Cytosine Arabinoside; Ara-C; (Cytosar, Alexan)

Chemical Characteristics. It is a substituted pyrimidine 1-β-D arabinofuranosyl-cytosine an analogue of deoxycytidine and closely related to azacytidine.

Action. It is converted to an active form which functions as a competitive inhibitor of DNA polymerase. It is S phase specific and is largely degraded by two enzymes, cytidine and deoxycytidylate deaminase.

Administration. Usually given intravenously either as a rapid injection or as an infusion lasting from 30 min to 24 hours. The half-life is brief and slow infusion increases its cytotoxic effect. Sometimes given subcutaneously. Intrathecal cytosine is an alternative to methotrexate for the treatment of meningeal leukaemia, the disappearance time from the CSF being slow because of the paucity of the relevant degradative enzymes in the CSF.

Indications

1. For induction of AML in combination with other drugs (DAT).

2. In AML maintenance.

Toxicities

1. Marrow suppression.

2. Moderately severe nausea and vomiting.

3. Stomatitis.

4. Hepatic damage.

5. Potentially teratogenic and carcinogenic since it produces chromosome breaks.

5-Azacytidine

Chemical Characteristics. Single nitrogen substitution in the pyrimidine ring of cytidine.

Action. Undergoes conversion to an active triphosphate and has action similar to cytosine arabinoside. It is cell-cycle phase specific.
Administration. Intravenous by infusion or subcutaneous injection.
Indications. Acute myeloid leukaemia.
Toxicities
  1. Nausea and vomiting.
  2. Marrow suppression.
  3. Liver damage.
  4. Uncommonly rhabdomyolysis.
  5. Lethargy, weakness and confusion.

ANTIBIOTIC CYTOTOXICS

The antibiotic cytotoxic drugs are natural products of the soil fungus, strep-tomyces, and include daunorubicin, adriamycin, mithramycin, bleomycin, ac-tinomycin D and mitomycin C.

Daunorubicin (Daunomycin; Rubidomycin; Cerubidin)

Chemical Characteristics. Anthracycline antibiotic.
Action. It directly binds to DNA and inhibits DNA and RNA synthesis. It has a variety of effects on different phases of the cell cycle, with maximum effect on S phase, but also has some effect on non-proliferating tissues.
Administration. Given intravenously into a rapidly running drip. The urine may turn red.
Indications. Largely restricted to induction of remission in acute leukaemia.
Toxicities
  1. Severe marrow suppression.
  2. Cardiac toxicity. This appears to be dose related; the recommended maxi-mum dose being 550 mg/m². Arrhythmias may occur early in treatment. Unrespon-sive congestive heart failure occurs later after a high cumulative dose, often with no premonitory ECG or echocardiographic evidence of impairment. Fragmentation and lysis of myocardial fibrosis may be seen at post-mortem.
  3. Severe nausea and vomiting.
  4. Alopecia.
  5. Severe irritation of tissues if extravasation occurs from vein.

Adriamycin (Doxorubicin; Hydroxydaunomycin)

Chemical Characteristics. Closely related to 'daunorubicin' and differs from it only by the addition of a single hydroxyl group.
Action. As for daunorubicin (*see above*).
Administration. Given i.v. into a rapidly running drip. With adriamycin the patient's urine may turn a red colour. Adriamycin may act as a radiation sensitizer and care should be taken if the patient is receiving concurrent radiotherapy.
Indications. It has one of the widest spectra of antitumour activity seen with any one agent.

1. First-line drug in unfavourable prognosis non-Hodgkin's lymphoma as part of combination therapy.
2. For induction and consolidation of acute lymphoblastic leukaemia.
3. Second-line drug in Hodgkin's disease.
4. Soft-tissue sarcomas.
5. Wide variety of carcinomas.

Toxicities. As for daunorubicin, but also:
1. Renal failure.
2. Hyperpigmentation.
3. Skin rashes.

Mithramycin (Mithracin)

Chemical Characteristics. A complex long-chain compound originally synthesized by streptomyces.
Action. Potent inhibitor of RNA synthesis which inhibits osteoclastic activity and bone resorption.
Administration. Given i.v. by rapid infusion.
Indications
1. For hypercalcaemia in:
        1.1 Metastatic malignancy.
        1.2 Myeloma.
2. For bone pain in breast cancer and myeloma. The dose used is less than that used in hypercalcaemia.
Toxicities
1. Marrow toxicity, particularly thrombocytopenia.
2. Hepatorenal failure.
3. Malaise, fever and vomiting.
4. Neurological complications.
5. Hypocalcaemia.
Many of these toxicities are severe and unpredictable.

Bleomycin (Blenoxane)

Chemical Characteristics. An antibiotic complex originally derived from streptomyces which separates into many fractions.
Action. Directly binds to DNA, resulting in reduced synthesis of DNA, RNA and proteins. It is not cell-cycle specific but has maximum activity against cycling cells in G_2 and M phases.
Administration. Given i.v., i.m. or s.c. It may cause a reaction resembling anaphylaxis.
Indications
1. Second-line drug in lymphomas.
2. Testicular neoplasms.
3. Head and neck carcinomas.
Toxicities
1. Pulmonary fibrosis common with more than 400 mg total dose.
2. Moderate to severe skin reactions.
3. Mutagenic and probably teratogenic.
4. Fulminant acute reaction occasionally, consisting of fever, hypotension and cardiorespiratory collapse.

VINCA ALKALOIDS

Vincristine (Oncovin)

Chemical Characteristics. An alkaloid extracted from the common periwinkle plant.

Action. Binds to cellular microtubular proteins which are the essential component of the mitotic spindle of dividing cells and causes arrest of cell mitosis. Surprisingly there is high cytotoxic effect in S phase as well as mitosis.

Administration. I.v. with great care to avoid extravasation.

Indications

1. Drug of first choice in acute lymphoblastic leukaemia induction.
2. Drug of first choice in combination chemotherapy for Hodgkin's and non-Hodgkin's lymphoma.
3. Also used for sarcomas, brain tumours and other carcinomas.

Toxicities

1. Mixed sensory and autonomic neuropathy (much more likely than with vinblastine). Includes paraesthesiae of extremities, constipation and paralytic ileus.
2. Marrow suppression is uncommon and much less prominent than with vinblastine.
3. Alopecia.
4. Inappropriate secretion of antidiuretic hormone.

Vinblastine (Velbe, Velban)

Chemical Characteristics. Identical to vincristine except for the substitution of a CH_3 group for an $O=CH$ group.

Action. As for vincristine.

Administration. Given i.v. with great care to avoid tissue extravasation.

Indications

1. Hodgkin's and non-Hodgkin's lymphomas.
2. Testicular tumours.
3. Breast, head and neck cancer.
4. Brain tumours.

Toxicities

1. Marrow suppression.
2. Gastrointestinal symptoms.
3. Uncommonly peripheral neuropathy and other neurological problems.

Vindesine (Eldisine)

Chemical Characteristics. It is a derivative of vinblastine.

Action. Probably similar to vincristine and vinblastine, though tumours resistant to vincristine may still be sensitive to vindesine.

Administration. Given i.v. × 1/week.

Indications. Still to be determined, but may be useful in:

1. Malignant melanoma.
2. Lymphoma.
3. Oat-cell carcinoma of bronchus.
4. Resistant acute lymphoblastic leukaemia.

5. Blastic crisis of chronic myeloid leukaemia.

Toxicities
1. Leucopenia.
2. Alopecia.
3. Neurotoxicity (less than with vincristine).

Etoposide (VP16-213; Epipodophyllotoxin)

Chemical Characteristics. Semi-synthetic derivative of podophyllotoxin, a crystalline plant extract.

Actions. Similar to vinca alkaloids, but cells are arrested and destroyed in the premitotic phase.

Administration. Orally or i.v.

Indications
1. Acute myeloid leukaemia, particularly with a monocytic component.
2. Solid tumours, particularly oat-cell carcinoma of lung.

Toxicities
1. Marrow suppression.
2. Alopecia.
3. Oral ulceration.
4. Gastrointestinal symptoms.

HORMONES

Corticosteroids

Chemical Characteristics. Synthetic analogues of naturally-occurring adrenocortical hormones.

Action. Unknown, but may alter membrane permeability and also bind to specific cytoplasmic receptor proteins forming complexes which bind DNA. Unlike most cytotoxic drugs they are equally effective in all phases of the cell cycle.

Administration. By mouth, i.v. or i.m.

Indications (in haematology)
1. In autoimmune phenomena, e.g. autoimmune haemolytic anaemia to lyse B cells and suppress activity of phagocytes, immune thrombocytopenia, aplastic anaemia, and graft versus host disease.
2. In thrombocytopenia for its supposed capillary stabilization effect.
3. With other cytotoxic agents in acute lymphoblastic leukaemia. Hodgkin's disease and non-Hodgkin's lymphoma.

Side Effects
1. Salt and water retention.
2. Hypertension.
3. Diabetes mellitus.
4. Osteoporosis.
5. Myopathy.
6. Peptic ulceration.
7. Growth failure in childhood.
8. Mood changes.
9. Cataracts.

OTHER AGENTS

Procarbazine (Natulan)

Chemical Characteristics. Methylhydrazine derivative.

Action. Only active when it is degraded; the metabolites depolymerize DNA, and have some alkylating activity. Although not obviously cell-cycle specific a 'plateau' is achieved with increasing dosage. Originally devised as a psychiatric drug and has monoamine oxidase inhibitor activity.

Administration. Orally. Patients should be warned not to take foods or drugs with monoamine oxidase activities, e.g. imiprimine.

Indications

1. Hodgkin's disase (MOPP—mustine hydrochloride, vincristine (Oncovin), procarbazine and prednisone).
2. Less useful in non-Hodgkin's lymphoma and other carcinomas.

Toxicities

1. Nausea and vomiting.
2. Marrow suppression.
3. Disorder of consciousness.
4. Peripheral neuropathy potentiated by other monoamine oxidase inhibitors.
5. 'Flushing' with alcohol.
6. Allergic skin rashes.
7. Pulmonary reactions with fever.
8. Haemolytic anaemia.
9. Teratogenic.

Hydroxyurea (Hydrea)

Action. Inhibitor of ribonucleotide reductase. Specifically cytotoxic to cells in S phase.

Administration. Daily oral dose.

Indications

1. First-line drug in chronic myeloid leukaemia.
2. Other myeloproliferative disorders.
3. Some carcinomas.

Toxicities

1. Marrow suppression.
2. Megaloblastic anaemia.
3. Skin reactions.

L-asparaginase (Colaspase)

Chemical Characteristics. An enzyme synthesized by *Escherichia coli* or Erwinia.

Actions. It decreases the availability of L-asparaginine and if the neoplastic cell cannot synthesize it, cell death occurs. Probably cell-cycle phase non-specific.

Administration. Usually given i.v. but can be given i.m. A test dose must always be given intradermally before each course in case of severe allergic reaction. Medication for resuscitation must be immediately available.

Indications. Acute lymphoblastic leukaemia therapy during induction consolidation or relapse.

Toxicities
1. Can cause anaphylaxis.
2. Nausea and vomiting.
3. Hepatic toxicity.
4. Depressed clotting factors.

Appendix
Conversion Table

	SI units		Standard units
Serum iron and total iron binding capacity	μmol/l	$\xrightarrow{\times 5\cdot586}$ $\xleftarrow{\times 0\cdot179}$	μg/100 ml
Bilirubin	μmol/l	$\xrightarrow{\times 17\cdot1}$ $\xleftarrow{\times 0\cdot058}$	mg/100 ml
Urea	μmol/l	$\xrightarrow{\times 6\cdot024}$ $\xleftarrow{\times 0\cdot166}$	mg/100 ml
Uric acid	μmol/l	$\xrightarrow{\times 0\cdot017}$ $\xleftarrow{\times 59\cdot1}$	mg/100 ml
Radioactivity	kBq	$\xrightarrow{\times 0\cdot027}$ $\xleftarrow{\times 37}$	μCi
	MBq	$\xrightarrow{\times 0\cdot027}$ $\xleftarrow{\times 37}$	mCi
Radiation dosage	Gy	$\xrightarrow{\times 100}$ $\xleftarrow{\times 0\cdot0}$	rad

291

Index

ABO system, 230–1
  typing, 234–5
Acanthocytes, 8
Acanthocytosis, hereditary, 68
Achlorhydria, 30
Aciduria, hereditary orotic, 50
Acyclovir, 54
Addison's disease, 106
Adenosine triphosphate, 69
Adrenal disease, anaemia and, 106
Adriamycin, 285–6
Afibrinogenaemia, (*Table* 21.1) 203, 206
Aggregation, platelet, 188–9, 215
  red cell, 8
Air embolism, post-transfusion, 252–3
Albers–Schönberg's disease, 114
Albumin, blood group compatibility test, 236, 237
  dried, 243
  transfusions, 97, 242–3
Alder–Reilly anomaly, 11, 13
Aldolase deficiency, 73
Alimentary tract, blood loss from, 30
Alkylating agents, 279–82
Allergy related to blood transfusion, 250
Allopurinol, 284
Amaurotic familial idiocy, 24
Amegakaryocytic thrombocytopenia, 192
Aminoglycoside, 54
Amphotericin, 54–55
Amyloidosis, 176–8, 212
Anaemia, aplastic, 51–57
    bone marrow transplantation in, 52, 56–57
    chemical-related, 52
    chronic acquired, 51–52
    classification, 51
    clinical features, 53
    congenital, 51
    drug-related, 52
    idiopathic, 51–52
    irradiation-related, 52
    laboratory features, 53
    pathogenesis, 51–53
    pregnancy-associated, 53
    treatment, 54–56
    viral hepatitis-related, 52–53
  blood transfusion for, 239
  chronic disease and, 102–8
  classification, 1–3
  definition, 1

Anaemia (*cont.*)
  diagnosis, 3–5
  Fanconi's, 51, 57–58
  folate-refractory, 50
  haemolytic, 61–74
    acquired non-immune, 97–101
    autoimmune, 92–97
    clinical findings, 61
    general investigations, 63–65
    haemoglobin synthesis defects, 74
    hereditary, 66–74
    laboratory findings, 61–63
    malignancy and, 103
    membrane defects, 66–69
    microangiopathic, 100–1
    red cell enzyme defects, 69–74
  iron-deficiency, 27, 30–35
    aetiology, 30
    biochemical findings, 32
    bone marrow in, 32
    definition, 27
    diagnosis, 32
    differential diagnosis, 32–33
    incidence, 27
    peripheral blood picture, 31–32
    radiological findings, 31
    symptoms, 31
    treatment, 33–35
  leuco-erythroblastic, 2, 8
  macrocytic, 4–5
  megaloblastic, 40–50
    classification, 42
    clinical features, 40–41
    folic-acid deficiency in, 47–50
    laboratory features, 41
    in rheumatoid arthritis, 107
    vitamin B_{12} deficiency in, 42–47
  microcytic, 4, 31–32
  multiple mechanisms in, 3
  myeloma and, 169, 170
  non-Hodgkin's lymphoma and, 158
  normocytic, 4
  pernicious, 44–46
    juvenile, 43
  sickle-cell disease and, 86
  sideroblastic, 36–37
    hereditary, 37
    primary acquired, 38
    secondary acquired, 38–39
  traumatization of red cells, 99

293

Anaemia (*cont.*)
  vitamin B_{12} refractory, 50
Ancrod, 227
Androgens for aplastic anaemia, 55
Angiokeratoma corporis diffusum, 24
Anisocytosis, 6–7
Ankle ulceration, 86
Antibiotics, cytotoxic, 285–6
  for infection in aplastic anaemia, 54–55
Antibodies, blood group, 233
  cold, 93–95, 233
  complicating blood transfusion, 246–7
  drug-associated, 95–96
  Duffy, 233
  in adrenal disease, 106
  in haemolytic disease of newborn, 96
  Kell, 232
  to DNA, 271
  to Factor VIII, 190
  to intrinsic factor, 45
  to Lewis antigens, 231
  warm, 92–93, 233
Anticoagulants, 220–5
  for blood storage, 245
  heparin (*see* Heparin)
  oral, 209, 222–5
    contraindication to, 225
    dosage, 223
    indications, 223
    interactions, 224–5
    laboratory tests, 223
    monitoring, 224
    resistance, 225
    reversal, 225
    side effects, 225
Antigens, 234
  red cell, 230–3
Antiglobulin test, direct, (*Fig.* 7.2) 64, 65
  indirect, 236, 237
Antilymphocyte serum for aplastic anaemia, 56
Antimetabolites, 282–5
Antinuclear factor, 270
Antiplasmin, 184, 185, 215, 218
Antiplatelet drugs, 183–4, 227–9
Antiserum, anti-common ALL, 129
  for aplastic anaemia, 56, 57
  thymocyte and T cell, 129
Antithrombin III, 185
  assay, 190, 218
  deficiency, 212, 214
  heparin and, 220
Antithrombotic drugs, 220–9
Aplasia, pure red cell, 58–60
  see also Anaemia, aplastic
Apoferritin, 27–29
Arterial occlusion, heparin for, 222
Arteriovenous shunt maintenance, 228, 229
L-Asparaginase, 289–90
Aspirin, 196, 218, 228
Auer rods, 19, 133
Autoagglutinin tests, 268

Auto-antibodies, organ-specific, 271
Autohaemolysis test, 266
5-Azacytidine, 284–5
Azathioprine, 284
Azlocillin, 54

B cells, classification, 140
  deficiency, 145
  examination, 12–13
  in non-Hodgkin's lymphoma, 159, 163
  maturation and corresponding malignancies, (*Fig.* 17.1) 150
  prolymphocytic leukaemia, 167
  rosetting, (*Table* 28.1) 257
Bacteraemic shock, 250–1
Basopenia, 12
Basophilia, 12
  punctate, 8
Basophils, examination in blood film, (*Fig.* 2.2) 9, 12
  in marrow, 23
  function, 111
BCNU, 282
Behçet's disease, thrombotic risks in, (*Table* 23.1) 215, 217
Bence Jones protein, 171, 269
Benzene, aplastic anaemia from, 52
Bernard–Soulier syndrome, 15, 192, 198
  platelet aggregation in, (*Table* 19.3) 189
Betalipoprotein, 68
Biguanides, therapy with, 226
  vitamin B_{12} deficiency following, 44
Bilirubin levels, in cord in haemolytic disease of newborn, 97
  in haemolytic anaemia, 61
Bishydroxycoumarin, 222
Bleeding disorders, screening tests for, (*Table* 19.2) 187
  see also under specific disorders
Bleeding time, 188
Bleomycin, 286
Blood, cell differentiation, (*Fig.* 3.1) 17
  count, in prothrombotic state, 218
  donors, rhesus grouping in, 235
  film examination, 6–15
    in acute lymphoblastic leukaemia, 128
    in acute myeloid leukaemia, 132
    in anaemia of chronic disease, 102
    in autoimmune haemolytic anaemia, 93, 94
    in chronic granulocytic leukaemia, 117
    in essential thrombocythaemia, 123
    in haemolytic anaemia, 65
    in haemolytic uraemic syndrome, 100
    in hereditary spherocytosis, 66–67
    in Hodgkin's disease, 153–4
    in infectious mononucleosis, 144
    in liver disease, 106
    in malignancy, 103–5
    in polycythaemia rubra vera, 120

Blood, film examination (*cont.*)
 in preleukaemia, 137
 in sickle-cell disease, 87
 in β-thalassaemia, 81
 preparation, 6
 staining, 6, 255–6
 formation, 142
 groups, ABO system, 230–1, 234–5
 antibodies, 233
 compatibility testing, 234–7
 D-subgroups, 232
 Duffy system, 232–3
 Ii system, 231
 incidence, (*Table* 25.1) 230
 Kell system, 232
 Kidd system, 233
 Lewis system, 231
 Lutheran system, 233
 MNS system, 233
 P system, 232
 rhesus system, 232, 235
 infected, 250–2
 loss, anaemia from, 2
 due to drugs, 107
 in hepatic disease, 105–6
 in renal disease, 105
 iron deficiency from, 30
 quantitation, 238
 whole blood for, 238
 products, use of, 238–44
 see also Blood transfusion
 storage, 142, 234, 245–6
 transfusion, air embolism, 253
 allergic reaction, 250
 bacteraemic shock, 250–1
 circulatory overload, 248–9
 compatibility testing, 236–7
 drug effects, 254
 febrile reactions, 249–50
 for haemolytic disease of newborn, 97
 for liver disease, 209
 for sickle-cell disease, 87
 for β-thalassaemia, 81
 for vitamin B_{12} deficiency, 47
 haemolytic reactions, 246–8
 hazards and complications, 245–54
 immunological sensitization, 253
 incompatibilities, 231, 247
 infections following, 251–2
 massive, 254
 platelet concentrates, 241
 potassium and citrate toxicity, 252
 red cell concentrates, 239
 siderosis, 253
 thrombophlebitis from, 253
 whole blood, 238–9
 whole, 238–9
 see also Coagulation; Haemoglobin; Haemostasis; Red blood cells; White blood cells
Bloom's syndrome, 126
Bone, changes in iron deficiency, 31

Bone (*cont.*)
 marrow, culture studies in AML, 135
 cytogenetic studies, 258–9
 description, 16
 examination, 16–26
 in acute lymphoblastic leukaemia, 128
 in acute myeloid leukaemia, 133
 in aplastic anaemia, 53
 in chronic granulocytic leukaemia, 118
 in chronic lymphocytic leukaemia, 166
 in Diamond–Blackfan syndrome, 59
 in essential thrombocythaemia, 123
 in Fanconi's anaemia, 58
 in hairy cell leukaemia, 168
 in hereditary spherocytosis, 67
 in iron-deficiency anaemia, 32
 in liver disease, 106
 in megaloblastic anaemia, 41
 in myeloma, 170
 in polycythaemia rubra vera, 120
 failure in aplastic anaemia, 51–57
 in infections, 102–3
 pathogenesis, 51–53
 infiltration, 2
 iron in, 22
 malignant cells in, 25–26, 103, 105
 morphology, 18–21
 obtaining, 16
 parasites in, 26
 staining, 16–18
 stimulation, 55–56
 suppression by drugs, 52
 tissue typing, 56
 transplantation in ALL, 132
 in AML, 136–7
 in aplastic anaemia, 52, 56–57
Bradykinin production, 184
Brucellosis, post-transfusion, 252
Burkitt's lymphoma, 157, 160, 163
Burns, haemolytic anaemia from, 99
Burr cells, 8
Busulphan, 281
 for chronic granulocytic leukaemia, 118
 for polycythaemia rubra vera, 121
 for thrombocythaemia, 197

Carbenicillin, 54
Cardiac prosthesis, haemolytic anaemia and, 99
CCNU, 82
Cell cycle, 278–9
 markers, in ALL, 129
 in AML, 134
Cerebrovascular disease therapy, 223, 228, 229
Chagas' disease, 252
Chédiak–Higashi syndrome, 11, 112, 199
Chemotherapy, 278–90
 for ALL, 131
 for AML, 135–6
 for CLL, 166

Chemotherapy (*cont.*)
  for cutaneous T-cell lymphoma, 164
  for Hodgkin's disease, 156–7
  for myeloma, 172
  for non-Hodgkin's lymphoma, 161–2
Chloracetate esterase stain, 256
Chlorambucil, 195, 280–1
Chloramphenicol aplasia, 52
Cholelithiasis, 86
Cholesteryl ester hydrolase deficiency, 24
Christmas disease, 205, 244
  tests for, 186, 187, 223
Chromosomes, banding technique, 259
  in ALL, 129–30
  in AML, 134
  in Fanconi's anaemia, 58
  in G-6-PD deficiency, 71
  in non-Hodgkin's lymphoma, 158
  Philadelphia, 117, 119
Chronic granulomatous disease, 112
Circulatory overload, 248–9
  stasis, 216
Citrate toxicity in blood transfusions, 252
Clotting *see* Coagulation
Coagulation, activity and VIII C test, 187
  disorders, (*Table 19.1*) 186
    acquired, 208–12
    hereditary, 202–7
    increased concentration of activated
      clotting factors, 214
    increased concentration of clotting factors,
      213–14
    inhibitor deficiency, 214
    plasma transfusion for, 242
  extrinsic cascade, 180
  inhibition, 185, 212
    assay, 190
  intrinsic cascade, 179–80
  pathway, 181
  tests, 186–8
    heparin effects on, 220
  see also Disseminated intravascular
    coagulation
Cobalamin deficiency, 42
Coeliac disease, 30
Colchicine, vitamin B_{12} deficiency from, 44
Cold haemagglutinin disease, 92–93
Colitis, ulcerative, vitamin B_{12} deficiency from,
  43
Collagen disorders, 201
Committed myeloid progenitor cells, 19
Complement, deficiency disorders, 145
  storage, 234
Contraceptive pill, thrombotic risk from,
  (*Table 23.1*) 216
Coombs' test, (*Fig. 7.2*) 64, 65, 235
Coronary artery disease therapy, 228
Corticosteroids, 288
Co-trimoxazole for infection in aplastic
  anaemia, 54
^{51}Cr labelling, 272

Cranial arteritis, anaemia and, 107
Crenated cells, 8
Crohn's disease, thrombocytes in, 196
  vitamin B_{12} deficiency from, 43
Cryoglobulinaemia, 174–5
Cryoprecipitate, 202, 204–6, 211, 243
Culling, 143
Cyanosis, 90
Cyclophosphamide, 195, 212, 280
  for bone marrow transplant, 56
Cyclosporin A, for bone marrow transplant, 56,
  57
Cytogenetics, 258–9
Cytomegalovirus infection, post-transfusion,
  251–2
Cytosine arabinoside, 284
  DNA inhibition by, 50
Cytotoxic drugs, 278–90
  see also Chemotherapy *and specific drugs*

Dactylitis, 86
Daunorubicin, 285
1-Deamino-8-D-arginine vasopressin (DDAVP)
  for haemophilia, 204
Defibrination therapy, 227
Deoxyribose nucleic acid (DNA), antibodies,
  271
  impaired formation, 1–2
    by anti-DNA drugs, 50
    in megaloblastic anaemia, 40
Deoxyuridine suppression test, 46
Dermatomyositis, anaemia and, 108
Desferrioxamine, for iron overload, 36, 253
  for β-thalassaemia major, 81
Dextran, iron, 34
Di Guglielmo's syndrome, 138
Diabetes, platelet aggregation in, 215
  thrombotic risk with, (*Table 23.1*) 217
Diamond–Blackfan syndrome, 59–60
Dicopac test, 45–46
2,3-Diphosphoglycerate, 69
  estimations, 262
Diphosphoglycerate mutase deficiency, 73
Diphyllobothrium latum, vitamin B_{12} deficiency
  from, 44
Dipyridamole, 228
Disseminated intravascular coagulation, 210–11
  cryoprecipitate for, 243
  heparin for, 222
DNA *see* Deoxyribose nucleic acid
Döhle bodies, 10–11
Donath–Landsteiner test, 232, 267
Drepanocytes, 8
Drugs, acute leukaemia associated with, 126
  aplastic anaemia from, 52
  G-6-PD deficiency from, (*Table 8.1*) 72
  haemolytic anaemia from, 95–96, 101
  interaction with anticoagulants, 224–5
  platelet function disorders from, 201

Drugs (*cont.*)
  thrombocytopenia from, 193, 195–6
  with blood transfusions, 254
  see also Chemotherapy *and specific drugs*
DTIC, 281–2
Duffy system, 232–3
Dysfibrinogenaemia, congenital, 206
Dyshaemopoiesis, toxic, 2

EACA (*see* Epsilon aminocaproic acid)
Electrophoresis, haemoglobin, 76, 259–60
  protein, 268
Elliptocytes, 7
Elliptocytosis, hereditary, 67–68
Embden–Meyerhof pathway defects, 73
Endoperoxides, 183
Enolase deficiency, 73
Enzymes, defects, causing haemolysis, 2
    congenital, 49
    red cell, 69–74
  iron in, 29
Eosinopenia, 12
Eosinophilia, 11
Eosinophils, examination, in blood film,
      (*Fig.* 2.2) 9, 11–12
  in marrow, 23
  function of, 110
Epsilon aminocaproic acid for haemophilia, 204
Epstein–Barr virus, infectious mononucleosis
      from, 143
  non-Hodgkin's lymphoma from, 157
Erythroblasts, 134
Erythrocytes, *see* Red blood cell
Erythropoiesis, extramedullary, 8
  ineffective, (*Fig.* 4.2) 33, 35, 37–38
    iron-deficient, 27
    megaloblastic, 4
    normoblastic, 4
    sideroblastic, 103
    splenic, 142
Erythropoietin, inappropriate production and
      polycythaemia, 122
Etoposide, 288
Euglobulin lysis time, 188–9, 219
Evans' syndrome, 195
Extracorporeal circulation, heparin for, 222

Fabry's disease, 24
Factor II deficiency, 223
  stability, 246
Factor V deficiency, (*Table* 21.1) 203, 206, 242,
      244
  stability, 246
Factor VII deficiency, (*Table* 21.1) 203, 206–7,
      223, 244
  stability, 246
Factor VIII antibodies, 212

Factor VIII (*cont.*)
  assay, 190
  concentrates, 243
  increase, 217
  plasma transfusion for deficiency, 242
  production, 143, 180, (*Fig.* 19.2) 181
  stability, 246
  therapy, 203–4
Factor IX concentrates, 244
  deficiency, *see* Christmas disease
  purified preparation, 244
  stability, 246
Factor X deficiency, (*Table* 21.1) 203, 223
Factor XI deficiency, (*Table* 21.1) 203, 207, 242
Factor XII deficiency, 179, (*Table* 21.1) 203,
      207
Factor XIII deficiency, (*Table* 21.1) 203, 207
Fanconi's anaemia, 51, 57–58
Favism, 71
^{59}Fe for surface counting, 276–7
Felty's syndrome, 107
Femoral head necrosis, 86
Ferritin, 27–29
  in iron-deficient anaemia, 32
Ferrous fumurate, 34
Ferrous gluconate, 34
Ferrous hydroxide, 34
Ferrous sulphate, 34
Fibrin, clot formation, 181
  fibrinogen degradation products, 189, 217,
      218
Fibrinogen, abnormalities, 206
  conversion by ancrod, 227
  dried, 244
  storage, 246
Fibrinogen-thrombin reaction, 181
Fibrinolysis, 184
  abnormal, 211, 214–15
  inhibition, 185, 209, 218
  tests, 188–9
Fibrinolytics, 226–7
Fibrinopeptides assay, 217–18
Fibroblast proliferation, 124
Filariasis, post-transfusion, 252
Fitzgerald factor, 184
Fletcher factor, 184, (*Table* 21.1) 203, 207
5-Fluorouracil, DNA inhibition by, 50
Foam cells, 23–25
Folate, absorption, 48
  defective utilization of, 49
  deficiency, 43
    in rheumatoid arthritis, 107
  increased requirements for, 48–49
  malabsorption, 48
  metabolic functions, 48
  nutritional deficiency, 48
  sources, 47
  therapy, 49
Folic acid, deficiency, 47–49
Folinic acid therapy, 49
Formate, 42

Gallstones, 67, 86
Gangliosidoses, 24
Gastrectomy, folate deficiency following, 48
Gastric surgery, iron deficiency following, 30
Gaucher's disease, 23–24
Genes, regulation defects of, 76–77
Genito-urinary disorders in sickle-cell disease, 86
Gentamicin, 54–55
Glanzmann's disease, 15, 199
   platelet aggregation in, (*Table* 19.3) 189
Globin chain, abnormalities, 84–91
   genetic coding, 75
   synthesis, 77, 260
Glossitis, atrophic, 31
β-Glucocerebrosidase deficiency, 24
Glucocorticoids for aplastic anaemia, 55
Glucose metabolism, 69, (*Fig.* 8.1) 70
Glucose phosphate isomerase deficiency, 73
Glucose-6-phosphate dehydrogenase deficiency, 69–72, 267
γ-Glutamyl cysteine synthetase deficiency, 73
Glutathione metabolism defects, 73–74
Glycogen storage disease, 24
Goodpasture's syndrome, anaemia and, 2
Graft, failure, 57
   versus host disease, 57, 196
Granulocytes, abnormalities, 111
   concentrates, 240
   morphology, (*Fig.* 2.2) 9
   production, 109
   storage, 245
   transfusion in aplastic anaemia, 55
Granuloma, eosinophilic, 114
Granulomatous disease, chronic, 112
GVHD *see* Graft versus host disease

Haem, structure, 75
   synthesis pathway, (*Fig.* 4.4) 39
Haemagglutinin disease, cold, 93–95, 231
Haematocrit measurement, 4
Haematuria in sickle-cell disease, 86
Haemochromatosis, 33–36
   serum iron levels in, (*Fig.* 4.2) 33
Haemoglobin, absorption spectra, (*Fig.* 28.2) 261
   Bart's, 78
   C disorders, 88–89
   Chesapeake, 91
   Constant Spring, 77–78, 84
   cord level in haemolytic disease of newborn, 97
   D disorders, 89
   developmental stages, 76
   E disorders, 89
   electrophoresis, 76, 259–60
   F levels, 82, 260–1
   H disease, 78, 79

Haemoglobin (*cont.*)
   Hammersmith, 90
   Heathrow, 91
   Hereditary persistence of fetal, 82, 88
   high affinity, 91
   impaired formation, 1–3
   iron in, 29
   Köln, 90
   Leiden, 90
   Lepore syndrome, 79, 82
   M disorder, 90
   measurement, 3, 238, 259–62, 264–5
   oxygen dissociation curves, 261–2
   plasma, 264–5
   Rahere, 91
   S variant, 84
   S/β-thalassaemia syndrome, 83
   structure, 75–76
   tests, 259–62
   unstable, 90–91, 261
   variations with age, (*Table* 1.1) 1
   Zurich, 90
Haemoglobinopathy, 84–91
Haemoglobinuria, in haemolytic anaemia, 61
   march, 99
   paroxysmal cold, 95
   paroxysmal nocturnal, 30, 36, 58, 98–99
Haemolysis, classification, 2–3
   cold, 94
   from infections, 103
   in G-6-PD deficiency, 71
   in hepatic disease, 106
   intravascular, 30, 71
   investigation of, 262–8
   iron overload in, 35
   schematic representation, (*Fig.* 7.1) 62
   serum iron levels in, (*Fig.* 4.2) 33
   see also Anaemia, haemolytic
Haemolytic disease of newborn, 96–97, 238
Haemolytic reaction to blood transfusions, 246–8
Haemolytic uraemic syndrome, 100
Haemopexin determination, 263–4
Haemophilia, A, 202–5
   B, 205
   cryoprecipitate for, 243
   tests for, 186, 187, 190
Haemopoiesis, splenic, 142
Haemorrhage, anaemia from, 2
Haemorrhagic disease of the newborn, 209
Haemosiderin, decreased, 22
   formation, 29
   increased, 22
Haemosiderinuria, in haemolytic anaemia, 63
   tests, 265
Haemosiderosis, 35–36
   idiopathic pulmonary, 2, 30, 36
Haemostasis, laboratory evaluation, 185–90
   normal, 179–90
Hageman factor, 179, (*Table* 21.1) 203, 207, 246
Hair in iron deficiency, 31

Hairy cell leukaemia, 167
Ham's test, 267
Hand–foot syndrome, 86, 88
Haptoglobins, determination, 262
  levels in haemolytic anaemia, 61
Heart, failure, thrombotic risk in, (*Table* 23.1) 217
    therapy for, 223
  surface counting, 276–7
Heart–lung machines, priming, 239
Heavy chain diseases, α, 157, 174
  γ, 174
  μ, 174
Heinz bodies, 90
Heparin, oral anticoagulants and, 224
  effect on coagulation tests, 220
  for ATIII deficiency, 214
  for DIC, 211
  indications for use, 220–2
  mode of action, 220
  reversal, 222
  side effects, 222
  structure, 220
  thrombocytopenia with, 196
Hepatitis, viral, A, 251
  aplastic anaemia following, 52–53
  B, 251
  in haemophilia, 202, 204
  non-A non-B, 251
Hermansky–Pudlak syndrome, 25, 199
Hexokinase defects, 73
Histiocytes, abnormalities, 113
  function, 140
  proliferation, 151
  sea-blue, 24–25
Histiocytosis, sinus, 146
  X spectrum, 24, 113
Hodgkin's disease, clinical features, 152–3
  histology, 153
  incidence, 152
  investigations, 153–4
  pathogenesis, 152
  prognosis, 157
  staging, 154–5
  treatment, 155–7
Homocysteinuria, thrombotic risk from, (*Table* 23.1) 217
Hookworm, blood loss from, 103
Hormones, 288
Howell–Jolly bodies, 8
Hyaline membrane disease, 242
Hydatid disease, anti-P in, 232
Hydrops fetalis, 78
Hydroxycobalamin therapy, 47
Hydroxyurea, 289
  DNA inhibition by, 50
Hyperchromia, anaemia and, 4
Hypercoagulability, 213–19, 228
Hyperlipoproteinaemia, 24
  thrombotic risk from, (*Table* 23.1) 217
Hyperplasia, 21

Hyperplasia (*cont.*)
  erythroid, 22, 63
  myeloid, 21–22
  reactive, 113
Hypersplenism, 147
  anaemia and, 105
  in primary myelofibrosis, 124
  red cell defects and, 3
  surface counts in, 275
Hyperthyroidism, 106
Hyperviscosity, causes of, 216
  symptoms in myeloma, 169–70
Hypochromia, anaemia and, 4, 32
Hypogammaglobulinaemia in CLL, 166
Hypoplasia, 21
  erythroid, 22, 58, 102
  from chemicals, 52
  from viral hepatitis, 52–53
  myeloid, 22
  pregnancy and, 53
  trephine biopsy, (*Fig.* 6.1) 54
Hypoproteinaemia, serum iron levels in, (*Fig.* 4.2) 33
Hyposplenism, 148
Hypothermia, transfusion, 254
Hypovolaemia, plasma for, 242
  whole blood for, 238
Hypoxanthine-guanine-phosphoribosyl transferase deficiency, 50

Ii system, 231
Ileal disease, vitamin B_{12} deficiency from, 43–44
Imerslund–Gräsbeck syndrome, 44
Immune response, 140, 143
Immune thrombocytopenic purpura *see* Thrombocytopenic purpura
Immunocyte dyscrasia with amyloidosis, 176–7
Immunodeficiency diseases, 145
  non-Hodgkin's lymphoma from, 157
Immunoelectrophoresis, 269
Immunofluorescent technique, Hbf-containing cells studies, 261
  surface marker studies, 257–8
Immunoglobulin, determination, 269
  for immune thrombocytopenic purpura, 195
  IgA deficiency and blood transfusions, 250
  in autoimmune haemolytic anaemia, 93
  in cryoglobulinaemia, 175
  in macroglobulinaemia, 173
  in myeloma, 170–1
  red cell antibody classification, 233
Immunological sensitization, post-transfusion, 253
Immunoproliferative disorders, 169–78
  X-linked, 157
Immunosuppressives, for aplastic anaemia, 56
  for idiopathic thrombocytopenic purpura, 195
Infarction in sickle-cell disease, 86
Infection, chronic disease anaemia and, 102–3

Infection (*cont.*)
  following marrow transplant, 57
  granulocyte transfusions for, 240
  in aplastic anaemia, 53–54
  in haemolytic anaemia, 101
  post-transfusion, 250–2
  thrombotic risk in, (*Table* 23.1) 217
Infectious mononucleosis, 143–4, 194, 252
  post-transfusion, 252
Iron, absorption test, 275
  balance, 29
  deficiency, 27, 30–35
    in HbH disease, 78
    surface counting, 276
  deposition in sideroblastic anaemia, 36–39
  dietary, 27–29, 30
  haemoglobin, 29
  in bone marrow, 22
  metabolism, 27–29
  overload, 35–36
  plasma clearance of, 276
  plasma turnover of, 276
  stain, 256
  storage, 29
  surface counting after ^{59}Fe, 276–7
  therapy, 33–35
  tissue, 29
  utilization, 276
    defect in, 102
Irradiation, acute leukaemia following, 126
  aplastic anaemia following, 52
  for ALL, 131
  for Hodgkin's disease, 155–6
  for myeloma, 172
  for non-Hodgkin's lymphoma, 161, 162
  non-Hodgkin's lymphoma following, 157
Isotope investigations, 271–7

Jaundice, in G-6-PD deficiency, 71
  in haemolytic anaemia, 61
  in hereditary spherocytosis, 66

Kallikrein, 184
Kell system, 232
Kidd system, 233
Kleihauer acid elution test, 260–1

Lactic acid dehydrogenase determination, 265
Latex rheumatoid arthritis screening test, 271
Lazy leucocyte syndrome, 112
Lead poisoning, red cell injury from, 3
Leishmania donovani in marrow, 26
Leptocytes, 7
Lesch–Nyhan syndrome, 50
Letterer–Siwe syndrome, 114

Leucoagglutinins, 249
Leucocytes, lazy syndrome, 112
  surface marker studies, 256–8
Leucocytosis following splenectomy, 147–8
Leucocytotoxins, 249
Leukaemia, acute, aetiology, 126
  classification, 127
  clinical features, 127
  definition, 126
  incidence, 126
  pathogenesis, 127
  smouldering, 138
  acute lymphoblastic, bone marrow in, 128
    bone marrow transplantation for, 132
    cell markers, 129
    chromosomes, 129–30
    clinical features, 127–8
    differential diagnosis, 127–8
    incidence, 127
    morphology, 127–8
    peripheral blood, 128
    phenotypes, 129–30
    prognosis, 131–2
    treatment, 130–1
  acute myeloid, bone marrow, 133
    bone marrow culture studies, 135
    bone marrow transplantation, 136–7
    cell markers, 134
    chromosomes, 134
    clinical features, 132
    erythroid, 133–4
    incidence, 132
    megakaryoblastic, 134
    monoblastic, 133
    morphology, 133–4
    myelomonocytic, 133
    peripheral blood, 132
    prognosis, 136
    promyelocytic, 133
    treatment, 135–6
    undifferentiated, 133
  adult type chronic granulocytic, 119
  chronic granulocytic, 117–18
  chronic lymphocytic, 165–6
    T-cell, 166
  chronic myelomonocytic, 118, 138
  hairly cell, 167–8
  juvenile chronic granulocytic, 119
  megakaryocytic, 123
  Sezary syndrome, 164
  prolymphocytic, 167
Leukaemia-associated inhibitors, 127
Leukaemoid reactions, 118
Lewis system, 231
Liver disease, anaemia and, 105–6
  coagulation disorders and, 208, 209, 214
  Factor IX for, 244
  in acquired red cell membrane defects, 99
  platelet abnormalities and, 200, 208–9
  surface counting, 275, 276–7
Lung disorders in sickle-cell disease, 87

Lutheran system, 233
Lymph nodes, functions, 140
  structure, (*Fig.* 16.1) 139
Lymphadenopathy, 145–6
  immunoblastic, 157
Lymphatic system structure, 139
Lymphoblasts, in marrow, 20, 23
  morphology, (*Table* 15.1) 128
Lymphocytes, examination in blood film, 12–13
  in marrow, 20, 23
  in CLL, 165–6
  in immune thrombocytopenia, 194
  in infectious mononucleosis, 144
  relationship to splenic arterial circulation,
    (*Fig.* 16.2) 141
  rosetting, (*Table* 28.1) 257
  storage, 140, 245
Lymphocytopenia, 13
Lymphocytosis, 12–13
Lymphoid cell development, (*Fig.* 3.3) 19
Lymphoma, Burkitt's, 157, 160, 163
  childhood, 161, 163
  classification, 158–60
  cutaneous T-cell, 163–4
  diffuse small cleaved cell, 161
  follicular, 161
  histiocytic, 159
  Hodgkin's, 152–7
  large-cell, 161–2
  localized diffuse, 161
  lymphoblastic, 159, 162, 163
  lymphocytic, 159
  nodular, 159
  non-Hodgkin's, 157–63
  small non-cleaved cell, 162, 163
Lymphoreticular system, 139–49
  malignant disorders in, 150–68
Lyon hypothesis, 71

Macrocytosis, 4–5, 41
Macroglobulin, α_2-, 185
Macroglobulinaemia, Waldenströms, 173–4
Macrophages, abnormal, 23–25, 113–14
  function, 111
Malaria, disseminated intravascular coagulation
    in, 210
  parasites in red cells, 8
  post-transfusion, 252
  sickle-cell tract and, 84
Malignancy, anaemia and, 103–5
  disseminated intravascular coagulation in,
    210
  Factor VIII inhibitors in, 212
  thrombotic risk in, (*Table* 23.1) 217
Malondialdehyde, 218
Mast cells, 23
Mast cell function, 111
May–Grünwald–Giemsa stain, 255
May–Hegglin anomaly, 11, 15, 192

Mean cell haemoglobin, 4
  concentration, 4
  volume, 4
Mediterranean fever, familial, 177
Megakaryoblasts, 134
  deficiency, 192
  examination in marrow, 20, 25
Megaloblasts, 40
Melphalan, 281
Menorrhagia, iron deficiency from, 30, 106
2-Mercaptoethane sulphate (MESNA), 56
6-Mercaptopurine, 283
  DNA inhibition by, 50
Metamyelocytes, 20, 40
Metformin, vitamin B_{12} deficiency from, 44
Methaemalbumin determination, 265
Methaemalbuminaemia, in haemolytic anaemia,
    63
Methaemoglobin, absorption spectra, (*Fig.* 28.3)
    263–4
  determination, 262
Methaemoglobinaemia, 90
Methionine, 43
Methotrexate, 282–3
Methyldopa, autoimmune haemolytic anaemia
    and, 96
Methylprednisolone for graft problems, 57
Methylprednisone, 55
Metronidazole, 54
Micro-organism elimination, 110, 142–3
Mithramycin, 286
Mitochondria, iron deposition in, 37–38
MNS system, 233
Monoblasts, 20
Monocytes, abnormalities, 113–14
  examination in blood film, 14
    in marrow, 21, 23
  functions, 111, 140
  maturation and corresponding malignancies,
    (*Fig.* 17.3) 152
  production, 109
  rosetting, (*Table* 28.1) 257
Monocytosis, 14
Mononucleosis, infectious, 143–4
  post-transfusion, 252
Monosomy, 7, 119
Moschcowitz's syndrome, 100–1
Mouth hygiene prophylaxis against infection, 55
  in iron deficiency, 31
Mumps, thrombocytopenia in, 194
Mycoplasma infection, 231
Mycosis fungoides, 163–4
Myeloblasts, 19
  morphology, (*Table* 15.1) 128, 133
Myelocytes, 19–20
Myelofibrosis, idiopathic, 118
  primary, 124
  trephine biopsy, (*Fig.* 6.1) 54
Myeloid cells, rosetting, (*Table* 28.1) 257
Myeloid : erythroid ratio alterations, 21–22
Myeloma, cells, 22, (*Fig.* 18.1) 170

Myeloma (*cont.*)
  clinical features, 169–70
  definition, 169
  diagnostic criteria, 171
  incidence, 169
  laboratory investigations, 170
  prognosis, 172
  staging, 171–2
  treatment, 172
Myeloperoxidase deficiency, 112
Myeloproliferative disorders, 116–24
  platelet abnormalities, 15, 200–1
Myelosis, erythemic, 50
Myocardial infarction therapy, 223, 228
Myoglobin, iron in, 29
Myxoedema, 106

Nails in iron deficiency, 31
Neomycin, vitamin B_{12} deficiency from, 44
Neoplasm, bone marrow aspirate diagnosis of, 25
Nephrotic syndrome, 211–12
  thrombotic risk, (*Table* 23.1) 217
Nervous system, symptoms in iron deficiency, 31
  dysfunction in myeloma, 170
Neutropenia, 10
  cyclical, 111
  granulocyte transfusions for, 240
Neutrophil, abnormalities, 111–12
  alkaline phosphatase stain, 256
  development, (*Fig.* 3.2) 19
  examination, 9–11
  function, 110
    assessment, 113
  in megaloblastic anaemia, 41
Neutrophilia, 9–10
Nicoumalone, 225
Niemann–Pick's disease, 24
Nitrogen mustard, 280
  for Hodgkin's disease, 156
Nitrosoureas, 282
Non-Hodgkin's lymphoma, clinical features, 158
  histology, 158–9
  immunology, 158–60
  incidence, 158
  laboratory investigations, 158
  pathogenesis, 157–8
  prognosis, 162–3
  staging, 160–1
  treatment, 161
Non-specific esterase stain, 256
Normoblasts, 8
  acidophilic, 20
  basophilic, 20
  polychromatic, 20
Nutritional deficiency, anaemia and, 103
  folic acid, 48

Nutritional deficiency (*cont.*)
  iron, 27–29, 30
  vitamin B_{12}, 43

Oedema, angioneurotic, 242
Opsonins, 110, 112
Orotidylic decarboxylase deficiency, 50
Osmotic fragility, 265–6
Osteoblasts, 21
Osteoclasts, 21
Osteomyelitis, 86
Osteopetrosis, 114
Oxygen-dissociation curves, 261–2
Oxymethalone for aplastic anaemia, 55

^{32}P for polycythaemia rubra vera, 121
  for thrombocythaemia, 197
P system, 232
Pancreatic disease, anaemia and, 106
  disseminated intravascular coagulation in, 210
  vitamin B_{12} deficiency and, 44
  vitamin K deficiency and, 209
Pancytopenia, 21
Para-aminosalicylic acid, vitamin B_{12} deficiency from, 44
Paraproteinaemia, 201
Parasites, blood loss and, 103
  in blood film, 8
  in marrow, 26
  post-transfusion, 252
  vitamin B_{12} deficiency from, 44
Paroxysmal nocturnal haemoglobinuria (PNM) 51, 97, 98, 193, 267
Paterson–Kelly–Brown syndrome, 31
Pelger–Huët anomaly, 10
Pencil cells, 7
Penicillin, autoimmune haemolytic anaemia and, 95
  Factor VIII inhibitor caused by, 212
  for infection, 53
  thrombocytopenia with, 196
Periodic Acid–Schiff stain, 255–6
Peroxidase stain, 255
Phagocytosis, 140, 142–3
  decreased, 112
Phenformin, vitamin B_{12} deficiency from, 44
Phenindione, 222
Phlebotomy for iron overload, 36
Phosphofructokinase deficiency, 73
6-Phosphogluconate dehydrogenase deficiency, 73, 267
Phosphoglycerate kinase deficiency, 73
Phototherapy, 97
Pica in iron deficiency, 31
Pitting, 143
Pituitary hypofunction, anaemia and, 107

Plasma, cells, examination in blood film, 14
    examination in marrow, 20, 22
    in myeloma, 169, 170
    dried, 241
    fresh, 242
    frozen, 242
    haemoglobin determination, 264–5
    iron clearance, 276
    iron turnover, 276
    protein abnormalities, 169, 170–1
    protein fraction (PPF), 242–3
    storage, 234, 246
    therapy for liver disease, 209
    viscosity, 269
    volume, anaemia from increased, 103
        determination, 274
Plasmacytomas, solitary, 172–3
Plasmapheresis, albumin with, 243
    for Factor VIII inhibitors, 212
    for platelet antibodies, 195
    in Moschcowitz's syndrome, 100–1
Plasminogen, 184, 214–15, 226
Platelet, adhesion, 188, 215
    aggregation, 188–9, 215
    antibodies, 193–6
    bleeding time, 188
    coagulation cascade, 179
    concentrates, 240–1
    count, 188
    disorders, (*Table* 19.1) 186, (*Table* 19.3) 189,
        191–201
    examination, 14–15
    following splenectomy, 148
    formation, 142
    function, 182–4
    in haemolytic anaemia, 65
    in megaloblastic anaemia, 41
    increased destruction of, 193–6
    infusion in aplastic anaemia, 55, 57
        in liver disease, 209
    inhibition, 183–4, 227–9
    interactions with vessel wall, (*Fig.* 19.4) 183,
        215–16
    prostaglandin synthesis, 218
    release test, 218
    storage, 142, 241, 245
    structure, 182
    survival test, 218
Plummer–Vinson syndrome, 31
Pneumonia, interstitial, following marrow
        transplant, 57
Poikilocytes, 7
Polyarteritis nodosa, anaemia and, 107
Polychromasia, 8
Polycythaemia, hypoxaemic, 121–2
    rubra vera, 119–21
    secondary, 121–2
Polymyositis, anaemia and, 108
Pooling, splenic, 147, 148
Porphyria, erythropoietic, 2
Porphyrin ring, 75

Portugese nephropathy, familial, 177
Postcricoid web in iron deficiency, 31
Potassium, supplements, vitamin B_{12} deficiency
        from, 44
    toxicity in blood transfusion, 252
Pregnancy, aplastic anaemia, and, 53
    antiplasmins in, 215
    Factor VIII inhibitors in, 212
    haemolytic disease of newborn and, 96–97
    haemophilia and, 204–5
    heparin during, 221
    sedimentation rate and, 270
    serum iron in, (*Fig.* 4.2) 33
    sickle-cell disease and, 88
    thalassaemia and, 78, 83
    thrombotic risk in, (*Table* 23.1) 216
    von Willebrand's disease and, 205
Prekallikrein deficiency, 207
Preleukaemia, 50, 137–8
Procarbazine, 289
    for Hodgkin's disease, 156
Proerythroblast, 20
Promyelocytes, 19
Prostacyclin, 184
    assay, 218–19
    deficiency, 100, 215–16
    inhibition, 228
Prostaglandin, platelet synthesis, 218
Protamine for heparin reversal, 222
Protein, Bence Jones, 171, 269
    electrophoresis, 268
    investigations, 268–70
    synthesis, 77
Prothrombin, 181
    complex concentrates, 209
    time, 186, 223
Pruritus vulvae in iron deficiency, 31
Prussian blue reaction, 256
Pulmonary embolism, therapy for, 221, 223, 226
Purpura, post-transfusion, 195
    see also Thrombocytopenic purpura
Putative stem cell, 18
Pyridoxal 5-phosphate for sideroblastic
        anaemia, 38
Pyridoxine for megaloblastic anaemia, 50
    for sideroblastic anaemia, 37, 38, 39
Pyropoikilocytosis, hereditary, 69
Pyruvate kinase deficiency, 72–73

Quinidine, haemolytic anaemia with, 95
    thrombocytopenia with, 195, 196
Quinine, haemolytic anaemia with, (*Table* 8.1)
        72
    thrombocytopenia with, 196

Radiation, measuring equipment, 271
    types, 271

Radiotherapy *see* Irradiation
Rai staging system, 165
Rappaport classification, 159
Red blood cell, acquired membrane defects,
    98–99
  acquired non-immune disorders, 3
  agglutination, 233, 235
  antibodies, 233
  antigens, 230–3
  aplasia, 58–60
  circulation in spleen, 141–2
  concentrates, 239
  congenital disorders, 2
  development, (*Fig.* 3.4) 19
  distribution variations, 8
  enzyme defects, 69–74
  following splenectomy, 147
  formation, 142
    impaired, 1–2
  fragmentation, 30, 63
  grouping and compatibility testing, 234–7
  immune destruction, 2–3
  in aplastic anaemia, 53
  in Fanconi's anaemia, 58
  in G-6-PD deficiency, 71
  in glutathione metabolism defects, 74
  in haemolytic anaemia, 63
  in hereditary elliptocytosis, 67
  in hereditary spherocytosis, 66
  in hereditary stomatocytosis, 68
  in iron-deficiency anaemia, 32
  in megaloblastic anaemia, 40, 41
  in polycythaemia rubra vera, 120
  in pyruvate kinase deficiency, 72
  in thalassaemias, 78–79, 81
  labelling, cohort, 274
    random, 272–4
    with ^{51}Cr, 272, 274–5
  mass determination, 272
  measurement, 3–4
  mechanical lysis, 247
  morphology, 6–8
  osmotic fragility, 265–6
  removal, 143
  sedimentation rate, 269–70
  sequestration, 148
  splenic destruction, 66
  staining abnormalities, 8
  storage, 142, 245
    frozen, 239–40, 247
  survival, demonstration of reduction, 63
    reduction in chronic disease, 102, 105
    tests, 272–4
  thermal damage, 247
  transfusions in aplastic anaemia, 55
  traumatization, 99
  variation of indices with age, (*Table* 1.1) 1
  washed, 239
Reed–Sternberg giant cell, 152, 153
Reider cells, 19
Renal impairment, anaemia and, 103, 105

Renal impairment (*cont.*)
  in myeloma, 170
Renal tract, blood loss from, 30
Reticulocytes, iron granules in, 8
  stain, 255
Reticulocytosis, in haemolytic anaemia, 63
  mean cell volume, 4
  staining for, 8
Reticulosis, histiocytic medullary, 168
Reticulum cells, 21
Retinopathy, 86
Rhesus group system, 232
  typing, 235
Rhesus sensitization, 96
Rheumatic heart disease therapy, 223
Rheumatoid arthritis, anaemia and, 107
  immune thrombocytopenia in, 195
  iron deposition in, 36
  latex screening test, 271
Ristocetin, platelet aggregation with, 198, 199
Romanowsky stains, 6
Rose–Waaler test, 271
Rosetting technique, 129, 256–7
Rouleaux formation, 8
Rubella, thrombocytopenia in, 194
Russell bodies, 14

Sacrum surface counting, 276–7
Saline, blood group compatibility test, 236
Schilling test, 45, (*Fig.* 5.1) 46
Schistocytes, 8
Schistosomes, blood loss and, 103
Schumm's test, 265
Scintillation counter, 271–2
Sedimentation rate determination, 269–70
Serum test, acidified, 267
Sézary syndrome, 163–4
Sheep cell agglutinating titre, 271
Shock, albumin for, 243
Sickle cell, disease, clinical features, 85–86
    haemolytic anaemia and, 63
    laboratory findings, 87
    prevention of crisis, 87
    radiological findings, 87
    thalassaemia and, 79
    treatment, 87–88
    whole blood for, 239
  disorders with other haemoglobin defects,
    88–89
  screening test, 259
  trait, 79, 84–85
  see also Drepanocytes
Sickle fibril formation, 84, (*Fig.* 10.1) 85
Sideroblasts, 22
  ring, (*Fig.* 4.3) 36
Siderocytes, 8, 63
Siderosis, transfusion, 253
Skeletal destruction in myeloma, 169
Skin, T-cell lymphoma, 163–4

Sleeping sickness, post-transfusion, 252
Snapper–Schneid anomaly, 14
Sodium iron edetate, 34
Sorbitol, iron, 34
Spherocytes, 7
Spherocytosis, hereditary, 58, 63, 66–67, 266
Spleen, functions, 142–3
    assessment, 148–9
  in Hodgkin's disease, 154
  sinusoidal circulation, 140, (*Fig.* 16.3) 141
  structure, 140–2
  surface counting, 274–5, 176–7
Splenectomy, blood changes following, 147–8
  for hereditary spherocytosis, 67
  for immune thrombocytopenic purpura, 194
  for thalassaemia, 81
  infection following, 143
  platelet abnormalities following, 15
Splenomegaly, 146–7
  in essential thrombocythaemia, 123
Sprue, tropical, vitamin B_{12} deficiency from, 43
Stains, 6, 255–6
Steroids, anabolic, 226
  for immune thrombocytopenic purpura, 194
Still's disease, 107
Stomach, carcinoma in pernicious anaemia, 47
  pernicious anaemia affecting, 45
Stomatitis, angular, 31
Stomatocytes, 8
Stomatocytosis, hereditary, 68
Storage pool disease, 15, 199–200
  platelet aggregation, (*Table* 19.3) 189
Streptokinase, 226–7
Sudan black stain, 255
Sulphinpyrazone, 228–9
Surface counting, 274–5, 276
Surface marker studies, 256–8
Syphilis, post-transfusion, 252
Systemic lupus erythematosus, anaemia and, 107
  Factor VIII antibodies in, 212
  neutropenia in, 196
  thrombocytosis in, 196
  thromboses in, 216

T cell, chronic lymphocytic leukaemia, 166
  classification, 140
  cutaneous lymphomas, 163–4
  deficiency, 145
  examination, in blood film, 12–13
    in marrow, 20
  in non-Hodgkin's lymphoma, 159
  maturation and corresponding malignancies,
    (*Fig.* 17.2) 151
  prolymphocytic leukaemia, 167
  rosetting, (*Table* 28.1) 257
Target cells, 7, 63
Tay–Sachs' disease, 24
Terminal deoxynucleotidyl transferase (Tdt),
    129, 258

Testicular prophylaxis for ALL, 131
Testosterone in iron-overload, 36
Thalassaemia syndromes, alpha, 78–79
  sickle-cell disorder with, 88
  antenatal diagnosis of, 83, 260
  beta, classification, 79
    delta chain defects and, 81–83
    genetic mechanism, 77
    intermedia, 80
    major, 80
    management, 81
    minima, 80
    minor, 80
    peripheral blood film, 81
    radiology, 80–81
    sickle-cell disorders with, 88
  delta, 81–83
  diagnosis, 260
  genetic mechanisms, 76–78
  Lepore, 82
Thiamine for megaloblastic anaemia, 50
6-Thioguanine, 283–4
  DNA inhibition by, 50
Thrombasthenia, 199
Thrombin, production, 181
  time, 186–7
Thrombin–fibrinogen reaction, 181
Thrombocythaemia, 196–7
  essential, 122–3
Thrombocytopenia, acquired, 193
  amegakaryocytic, 192
  drug-induced, 193
    immune, 195–6
  immune, 15, 194–6
  in Moschcowitz's syndrome, 100
  increased platelet destruction in, 193–7
  isoimmune neonatal, 195
  platelet transfusion for, 241
  production, 191–3
Thrombocytopenic purpura, immune, 194–5
  thrombotic, 100–1
Thrombocytosis, 196–7, 215
  following splenectomy, 148
β-Thromboglobulin, 218
Thrombophlebitis, post-transfusion, 253
Thromboplastin time, partial, 186
Thrombosis, arterial, therapy for, 226
  circulatory stasis and, 216
  coagulation abnormalities and, 213–14
  fibrinolytic abnormalities and, 214–15
  laboratory tests in prothrombotic states,
    216–19
  platelet-vessel wall interaction abnormalities,
    215–16
  predisposition to, 213, (*Table* 23.1) 216–17
  venous, in paroxysmal nocturnal haemo-
    globinuria, 98
    patient selection with DVT, 219
    prophylaxis, 221
    therapy, 221, 223, 226, 228
Thromboxane, 183

Thymomas in pure red cell aplasia, 60
Thyroid disease, anaemia and, 106
Tissue, anoxia in iron deficiency, 31
  typing, 56
Tranexamic acid for haemophilia, 204
Transcobalamin II deficiency, 44
Transferrin, 27–29
Transplantation *see* Bone marrow
Triglyceride lipase deficiency, 24
Triosephosphate isomerase deficiency, 73
Trypanosomiasis, post-transfusion, 252
Tumours, metastasizing to marrow, 26

Uraemia, 200
Urinary light chain in myeloma, 171
Urobilinogen levels, in haemolytic anaemia, 61
  in hereditary spherocytosis, 67
Urokinase, 227

Varicella, thrombocytopenia in, 194
Vaso-occlusive crises in sickle-cell disease, 86
Venom, for defibrination, 227
  haemolytic anaemia from, 101
Venous thrombosis, recurrent, 215
Vinblastine, 287
Vinca alkaloids, 287–8
Vincristine, 287
Vindesine, 287–8
Viruses, acute leukaemia from, 126
  non-Hodgkin's lymphoma from, 157
  thrombocytopenia from, 193
Vitamin B_{12}, absorption, 42
  deficiency, aetiology of, 43–44
    in pernicious anaemia, 44–47

Vitamin B_{12} (*cont.*)
  increased requirements for, 44
  malabsorption, 43–44
  metabolic functions, 42–43
  sources, 42
  storage disorders, 44
  tests for deficiency, 45–46
  therapy, 47
Vitamin E deficiency in acquired red cell
    membrane defects, 99
Vitamin K deficiency, 209
  therapy for, 209, 222, 225
von Gierke's glycogen storage disease, 24
von Willebrand's disease, 198–9, 205
  characteristics, (*Table* 21.1) 203
  cryoprecipitate for, 243
  diagnosis of, 187, 188
  plasma for, 242
von Willebrand's factor, 180, 182

Waldenström's macroglobulinaemia, 173–4
Warfarin, 222–5
Westergren method for ESR, 269
Whipple's disease, 25
White blood cells, examination, 9–14
  following splenectomy, 147
  formation, 142
  in haemolytic anaemia, 65
  in megaloblastic anaemia, 41
  storage, 142, 245
Wiskott–Aldrich syndrome, 15, 192, 199
Wolman's disease, 24

Zieve's syndrome, 99, 106
Zollinger–Ellison syndrome, 43